WOUNDED

FOR LIFE

WOUNDED FOR LIFE

Seven Union Veterans of the Civil War

ROBERT D. HICKS

INDIANA UNIVERSITY PRESS

This book is a publication of

Indiana University Press
Office of Scholarly Publishing
Herman B Wells Library 350
1320 East 10th Street
Bloomington, Indiana 47405 USA

iupress.org

First printing 2024

Library of Congress Cataloging-in-Publication Data

Names: Hicks, Robert D., author.
Title: Wounded for life : seven Union veterans of the Civil War / Robert D. Hicks.
Other titles: Seven Union veterans of the Civil War
Description: Bloomington, Indiana : Indiana University Press, [2024] | Includes bibliographical references and index.
Identifiers: LCCN 2024001340 (print) | LCCN 2024001341 (ebook) | ISBN 9780253070760 (hardback) | ISBN 9780253070784 (ebook)
Subjects: LCSH: United States—History—Civil War, 1861-1865—Medical care. | Soldiers—Medical care—United States—History—19th century. | United States—History—Civil War, 1861-1865—Veterans. | Disabled veterans—United States—Social conditions—19th century. | Disabled veterans—United States—Social conditions—20th century. | Disabled veterans—Care—United States—History—19th century. | Disabled veterans—United States—History—20th century. | Body image—United States—Care—History—19th century. | Body image—United States—History—20th century. | Masculinity—United States—History. | BISAC: HISTORY / United States / Civil War Period (1850-1877) | HISTORY / Military / Veterans
Classification: LCC E621 .H539 2024 (print) | LCC E621 (ebook) | DDC 973.7/75—dc23/eng/20240321
LC record available at https://lccn.loc.gov/2024001340
LC ebook record available at https://lccn.loc.gov/2024001341

To the memory of:

JOHN ANDERSON DAVIS
US Army, World War I; US Navy, World War II

THOMAS I. DAWSON
US Merchant Marine, World War II; US Army

ROBERT D. HICKS JR.
US Army Air Force, World War II; US Air Force, Korean War

STEPHEN E. SQUIRE
conscientious objector, Vietnam era

CONTENTS

ACKNOWLEDGMENTS

THIS BOOK BEGAN TO GERMINATE in 2012 as the Mütter Museum of the College of Physicians of Philadelphia was preparing to launch a long-term exhibition to coincide with the sesquicentennial of the Civil War: *Broken Bodies, Suffering Spirits: Injury, Death, and Healing in Civil War Philadelphia*. The stimulus for the exhibition derived from my discovery of Dr. S. Weir Mitchell's questionnaires and related correspondence with war veterans, particularly a letter from Henry S. Huidekoper (the subject of chapter 7) to Mitchell about his phantom arm. Although it was not possible to spotlight the questionnaires in the exhibition, their theme—a history of the body, focusing on what harms, heals, or kills the soldier's body—informed the research for this book. In the early stages, I benefited from several conversations and subsequent correspondence with scholar and poet Lindsay Tuggle. She was awarded three F.C. Wood Institute Travel Grants to conduct research at the Historical Medical Library, College of Physicians of Philadelphia to support *The Afterlives of Specimens: Science, Mourning, and Whitman's Civil War* (University of Iowa Press, 2017). Her work influenced mine as I thought about the lives of the men portrayed in my book.

The Civil War–related holdings of the Historical Medical Library in Philadelphia anchored this study. Without those resources, this book would not have been possible. I owe a huge debt to Beth Lander and Heidi Nance, former librarians; former reference librarian Caitlin Angelone; and archivist Chrissie Perella Clement. Library intern Cora Johnson-Grau and volunteer Cindy Markushewski conducted essential biographical research. I thank George M. Wohlreich, MD, former president and CEO of the college, for his interest, support, and encouragement.

Librarians, archivists, and the stewards of the many invaluable collections in local history societies contribute the gems of historical inquiry that support important themes. Key insights that inform my chapters derive from these collections, which, in most cases, cannot be searched online but require on-the-ground inspection. The stewards of these collections are usually volunteers. I hereby praise former archivist Theresa Altieri Taplin, Union League Legacy Foundation, Philadelphia; the National Park Service library staff at Gettysburg National Military Park; Anna Kimball, Belleville Public Library, Illinois; Pam Robinson, Hunterdon County Historical Society, New Jersey; and Patricia A. Martinelli, Vineland Historical & Antiquarian Society, New Jersey. While the Caroline County Historical Society, Maryland, was closed during the COVID-19 shutdown, I benefited from telephone and email exchanges with its director, Jack Walsh, who introduced me to genealogical researcher Patricia Guida. Pat voluntarily searched for details of Prestley Dorsey/Dawson's (chapter 6) prewar and postwar life in Maryland and greatly illuminated his sojourn and community there.

Closer to home, my study benefited from insights and information provided by colleagues. A shout-out to historian James Paradis, who suggested that I examine the life of Thomas Hawkins (chapter 8); historian James E. Johnson, whose expertise on United States Colored Troops filled in the crevices and interstices of my research; Joyce Werkman, head of Citizens for the Restoration of Historic LaMott and Camp William Penn; local history researchers David Harrower and Thomas Wieckowski, whose work in researching and making public the history of the first and largest federal training camp for black soldiers during the Civil War proved indispensable; the late Thomas Dawson, grandson of the subject of chapter 6, and his daughter, Professor Gail Dawson, the Dawson family's genealogical torchbearer. Filmmaker Carole Adrienne Murphy, author of the popular *Healing a Divided Nation* (Pegasus Books, 2022), through discussions and email contributed useful nuggets of medical history.

For over a decade, Mary Ellen Donatelli, F.C. Wood Institute Associate at the College of Physicians of Philadelphia, has provided invaluable support for my diverse projects. She proved to be an enthusiastic historical researcher, and throughout this project, she has indefatigably taken clues and run them to ground to ferret out valuable biographical details of the seven veterans profiled in this book. A rigorous and superb organizer, Mary Ellen enabled me to be systematic and thorough in sifting through an enormous stew of evidence, mostly in shreds and patches in the historical record. My debt to Mary Ellen is incalculable.

To Kathleen R. D. Sands, author of sixteenth- and seventeenth-century histories and now a writer of fiction, and my spouse, effusive gratitude for endless discussions about the subjects of this book and merciless, exacting, and indispensable editing. In writing, in editing, and in being life's partner, she knows how, as Walt Whitman wrote, "to mystify the familiar and familiarize the strange."

I am grateful to Dan Crissman of Indiana University Press for recognizing the worth of this book and offering to publish it. Indiana University Press published my last book in 2019, *Civil War Medicine,* and has again demonstrated its staff's multifarious talents in bringing the manuscript to publication. Particular thanks to Lesley Bolton, Anna C. Francis, and Vickrutha Sudharsan of Amnet. All people associated with publishing this book at Indiana have ever been responsive to questions or difficulties, speedy, thorough, exacting, and supportive in all important ways. I cannot recommend Indiana University Press too highly.

A book of this kind is useless without a comprehensive index. Susan Certo, Mark Your Words Indexing, grandly provided this indispensable ingredient.

A generous travel grant from the Bakken Museum in Minneapolis furnished me with an essential understanding of electricity in nineteenth-century United States. The Bakken's collection of electrical instruments and the library cannot be praised too highly.

Finally, I acknowledge the soundscape of writing that ushered this project forward: gratitude and praise be unto Robert Hakalski and Ludovico Einaudi.

WOUNDED
FOR LIFE

ONE

LISTENING TO ANOTHER'S WOUND

HALLUCINATORY BODIES

Having "heard of the delightful feelings produced by Ether, and [having] a strong desire to inhale it," a soldier at the largest army hospital in Philadelphia, Pennsylvania, during the Civil War drew its fumes through a mask, "intoxicating draughts of what seemed to [him] a delightful beverage." Thus began a hallucinatory journey: "I commenced passing through regions of space with incredible velocity. Everything was colored with the nicest regard to shade and effect." From his hospital bed in 1863, the soldier imagined traveling to New York City and then out to sea, and upon hearing a voice, he turned into a statue. Finally, he arrived at a vision of himself in an infinite cosmos: "One single idea possessed my mind all the time, and that was—that everything progressed in the next world as it does in this; and that world succeeded world, each one growing larger and larger, until at last they grew to the size not to be conceived by human minds. This was the third world, and compared to some in progress, was as an orange is to the earth."[1]

After being told by a physician that surgery was required to remove bone fragments embedded within a bullet wound to his shoulder, another soldier in the same hospital agreed to an operation that evening when the air would be cool. As the surgeon and one or more assistants placed him on a table, the soldier, identified only as E. S., gave himself over to the circumstances "with a total indifference as to the result, and a passive carelessness." He "reveled in [his] helplessness" and, disregarding all other cares, focused "around one exclusive object—self." With the application of ether, E. S. observed that "the odor was as sweet and pleasant as the perfume of the orange blossom." In his hallucination, E. S. became invigorated, "all aglow," and his "blood danced and coursed . . . with lightning pace." "My head was like a vast hive, with bees singing a wild, melodious chant, that now rung out fine, clear and distinct; now rose in sharp, shrill tones; and now drifting in harmonious cadence, sank slowly and more slowly into a low indistinct buzz. Then all sound was hushed; I was alone, all alone; my body was below; I was a vapor . . . but still retaining individuality. That *frame* was mine, but was not *I*: I was sailing in space, reveling in the joys of unbounded freedom, without a want to satisfy, and utterly alone."[2]

His ether journey led not only to involuntary introspection but also to terror as E. S. coursed through "a mental panorama of [his] life" in acute detail, surveying "burning mind-pictures" of all his experiences and actions, joyous and despairing: "Nothing was omitted." Unlike the pleasant ether experience described previously by the anonymous soldier-author, in his hallucination E. S. was trapped in a fire, engulfed in flames, and dashed to rocks into unconsciousness. Upon awakening after surgery, he discovered that his actual ether exhalations had caught fire from a nearby lamp, and as the hospital attendants worked to extinguish the flames, the unconscious E. S. had struggled and fallen off the operating table onto the floor.[3]

Both of these Union soldiers were recovering from wounds at West Philadelphia Hospital, Pennsylvania—also known as Satterlee Hospital—and recorded their experiences in the hospital newspaper. Both accounts appear to contradict the common

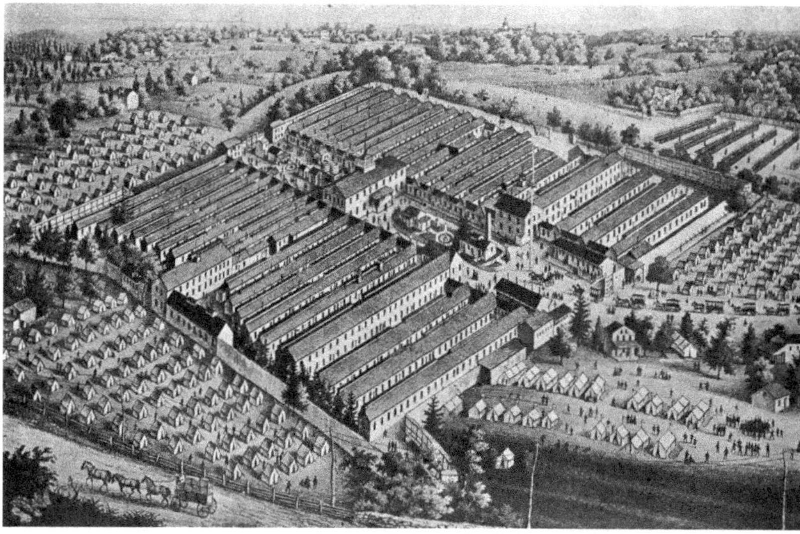

From its opening in 1862 until its closure in 1865, West Philadelphia Hospital—also known as Satterlee—treated approximately fifty thousand soldiers. Based on a pavilion model promoted by Florence Nightingale, wards were clustered near administrative, supply, and kitchen buildings. *Credit: Frank Taylor,* Philadelphia in the Civil War. *Philadelphia, 1913.*

perception of manly behavior in the mid-nineteenth-century United States that men do not share or publicize their innermost thoughts and that self-control and disciplined, logical, and practical actions are expected, even demanded. Manhood did not allow for voluntary hallucinatory journeys beyond conscious bodily control. The soldiers' accounts also reveal that the hospital served multiple purposes, not only allowing patients to heal and have the time and means for self-discovery but also, based on these men's experiences, freeing them from gender boundaries.

A common narrative of manhood permitted few digressions for the postwar lives of veterans. Most published narratives of soldiers' personal experiences from the Civil War conclude either with mustering out and then returning to civilian life or with medical discharge due to wounds or illness. Ex-soldiers returned to home communities or new urban environments, married, had children, and resumed old trades in farming or business. Or they tried to live with dignity working unskilled jobs if they had been "limbed," the common wartime term for bodies subjected to amputation. Or they drifted into relative anonymity except when they banded together at veterans' meetings to raise the banner of public awareness of wartime service and demand recognition. Except for intimate histories of the soldiers' bodies found in wartime medical reports and postwar pension records, in most accounts, veterans' bodies cease to be objects of anatomical scrutiny as veterans themselves dispersed throughout the country and new generations came forth with no experience of the Civil War.

The two ether narratives suggest a more complex picture. Both hospitalized soldiers publicly exposed their journeys as kings of infinite space. Both soldiers had developed intimate partnerships with surgeons and their assistants, hospital stewards, and nurses and collaborated in making decisions about their therapies. Wounded soldiers often became fascinated by the behavior of their bodies with new sensations and thoughts, transformations of skin and movement, and manifestations of healing. They became articulate about their bodies in ways they could not have anticipated in civilian life. Because of their severe wounds or illnesses, ex-soldiers became both spectators of and partners with their bodies in exploring new phenomena from extreme, uncommon pain to apparently irrational behavior of nerves and muscles.

As observant students of their bodies, these ex-soldiers created a view of self that merged attributes of manhood as defined by their era with those ascribed to the feminine sphere. They redefined themselves based on how wounds, disease, and healing altered their bodies. In public, they bore themselves accordingly as a matter of distinction or pride in what their bodies had endured despite long-term pain or debility. Partners in understanding veterans' infirmities, physicians helped to build these new identities, giving them a language with which to understand and manage their recovering bodies. Doctors' assessments of veterans' conditions could be at odds with the views of pension examiners and government bureaucrats who determined what compensation was appropriate.

SEEING THE ELEPHANT, SEEING THE BODY

A recitation of wartime tactics and battlefield sagas can be found elsewhere. In this work, my focus is on the veteran's body as shaped by the trauma of the battlefield, the construction of a postwar identity in relation to that trauma, and the changing social circumstances of the last quarter of the nineteenth century as they impacted a traumatized body. The historical record does not permit a consistently intimate examination of these soldiers' lives over time, but with the available evidence, we can explore "the very possibility and surprise of listening to another's wound," as suggested by literature professor Cathy Caruth. Unlike their dead comrades, these soldiers were indeed "sentenced to life" and believed they were obliged to elucidate the sufferings of less fortunate veterans and to own the national narrative of the war by reminding the public of their sacrifice.[4]

This book explores the postwar lives of six Union veterans of disparate backgrounds: four white—Henry A. Kircher, Richard D. Dunphy, Henry S. Huidekoper, and John Shields—and two black—Thomas R. Hawkins and Presley Dorsey/Dawson—as intimate encounters with the bodies of men who suffered severe wounds, injury, or disease.[5] All had "seen the elephant," war vernacular for experiencing combat, and three were later awarded the Medal of Honor. In parallel, I examine the work of another veteran of Union wartime service, a physician—S. Weir Mitchell—who links the four white soldiers. Two of the men submitted a health questionnaire to Mitchell, one wrote him a letter (accompanied by a letter from his physician) and was examined by him, and the fourth wrote him an account of his war wounds in response to a conversation between them. The experiences of the two African American soldiers, who did not have the benefit of specialized medical care or any long-term relationship with army surgeons, contrast with those of the white soldiers. In the 1890s, Dr. Mitchell, who paid close attention to veterans and their health throughout the decades of his career, with his son, John K. Mitchell, MD, circulated a questionnaire to elicit personal data about veterans' bodies, perhaps the only longitudinal survey of the health of ex-Civil War soldiers conducted. The survey responses present a snapshot of veterans' bodies decades after the war.

The veterans examined here experienced lifelong maladies because of the indeterminacy of healing. An amputation left a stump, but although a scar appeared to seal the wound, a moment never arrived when veterans deemed healing to be complete. Nerves continued to alter sensation or evoke pain, tumors appeared, and unremoved bullets or bone fragments continued to torment. There was no finality or completion to healing. That healing remained a dynamic feature of the body influenced veterans' conception of their manhood, combining prewar notions with ideas born of changing circumstances. The redefinition of manhood was based on a joint exploration of healing with various physicians over time, some of whom became long-term partners. The veterans appeared to care little for demarcating the traditional spheres of men and women in their recovery and combined both spheres if doing so served their needs at any given moment. The trajectories of white and black soldiers were similar in some respects, divergent in others. A study of each veteran reveals adaptability and resilience, lonely suffering, attempts to improve knowledge of his body, and an ongoing appraisal of what he could expect from the world.

While our veterans lived their lives, their relationship to the medical world changed over time. Medical ideology and therapeutics introduced new concepts while older ideas were discarded. Mitchell's atypical therapies and experiments with drugs—including morphine and atropine, massage, hydrotherapy, and particularly "electrization"—explored new pathways in comprehending the human body and required ongoing intimacy with veterans' bodies. In particular, the use of electricity forced new dimensions of manhood through a doctor-patient collaboration in mapping anomalies of the nervous system. Mitchell's case studies, clinical notes, and publications reveal his deep respect for a peculiarly American notion of manhood he championed and helped engender in his white patients.

The physical examinations found among pension records and Mitchell's questionnaires and related correspondence present a wound's-eye history of the body that anchors veterans' health to discrete moments in the late nineteenth century. These documents allowed each veteran to appraise his body in relation to the original moment of wounding or injury and evaluate his healing over the decades. The examinations and surveys allow us to glimpse the identity each ex-soldier created for himself. As veterans met with physicians in later years, they saw a new professional subclass of medical professionals—specialists—who "promised innovation through medical research, which translated into acceptance and even demand for these treatments from some of the soldier population and, by extension, the larger public."[6]

Three recent works—two historical studies and one literary-historical title—influenced the present study. Historian Brian Matthew Jordan's *Marching Home: Union Veterans and Their Unending Civil War* outlines the spectrum of soldiers' postwar lives and discusses how veterans were challenged to live up to contemporary notions of manhood. We learn of penurious veterans in asylums with neither work nor prospects who were conscious of the erosion of their wartime identities. Other veterans may have suffered wounds but found support through employment, family, or fraternal organizations, and yet all veterans' lives were shaped by the health consequences of wartime suffering. These insights take us only so far in understanding veterans recovering from trauma (from the Greek for "wound").[7]

Poet and critic Lindsay Tuggle's *The Afterlives of Specimens: Science and Mourning in Whitman's America* examines the wartime writing of Walt Whitman regarding dead and dying soldiers as "specimens" who, as men languishing in hospitals, occupied a threshold between corporeal existence and oblivion. Meditating on these men, Whitman's wartime poems, suffused with "melancholic attachment," explore individual identities against the incomprehensible mass mortality of the battlefield dead. With Whitman as a lens, Tuggle examines the pathological narratives of the war dead and wounded as enshrined within the Army Medical Museum in Washington, DC, as scientific specimens. Tuggle's pairing of Whitman's intimate encounters with soldiers as a hospital visitor and the Union Army's creation of the Army Medical Museum parallels the decades-long recovery of severely wounded or amputee veterans and Mitchell's intimate probing of their bodies to understand and treat damage to the nervous system.[8]

Historian Sarah Handley-Cousins's *Bodies in Blue: Disability in the Civil War North* "explore[s] the ways in which soldiers, civilians, and institutions grappled with disorders that did not easily fit into existing cultural narratives of manhood and sacrifice." Handley-Cousins provides an intimate analysis of Union Brigadier General Joshua Lawrence Chamberlain's experience in managing his Gettysburg hero persona while suffering from incomplete healing of his war wounds. Paralleling her approach, I construct intimate biographies of veterans' bodies in relation to the physician and his anatomical invasions (and associated violence) of treatment, a mutual exploration that created new identities.[9]

Posttraumatic stress disorder (PTSD) does not appear in the discussions of the soldiers portrayed in this book. Retro-application of a modern psychiatric designation to Civil War veterans presents interpretive difficulties and risks ahistorical characterizations of their experiences. Military psychiatry originated later, during World War I. Our understanding of mental illness is conditioned by a cultural milieu unknown to Civil War–era people. There is no one-to-one correspondence between markers of mental illness today and those used by doctors in the late nineteenth century.

PTSD is defined in the *Diagnostic and Statistical Manual of Mental Disorders-5* (*DSM*), the inventory of named pathologies and their behavioral symptoms published by the American Psychiatric Association. The disorder "reflects the direct imposition on the mind of the unavoidable reality of horrific events, the taking over of the mind, psychically and neurobiologically, by an event that it cannot control. . . . [It is] the most destructive psychic disorder." The *DSM*'s description states that exposure to combat violence and death constitutes a stressor that may result in "intrusion symptoms" such as nightmares and flashbacks. The sufferer may therefore strive to avoid experiencing situations that evoke similar trauma and may feel "negative alterations in cognition" such as self-blame, sense of isolation, and negative thoughts about oneself, possibly leading to suicidal or other self-destructive behavior.[10]

The language of mental suffering during and after the Civil War differed from that of the *DSM*. Wartime and later pension doctors described aberrant symptoms as *melancholia, nostalgia, hysteria,* or even *insanity*. Persons labeled as insane were removed from familial and working environments and placed in asylums if violent or incapable of labor. Originally, *hysteria* referred to a belief that uteruses traveled through women's bodies, causing distress. Unusually, Mitchell adapted that term to denote extreme pain in soldiers.

By the late twentieth century, nervous system disorder replaced hysteria. Similarly, the medical literature following the war identified trauma due to "catastrophic effects of improved warfare technology," a phenomenon that gained definition and elaboration following each subsequent war to become *combat fatigue* or *shell shock*. The other Civil War labels underwent similar changes over time.[11]

This introductory chapter places my study within histories of Civil War disability, gender studies, and the body. It circumscribes key themes governing the exploration of the six veterans' bodies in relation to physicians, identity and its subcategory manhood, disability and its representations, the material culture of the body, and the experience of pain. My investigation of six veterans also shows that the boundary between what was considered masculine and feminine spheres of appearance and behavior proved to be permeable.

Chapter 2 considers the work of S. Weir Mitchell, MD, founder of medical neurology. Mitchell was a contract assistant surgeon during the war who, together with two fellow physicians, supervised a special Philadelphia ward to treat extreme wounds of the nerves. A veteran of the immediate aftermath of the Gettysburg battle, Mitchell coined the phrase *phantom limb* to name the sensation of a ghost arm, leg, foot, or finger following amputation. His work creates a benchmark for explaining or managing pain following wounds or amputations. Army surgeons did not investigate pain; they were concerned only with maladies anchored in verifiable "lesions." Mitchell found pain's seat in the nerves and coined a name for specific, extreme pains of the nerves, *causalgia,* known today as complex pain syndrome. His insights provided veterans with an acknowledgment of the reality and possible causes of the chronic pain they endured for decades.

Mitchell's most unusual therapy, electrization, his electrical treatments to gauge the functioning of nerves and to treat the lack of nervous response by purposely inducing pain, is the subject of chapter 3. Through this especially intrusive and painful therapy, Mitchell relied on conversations with his soldier-patients to understand what was happening to their bodies. The use of electricity to heal disabled nerves was otherwise unknown in army practice. At the time, no standards existed for the use of electricity, its measurement, or its medical application. Electrization could activate deadened limbs, stimulate painful phantom sensations, and supply a language for articulating nerve damage and pain.

Chapters 4 through 9 each focus on one veteran's body: how it was injured, wounded, or diseased; how the body became a medical subject; how medical therapies were applied to the body and to what effect; how the veteran's body became a contested commodity concerning public benefits and the war's legacy; and how federal pension officers[12] compensated the body through monthly payments according to schedules of fixed amounts.

Chapter 4 examines the experience of Captain Henry A. Kircher, Twelfth Missouri Infantry, who suffered three bullet wounds in 1863 that led to the amputation of an arm and leg. Kircher's experience permits examination of his longtime patronage of a particular physician, his negotiation about the types of amputations conducted on his body, and his subsequent use of prostheses. As a son of German immigrants, Kircher's identity shaped his view of his own suffering and healing. His Saxon body (as he described it), with its wartime disfigurement, imbued his American identity with a superior intelligence beyond that of most Americans who served during the war. Although evidence suggests that Kircher did not display his veteran's body to other veterans, in his pension body, he engaged in continuous arguments with governmental authorities. In his civic body, he built a home, married, and became a well-known business professional and leader.

Coal heaver Richard D. Dunphy is the focus of chapter 5. An Irish immigrant and member of the crew of USS *Hartford,* the flagship of Admiral David Farragut, Dunphy sustained wounds from a fight with Confederate shore and ship artillery at Mobile Bay in 1864, resulting in the amputation of both arms and a subsequent award of the Medal of Honor. Dunphy is a lens for discussing the meaning of disability during the war and the public view of amputees. As a postwar cultural phenomenon, amputees sometimes discomfited civilians by their scarred bodies, which were viewed as morally dangerous, and could be shunned by so-called ugly laws that regulated their public appearances. Amputees' need for surrogate bodies to accompany them could disorient or confuse the public. Dunphy's public tag as the "armless veteran" demonstrates that even within the population of disabled persons, some forms of abnormality were accepted, and others were shunned with a taint of immorality. In the public's view, the amputation of both arms was worse than any other combination of missing limbs. Dunphy, however, viewed himself as a self-sufficient working man with a family and home. This view was increasingly at odds with that of his family, who tried to manage both his alcoholism and his pension.

Chapter 6 explores the life of Presley Dorsey/Dawson, who served as a private in the Forty-Third Regiment, United States Colored Infantry. He inhabits the shadows at the margin of society. Possibly a former enslaved man and nonliterate, he is unique among the soldiers profiled in this work because he never received a bullet wound. Rather, he was maimed by a portion of trench fortification collapsing on his body while under fire, which caused permanent lameness. More serious, though, was his contraction of malaria, which resulted in two long hospital stays. This chapter speculates on what his postwar life as a veteran looked like, the importance of claiming identity as a patriot who sacrificed his health to the Union cause, and the possibility that his postwar health intersected with various medical traditions, whether the allopathic ideology of military doctors or the health practices of the enslaved. Unlike the white veterans, Dorsey/Dawson waited years before approaching the pension office through a hired pension agent, and his nonliteracy—and that of his friends and neighbors—had consequences for his widow's unsuccessful attempt to receive a pension. Black bodies emerging from enslavement without an understanding of the white bureaucratic infrastructure faced huge obstacles to receiving pensions for disabilities.

Chapter 7 focuses on Irish-born Captain John Shields, who served with the Fifty-Third Pennsylvania Infantry. He suffered a thigh wound from a bullet at Fredericksburg in 1862 and another through the neck at Gettysburg, Pennsylvania, in 1863. Owing to the latter wound, Shields was discharged for medical disability, but he found an identity as a rising businessman. Following the war, he magnified his veteran body through active participation and leadership in the Grand Army of the Republic (GAR), the influential fraternal organization of Union veterans. Suffering a business failure in middle age, Shields ran a home for disabled and impoverished veterans that may have been arranged by the GAR. He fashioned an identity around his wounded body that advertised his status as a patriot who made sacrifices to save his adopted nation. Throughout his postwar years, despite changes in public sentiment and politics, he used his body to champion a fixed identity, represent patriotic manhood, and act as a spokesman for less fortunate veterans.

Chapter 8 scrutinizes Sergeant Major Thomas R. Hawkins, a paid substitute who served in the Sixth Regiment, United States Colored Infantry, and received a bullet wound near Petersburg, Virginia, in 1864 and, months later, three more within the space of minutes at New Market Heights, Virginia. Discharged for wounds and illness, he never recovered. Despite his wounds, he got married and fathered a child. He received the Medal of Honor only weeks before he died, five years after the war's end. In addition to the ongoing debilitation of his body due to the bullet wounds, Hawkins struggled to place himself—and his family—within a rising black middle class in the nation's capital. Despite the position and privilege of an army sergeant major, the highest-ranking enlisted man in the regiment, Hawkins's former role did not advance him professionally in civilian life, although he evidently made inroads into a higher echelon of social life. Sympathetic physicians monitored and aided his short postwar life, but no specialized medical help was available to ameliorate his increasing pain and debility.

Chapter 9 introduces Lieutenant Colonel Henry S. Huidekoper, initially second-in-command of the 150th Pennsylvania Infantry Regiment, and later its commanding officer. A severe bullet wound to his right arm at Gettysburg led to amputation and brief captivity. Although he later returned to duty, his wound forced his resignation within months. He did not receive a survey from Mitchell, but he wrote to him about his wartime experience and evocatively described how his dreams induced phantom limb pain. Huidekoper's story connects to the idea of the phantom body as depicted in Mitchell's first published description of the phenomenon. In his postwar life, Huidekoper campaigned to keep the Gettysburg battle, later considered to be the war's turning point, memorialized. His pinned-up sleeve constituted a flag-draped coffin for his sacrificed limb, reminding others that his stump, a stigma, perpetually, if figuratively, bled for the nation.

In conclusion, chapter 10 generalizes the veterans' management of their wounded or diseased bodies to the ends of their lives. This group of veterans reshaped their identities in various ways as society moved on, trying to adjust their views of manhood as they aged and became progressively more disabled. To a

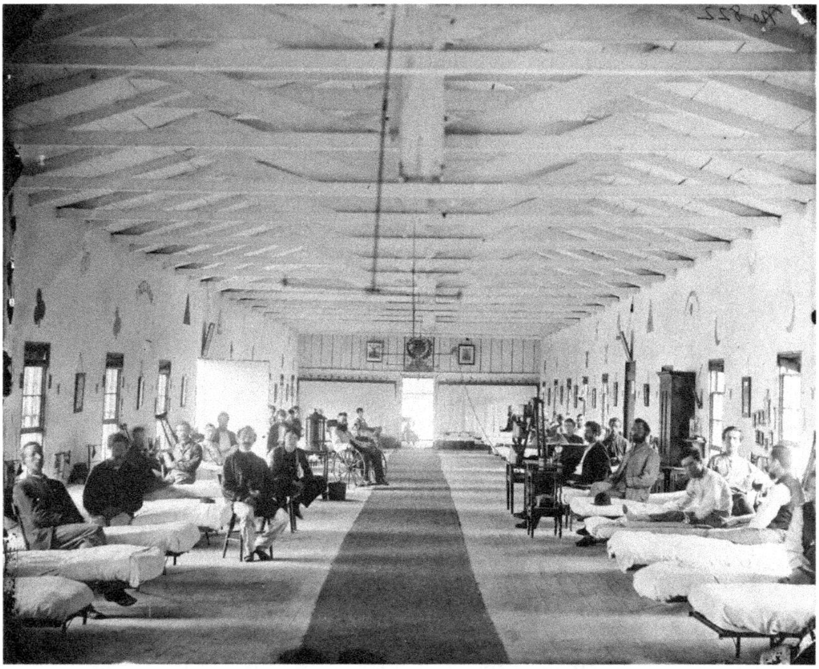

Interior view of Ward K, Armory Square Hospital in Washington, DC, around 1865. An example of a pavilion-style hospital ward, the whitewashed interior features large windows for ventilation and fresh clothing and bedding for patients. *Credit: Library of Congress (LC-DIG-cwpb-04246).*

degree, each tried to keep the suffering, patriotic soldier and the stigmata of his visible wounds in the public eye. All six soldiers presented three postwar bodies: the fraternal veteran, the veteran among veterans; the pensioned veteran, who negotiated compensation for his damaged body with government officials and physicians; and the civic veteran, who negotiated employment and social life after the war. As veterans aged, the nation that awarded pensions valued their individual stories less and transformed their bodies into statistical data, charts, and graphs that supported industrial insurance underwriting and generalized the veterans' experiences in limited ways. Veterans' persistence in sharing their narratives of healing or continued suffering forced others to "listen" to their wounds.

AMERICAN MANHOOD

The terms *manhood* and *masculinity* occur frequently in this study. This section defines and distinguishes the terms as they apply to the veterans profiled. A soldier's identity consists of an innate character that comes to embrace beliefs shaped by an unfolding sequence of events and reactions to and introspection about those events and the personal meaning attached to them. These beliefs, which encompass values, ambitions, and attitudes, are further shaped by biology; that is, one's physical abilities, bodily functions, and—as we now know—biochemical reactions. *Manhood,* a dynamic cluster of beliefs about how biological males guide their lives in a social context, evolves as beliefs change through time. The impact of manhood, or its synonym *masculinity,* on soldierly identity is not static. "There is no inevitable association between the male body and masculinity. Historical representations and individual embodiment often become confused. Anatomy may not be destiny, but the *belief* that it is moulds most lives." Civil War soldiers and the veterans they became discussed manhood frequently, whether in correspondence or other writing, and physicians also took up the theme as if the cultural was biological and deterministic. Discussions of manhood became explicit among soldiers because the war furnished a rite of passage.[13]

A soldier in Ward Z at West Philadelphia Hospital, doubtless debilitated by illness or wound, published a manifesto about manhood to affirm its essential characteristics. Not surprisingly, the soldier posited attributes within a discourse of war. *True* manhood means the following: "Does he possess the power by which to prove successful in every struggle those attributes essential to succeed triumphantly in every contest?" The author then listed the attributes that supply that power to include cultivation of the mind: inherent goodness (with attendant restraint of passions and desires); the ability "to hold in check the impulses of his nature"; "not . . . being controlled by the caprices of the multitude"; and "not . . . subjecting the spirit to the perpetual bondage of the flesh." To realize any of these, the soldier must exercise *energy* to maintain self-control and vigilance "and manful resistance to beat back those colloiding influences" that can destroy the weak. If a man succeeds in these contests, then "he becomes a being noble and God-like, the perfection of his Creator's ideal, crowned with honer [*sic*], dignity and excellence." "God-like" includes Christ's bodily suffering. This description of manhood does not address physical suffering due to disease, injury, or wounds. Nor does the essay discuss the endurance of pain, repeated operations to repair the body, or emerging from the hospital unfit to return to duty within the chart of manhood.[14]

The ideal espoused by the soldier in Ward Z is found throughout most discourses of Victorian manhood. As soldiers in hospitals revisited these ideals, however, they raised questions about their interpretation in the context of war's depredations on the body. To contemporaries, manhood was something to be achieved or won, not an innate attribute of being a male. In damaging bodies, war disorganized the attributes of manhood. In the public view, wounded and diseased bodies signified morality and character. If war could alter the body, it could also alter morality and character; thus, war could threaten gender. Women were not present in the military to balance wartime influences on manhood, but virtues ascribed to the feminine infused hospital care even where women nurses were not present. Without the ubiquity of women in civilian life, the forced intimacy created by military order opened new possibilities for introducing intimacy in relationships with other men, especially when those men were wounded or ill.[15]

That feeling of brotherhood and the emergence of soldierly identity began once the recruit entered a training environment and joined a regiment with a distinctive local identity (the emblem of which, the regimental colors, functioned as the holy banner under which the soldier crusaded). Through participation in a regiment, a collective body, personal identity enlarged for the soldier to create comradeship in a cause. "It was the regiment, more than anything else, that gave the soldier . . . his primary identity, and in the regiment 'the colonel, as a father, should have a personal acquaintance with every officer and man.'" Officers, then, performed in loco parentis when necessary in extending feminine (maternal) interest in their men's bodies.[16]

The national ideal was essential in eliciting the soldier's patriotism and soldierly duty, but in military service, the soldier was deprived of home, hearth, and family. Because most soldiers joined volunteer regiments formed in their home communities, camp life exhibited a combination of the culture of home (including other soldiers who were neighbors and acquaintances) and the new regimen of military life. Each soldier found his balance between the values of home—less the physical appearance of family and home—and his new life. Soldiers managed their bodies according to this amorphous zone of influences, conditioned by the behavior of comrades.[17]

As the country entered the war, communal manhood framed the preeminent version of manhood that functioned as a motivating psyche to the Union soldier. The family served as the "primary unit of production" for the nation, thus cementing an obligation to the family patriarchs to perform a key social role expected by that nation: to become a soldier. "Duty was a crucial word for manhood . . . each role was governed by a set of duties owed to the others." The majority of serving soldiers were volunteers, a central quality of military service to these men: "He was to be brave but not reckless, pious but not a zealot, disciplined but not authoritarian, and dutiful but not obsequious."[18]

The experience of soldiering within an ersatz family of the regiment, in a much larger military organism of brigade, division, and corps promoted a national identity that intensified in hospitals and demonstrably informed the lives of veterans who "willingly, often enthusiastically, committed to embracing an all-encompassing national identity . . . an identity as Americans, one and all." For veterans, this identity was challenged to change with the times as the cultural environment with subsequent generations found new meanings in the war. Nevertheless, veterans, strengthened by their fraternal veterans' organizations, "preserved the memories of their sectional ideals, their trials, and their respective causes."[19]

From the war forward, veterans' patriotism championed an "abstract notion of 'America'" that bent to the original ideals that formed the basis of the United States. This abstraction included battlefield experiences transformed over time from distinct sights, sounds, and smells of powder, artillery fire, and voices taking up the charge to narratives of participation in a crusade of transcendent proportions in which the individual veteran had a role. The veteran's personal experiences, then, expanded to a "whole story—thus picked up and patched together—until . . . after a while, [they] swear to being an eyewitness to every scene and movement of that battle." Their individual bodies stood in for the bodies of their lost comrades.[20]

In addition to identifiable, discrete signs of manhood in bodily appearance, emotions and beliefs could also manifest in the body, if indirectly. Much has been written about how Protestant Christianity formed a component of soldierly manhood in the North. This religious stratum in civilian life became, for some veterans after the war, a form of "muscular Christianity," a union of "metaphors of fitness and body-building" with "a strong, forceful Jesus with a religion to match." Some historians generalize that after the war, veterans carried forth an emotional complexity that incorporated Christian identity with attitudes about bodily suffering and endurance. Untangling emotional responses to circumstances and their impact on the body is difficult not only because of the dearth of primary documents that include interpretations about emotional life but also because of the challenge of overcoming a twenty-first-century view that "emotions are taken for granted as psychological phenomena."[21]

For the comrades of the slain, death did not conclude a preoccupation with manhood. Soldiers, medical professionals, and volunteers sometimes gazed at and admired soldiers' corpses. As both soldiers and medical workers became inured to the sights, sounds, and smells of the battlefields, they could set aside grief and horror at the misery surrounding them and contemplate the dead body as aesthetic, even beautiful. After seeing violently destroyed bodies in this way, a soldier could only confide to fellow soldiers or trusted others. In a letter to her niece, volunteer nurse Cornelia Hancock acknowledged that "one can get used to anything. One of my favorite resorts is our dead house, some such fine looking men die. Sometimes Dr. Dudley embalms them and keeps them quite a while just to look at. Men are put into neat coffins and buried very decently from this hospital." Before a body decayed and required burial, corpses were made to appear manly; the attitude of the body in death was a statement of the soldier's manhood when alive.[22]

Other soldiers seemed to disconnect themselves from the suffering to contemplate exposed human anatomy. Doing so reflected a manly scientific detachment. A Union soldier ate his dinner within "six paces of a rebel in four pieces." The trunk and upper body had detached from the pelvis and both legs, evidently from an artillery shell. When the Union soldier was at leisure, he and his companions "examine[d] the internal structure of man ... [including] brains, heart, stomach, layers of muscle, structure of bones ... for there was every form of mutilation." Mutilation horrified but also proved instructive with an aesthetic that civilians would not comprehend.[23]

Dead bodies in uniform also created a crisis of manhood for the living. During the Civil War, stories circulated of Confederate desecration of Union corpses. White soldiers may have made up the Confederate and a large proportion of the Union armies, but distinct and opposing cultural viewpoints widespread in both armies led many soldiers to characterize each other as aliens. Human trophy hunting during the war was an activity tangent to "some important developments taking place in the fields of medicine, comparative anatomy and racial science." Human remains were not only removed as trophies; physicians also retained specimens that documented battle wounds and surgical responses to them. The surgeon general of the army required field surgeons to package and ship to Washington specimens of interest that were eventually stored or displayed at the Army Medical Museum.[24]

Whether bones were removed as personal trophies or medical specimens, they represented "the new significance given to these parts of the body as material evidence of the naturalness of racial hierarchy and the permanence of differences." The soldier's anxiety about death in combat, then, embraced apprehension about the destination of his body after death: A soldier might fear being forgotten in an unmarked grave, dismembered, or dissected. Even a battlefield photograph of a dead soldier evoked anxiety among the living, who saw the corpse as out of control, in grotesque poses, possibly comical, certainly shorn of manhood.[25]

The concept of the manhood of combat-damaged veterans was clearly formed from a variety of sources. My focus is on veterans' bodies through the evolving cultural shell of manhood, how they cared for themselves, evaluated their wartime wounds of injuries over time, and developed strategies to coexist with them and their marriages, families, careers, and the esteem of their communities. Veterans' bodies and their evolving identities were intimately linked to medical observation, intervention, and influence.

MAKING MILITARY BODIES

Before the new soldier was allowed to wear the uniform, his body had to be prepared. Wearing a uniform required the body within it to be approved for military service and shorn of civilian identity. The military redefined the boundaries of personal intimacy, beginning with the recruitment examination. The recruit, in his nakedness, was forced to tolerate intimate touching.

Physicians and army comrades came to view each other's nude bodies in ways unknown in prewar life. As in other wars with mass conscription and volunteering to join the military, "men took on a new attractiveness for each other." In *A Manual of Instructions for Enlisting and Discharging Soldiers,* Dr. Roberts Bartholow recognized the transition of the body from a private, protected space to the opposite: transitory camps, multiple tent mates, and group hygiene, including occasional common baths in streams and rivers. He encouraged the examining surgeon to coax recruits reluctant to undress to exercise sensitivity and respect for privacy when possible. Observed Bartholow, "It is important that this first unpleasant experience of his new military life may be rendered as little unpleasant to the drafted man as possible; that in undressing and dressing he may not be exposed to the curious gaze of bystanders, and that he may feel that the persons whose duty it is to examine him do it in their official capacity in conformity to law."[26]

The surgeon then observed the recruit walk around the room, gradually increasing speed until he was commanded to halt, then to hop on one foot and then the other. After this vigorous exercise, the surgeon placed "his hand upon the praecordial region to detect an abnormal action of the heart." Next, the recruit stood as "a soldier under arms, with heels together and the knees about an inch apart," standing still as the physician began a systematic inspection of his body, beginning with the head, mouth, nose, eyes, and ears and noting characteristic signs of trauma such as "fractures, depressions, cicatrices [scars], or diseases of the scalp." The head received particularly careful inspection "to detect the physiognomy of epilepsy, imbecility, or insanity." The examination became progressively intimate and intrusive and included peering into the ear and the "auditory canal . . . for foreign bodies, for discharges, for vegetations or tumors; the tongue, posterior fauces [pharynx or throat], palate, and teeth, for defects, loss of substance, mutilations, or tumors."

Eventually, the surgeon peered at (or into) the genitals and rectum. "The testes and cords should be examined for chronic enlargements, varicocele [varicose dilation], cirsocele [dilation of spermatic veins], hydrocele [swelling due to fluid buildup], or sarcocele [swelling or tumor]." Finally, as twenty-first-century army inductees can relate, the recruit was told to spread his legs and bend over so that the physician could check for "hemorrhoids, fissures of the anus, fistula in ano [abnormal opening involving the anal canal], or urinary fistula [opening between an organ and the surface of the skin]." Bartholow's examination procedure applied only to enlisted men. If officers were subjected to such tests, they were conducted in private. Officers and enlisted soldiers did not expose their nude bodies to one another. Fraternization between officer and enlisted ranks was forbidden; the mixing of nude male bodies with no visible signifiers of rank threatened discipline.[27]

The army's recruiting guidelines for physicians and postwar studies of soldiers explicitly frame manhood in relation to traits that can be observed or measured on the body. Writing after the war, physician Sanford Hunt, based on his analysis of soldierly qualities during the war, opined "that the American, in founding a new nationality, has also established a new type of manhood." In a comparison of the physical attributes of white American soldiers with those of French and British soldiers, he found that the American soldier was the tallest, at 5 feet, 8 1/2 inches, and also the heaviest. While white men's measurements had expanded in all ways in North America, however, the same measurements of African men in the New World either remained static or were physically diminished. The African was not alone, though: Southern white men showed reduced brain size. Hunt noted that education could modify brain size and shape "and that the competitive success of the freedmen of this country rests upon the effort that may be devoted to their mental and moral elevation." Manhood, therefore, could be measured; it could go up or down.[28]

Outside of white men who had been born in the United States, the other nationalities that were best represented among recruits were German and Irish. Dr. Bartholow identified specific deficiencies of manhood that surfaced during physical examinations of soldiers for possible malingering. To twenty-first-century readers, Roberts's study presents vexing arguments about national proclivities as he conflates cultural and biological characteristics. Of the three nationalities, Germans feigned illness more than Americans or Irish, despite their patriotism and natural "devotion to unity and liberty," but love of "ease and money" resulted in a lack of discipline. The physician, however, would have known that Germans most often feigned chronic rheumatism, incontinence, diarrhea, and hematuria (blood in urine). Roberts's implicit argument is that while each ethnic group can be characterized by distinct bodily phenomena, national characteristics may also dictate what diseases are faked.[29]

By contrast, disorders "of the respiratory organs, of the urinary and genital organs, diarrhea, dyspepsia, heart-disease, and epilepsy, were the disabilities usually feigned by Americans." "Sunstroke, chronic rheumatism, and 'pain in the back' are the favorite diseases of the Irish." Nevertheless, the Irish faked illness less often than Americans or Germans. These stereotypes may have informed the medical examinations conducted on the bodies of the veterans profiled in this book. Despite the generalizations made about different ethnicities, as a rule, the military doctor cautioned fellow doctors to beware of feigning among soldiers whose bodies appeared to be ruled by specific temperaments: "the bilious and melancholic or hypochondriacal, the nervous, the lymphatic; whilst the sanguine is least of all disposed to it. The typical malingerer has dark brown or hazel eyes, dark hair, and dark complexion; his face is stealthy, dogged, lowering; his eyes suspicious, furtive, restless; and his manner habitually constrained and exhibiting violent attempts at composure."[30]

Not only did the recruitment physical examination signify a transition into military discipline and the army's possession of the body; it also marked the first assertion of physicians' authority over it. Thereafter, the physician attended to a soldier's wounds, injuries, or diseases and certified him fit for duty or infirm and unfit for duty. The physician recommended discharge from the military, signifying the army's abandonment of the body. The physician was the ultimate arbiter of what was normal or abnormal, categories that were not static. By selecting recruits deemed normal by the physician, his goal was to keep the soldier normal in body and mind. The physician constituted the regimental body police.[31]

A focus on the body necessarily includes objects that enfold and protect it, confer identity and status, or violate it through injury, death, or healing, namely, the uniform, weapons, and other equipment. Objects on, in, or otherwise attached to bodies "act, [they] have effects in the world." Objects do not have to be actively contiguous to bodies to have meanings; even after they cease to exist with the body, their influence remains identifiable. "A rifle, flag, tent, uniform, canteen, and haversack could fill a man with a range of emotions and meanings, but these things were not just containers of memories. They could shape behavior, filter perceptions, and serve as conductors of action." As postwar guardians of the national democratic ethos, veterans were responsible for "the afterlives of things," hence the museums of relics found at GAR posts in later years.[32]

The soldier's uniform represents the soldier's body. The purpose of a uniform is to diminish individualism and promote the synchronous functioning of a large group of soldiers. The uniform of the newly minted soldier created a masculine ideal because it "enhanced men's masculine appearance: a well-designed headdress made them look taller, stripes on trousers have the illusion of length in stocky legs, epaulets exaggerated the width of shoulders." Following months of campaigning, soldiers' uniforms degraded from sweat, heat, cold, rain, ice, and dirt and assumed an idiosyncratic character unique to the soldier. The uniform thus became a dependable ally, sleeping clothing, and a commodity. Soldiers removed buttons and insignia from defeated foes to sell or trade, or they perhaps traded some of their own gear.

The uniform was not just a benign covering that identified the soldier's cause. Both physicians and soldiers considered the health challenges posed by clothing. Clothing concealed disease-causing fomites or other minute agents of disease, but it could also protect against disease. A soldier might provide extra body covering to protect against mosquitoes or wear red flannel underwear to avoid colds, coughs, or backaches. Soldiers accommodated their clothing to their own beliefs about maintaining health in small ways, from their choice of underwear to repairing or slightly modifying their government-issued garments. Although soldiers traded, loaned, or at times discarded items of clothing or equipment, they exchanged information with their comrades about healing and maintaining their bodies. Because of the uniform they wore in common, soldiers formed a common mess to share cooking and food, worked to control threatening or interfering animals or insects in camp, foraged together to find fresh food, and collaborated to define how, when, and where to evacuate bodily waste.[33]

In considering its manifestations of manhood, the soldier's body must be observed in its totality with uniform, rifle, knapsack, and other paraphernalia, both military and personal. Indeed, soldiers viewed their weapons and uniforms as emblems of masculinity. On the march and in camp, soldiers developed a respect for their uniforms and adjusted personal appearance—hairstyles and posture, for example—to comport with a military self-image. Soldiers wasted no opportunity visiting photographic studios to have their uniformed bodies memorialized in tintypes, cabinet cards, and cartes de visite (a small portrait used as a visiting card). These images served not only as mementos for self and family; soldiers also created albums of images of comrades to remember their bodies.

A striking example of photograph albums created for that purpose was that of Lieutenant T.F. Wright, 108th Regiment, United States Colored Infantry. Lieutenant Wright—a white company officer—obtained and placed in his album cartes de visite of African American enlisted men and annotated each photograph with the subject's name and a description of duties performed and his manly qualities. For instance, Corporal Rendwick Allen "commands obedience"; Sergeant Samuel Martin has "very light eyes and hair and light complexion [and] uses no tobacco or stimulant" and is appreciated by officers for his "soldierly bearing"; and Drummer James Roberts who appeared to challenge officers by asserting himself, "a freeman, hard to manage [and] stubborn and reckless."[34]

Cartes de visite portraits employ common backgrounds and furnishings and served not only for formal portraits but also to document ravaged bodies. Some physicians and the army surgeon general's office took portraits of wounded or injured soldiers as clinical documents. Whether viewers of these images were fellow soldiers, the public, or physicians, these photographs were inspected for clues about health, bearing, attitude, courage, and moral rectitude; in short, manhood.[35]

HOSPITALIZED BODIES

"The Civil War . . . produced the largest biological crisis of the nineteenth century, claiming more soldiers' lives and resulting in more casualties than battle or warfare and wreaking havoc on the population of the newly freed." Recently, the tally of soldier mortality from that war has been revised upward, although the actual number will never be known. The veteran who died twenty years after the war from complications of a bullet wound may not have been part of an official count but was a war fatality nonetheless. Given the human devastation, it seems unthinkable that soldiers' experiences with wounds, injuries, and diseases and the intervention of medical practitioners to keep them healthy should not alter, embellish, or enlarge men's identities as veterans.[36]

Soldiers recovering in hospital beds adjusted concepts of manhood to align with the presentation of their wounded, ill, or injured bodies. They had plenty of time to recognize what soldiers in other wars had discovered, that men's bodies were "*intended* to be mutilated." While in hospitals, soldiers expected a dialogue with doctors and other medical workers about their bodies, a conversation accompanied by the touching and probing of recovering (or failing) parts. Diagnosis proceeded "according to the interpretation of a number of sensory signs (visual, aural, and haptic) by which the inner body was understood." For soldiers, owning and articulating one's malady constituted an exercise in exhibiting manhood. Dr. S. Weir Mitchell gratefully cited soldiers' ability to articulate their maladies as an exceptional quality that enabled him and his colleagues to develop "so full a knowledge of these early phenomena [of the nervous system]." Indeed, he engaged patients as partners in bodily exploration who had "a very natural curiosity as to the condition of the wounded part, and are apt almost immediately to handle it, and to try to move it."[37]

Extended hospital stays for serious injuries, wounds, or illnesses created new communities for soldier-patients that contributed narratives of recovery or death. These narratives blended conventional attributes of manhood with those articulated by comrades, medical practitioners, and the soldiers themselves. Doctors, nurses, and ward mates—fellow sufferers—observed ailing (or recovering) comrades not only to follow the progress of healing but for comparative self-reflection. Even if soldier-patients ultimately died, surviving friends felt obligated to inscribe the deceased's identity in some fashion that blended personal biographies, medical narratives, and eyewitness accounts with a spiritual dimension. The uncensored West Philadelphia Hospital newspaper attests to identity formation in this way.

For example, the newspaper featured an account by an anonymous patient who observed medical interventions to heal two diseased soldiers, Marion C. Frost and Charles Chadbourne. Writing on behalf of his ward companions, he described the suffering of Frost and Chadbourne, both residents of the same ward. The pair appeared to suffer the same illness. Both men were about nineteen years old with similar upbringings supervised by "pious mothers. They were trained in youth with assiduous care, and moulded by the plastic hands of those who most do give tone and shape to manhood." Although their temperaments were different, they made friends easily, enjoyed wide comradeship, "and secured the favorable regard of strangers." Comrades commented on Frost's childlike traits, a soldier whose "loving, tender disposition that could not be comforted in the absence of his mother" who was summoned to attend his last days. Because of their incapacitation, soldiers in hospitals became feminized in relying on the ministrations of doctors, nurses, orderlies, and cooks. Nevertheless, Frost commanded respect despite this feminine characteristic. It made no difference to his comrades; perhaps they prized his femininity.[38]

Chadbourne, by contrast, "was a manly character." He was a quiet man "who was a favorite with all who knew him, and enjoyed the confidence of all." As he neared death, he exhibited what were considered feminine characteristics of resignation and increased dependence on nurses. His pain and suffering increased, leading to "constant groaning for days and nights," yet he endured patiently and became "anxious for his soul's welfare." The sincerity of his desire to live for God impressed his ward mates.

The soldier who recorded these stories wanted them known and understood. In this memorial, the deceased soldiers' parallel lives highlighted their final weeks as crucial capstones of identity, as if prewar identity served as a preamble to that formed around the struggle for life in a hospital. Hospital stories attest that the formation of identity was never fixed at a discrete point in adult life, but the horrific experience of battles, wounding, disease, and continued suffering stimulated the creation of new narratives of identity and its main ingredient, manhood. Identity formation in Civil War hospitals blurred genders, plumbed the psyche for dreams and hallucinations, and explored one's reservoir of impulses and thought as mediated through suffering and therapeutic drugs, characteristics that prevailing social standards defined as unstable and unmanly.[39]

The circumstances of the hospitalization and eventual demise of Private George Dash, Company D of an unnamed New York volunteer regiment, led to a narrative of identity less informed by thoughts, dreams, or hallucinations than by Dash's response to a series of medical interventions to save his life. At Chancellorsville, Virginia, in May 1863, a Confederate musket ball nearly tore off Dash's left arm near the head of the humerus and opened the subscapular artery. At the field hospital, the arm was amputated using the flap method,[40] followed by the application of various dressings and bandages.[41]

Because the amputation site was so close to the trunk of Dash's body, his recovery did not appear promising. The surgeon initially reported some improvement, but then gangrene appeared around the wound. The skin flaps were insufficient to close the wound, and the surrounding tissues looked diseased. Dash lost his appetite and developed bedsores. One night, around midnight, the wound began to bleed. As the wound site could not be repaired, doctors decided to cut the flesh higher up into the shoulder to tie off the artery there. Dash remained conscious through the operation and expressed relief "at the protection he has thus gained from future accidents."[42]

Dash worsened. His pale face, cold sweat, and changes in respiration "showed how near to 'the valley of the shadow of death' he had been." After six days of anxiety in hopes that the wound would begin healing, "jets of bright scarlet blood shot out from the spot where the artery had been last tied, and the hemorrhage was only stopped by pressing the finger hard upon the bleeding vessel." Dash's physician arranged to have fourteen medical cadets take shifts to apply pressure to the exposed artery in the hope that a clot would form and close the wound. "Here was a veteran who had fought in seven battles and had risked his life dozens of times in the excitement of action. Now he was more helpless than a puny babe; for a misapplication of the finger upon the proper spot—a slip of the artery under the pressure—and in two minutes he would be dead!" Another volunteer, the anonymous author, not only chronicled Dash's precarious condition but also participated in the medical intervention and doubtless talked with medical staff about it.[43]

Dash remained aware of the necessity of rotating the job of placing pressure on the wound while contemplating "the uncertainty of his living to from hour to hour." Medical cadets assisted by the Sisters of Mercy rotated the pressure duty every half hour, but the messy wound made it "an extremely difficult matter to find the exact spot to place the finger upon." The wound was large—about three inches long and almost as deep—with dead tissue mingled with healthy, blood mixing with a discharge of bone-splintered exudate.[44]

Despite the efforts to force a clot, the artery opened again, spewing blood onto the bed, pillow, and wall. The author and other ward patients watched as Dash weakened, his eyes pleading "with appealing pity." As with Marion Frost, observers feminized

Dash's condition of helplessness but strove to determine how he might summon the resilience of his soldierly identity to come to terms with eternity. Would the capstone of Dash's identity be his nonverbal instruction to fellow soldiers on how to meet the mystery of death? The author's account does not answer the question, but the fact that it cannot be answered led the author to conclude that our lives are as "an atom in eternity—a breath gone as quickly as it has been exhaled, and soon lost in the immensity of space." Dash's companion, the author, depicted an identity that collected the expected virtues of manhood before wounding—the forbearance under great trials, the healthy youth who displayed courage and endurance—with his intense suffering as under medical direction, a procession of people inserted their hands into his body to heal. Dash was chronicled as a suffering Christ. The scene bears a striking similarity to the medieval preoccupation with Christ's Side Wound at his Crucifixion, as the attending Sisters of Mercy, who composed the hospital's nursing corps, might have thought: "The Side Wound . . . became a nuptial bedchamber and a refuge, offering protection, nourishment, and cleansing. Womb-like, it also suggested a place of rebirth. In each instance, senses are engaged, especially touch. Devotional literature often encouraged the faithful to taste, touch, suck, kiss, and enter into Christ's side wound."[45]

Not only is the Side Wound womb-like; according to its description in medieval manuscripts, it resembles a vagina. The wounded soldier is the feminized Christ.

Dash released his grip on life slowly over several days, but as he was known as an experienced, disciplined, and reliable soldier before he was fatally wounded, his weeklong precarious hold on life expanded his identity to include an experience few people face. Dash recognized his tenuous hold on existence just as his chronicler recognized the evanescent nature of all life. The people whose hands entered Dash's wound participated with Dash in his deconstruction into eternity within "the immensity of space."

Dash died in the hospital, but thanks to his friend who bathed his hands in his blood, Dash's identity did not disappear when he died but rather was enlarged in print to incorporate his ward disciples, doctors, medical cadets, and nurses, and his pilgrimage to the Cross.

Other wounded soldiers in the wards wrote that being in a hospital created an enhanced awareness of their thoughts, bodies, and environment. The wounded patient could cleanse "deep rooted prejudices" and release self-interest in favor of a larger, liberal view, as was shown in the ether hallucinations. Another soldier meditated on self-renewal in the hospital: "For every great convulsion recorded can be traced more or less directly to the shock when the onward progress of humanity comes into collision with deep rooted prejudices; and sooner or later these prejudices have been forced to yield." One anonymous hospitalized soldier contemplated the composition of the Union army in relation to its virtuous mission "to support the standard of moral and civil progress" of the nation, an army of American "hardy yeomen" whose ancestors had abandoned "the worn-out and crumbling systems of old-world life, to broaden and deepen in the free air of democratic America." The soldier-writer then turned his attention to the common experience of suffering in a hospital, a form of resilience that frames this new opportunity for identity formation: "In the camp, in the field, amid the roar of battle, the groans of the dying, the silent companionship of death, they have mingled, and fought, and fallen. On the painful couches where these lines are read they lie together and will clasp trembling hands as that feeling of brotherhood wells up to the hearts at the memory of past dangers shared, and sufferings endured."[46]

Fellow soldier-patients who chronicled the lives and deaths of their ward mates implicitly recognized that the soldier's body was "an almost infinitely flexible symbolic resource" that mirrored a larger damaged body, the ruined landscape. As a symbol, the soldier's body "is more than flesh and blood: it is a symbolic site invested with political as well as personal meaning." The examples of Frost, Chadbourne, and Dash attest to the prized attributes of self-denial, manly courage, and patriotic ideals while also achieving an apotheosis as feminine, generous souls who had discovered eternal truths. The ward mates who chronicled their travails scrutinized their behavior for signs and wonders, hoping for reassuring gestures or words that communicated the patients' contentment at sacrifices for their country and a vision of celestial reward, behavior that would embolden the onlooker and strengthen their faith. The ward scenes of surgery, suffering, and dying presented onlookers and participants with theater: "The wounded body was a 'theatrical site,' the object of civilian curiosity and entertainment, a signifier of authenticity, and a site of memory and mourning."[47]

Visibly wounded veterans may have been signifiers of authenticity, but they could also suggest a lack of physical courage or moral failure. People unable to "read" the disfigured or mutilated faces of veterans sometimes inferred damaged moral states. Disfigured bodies might also have connoted the presence of disease, particularly those conditions associated with immorality, such as syphilis. Disfigured bodies could be read as object lessons in punishment for sins. The abnormality of disfigured bodies sometimes disturbed people who did not participate in war, but abnormality did not represent moral deficiency to other veterans. Also, physicians proved to be ideal partners to wounded or ill soldiers who were trying to revise their sense of identity to cope with a future life decisively altered by war. Physicians' dialogue with debilitated veterans enabled the latter to "man up" to a form of conversation characterized by reason and manly authority, even when it included conversation about intimate bodily sensations.[48]

If hospitalized soldiers modified their view of manhood because of forced inaction and dependence, some were surprised that hospitals did not conform to the stereotype of being places where poor people came to die. The war's most famous hospital visitor, Walt Whitman, discovered sublimity in hospitals. He visited thousands of soldiers in the hospital, observing their impaired bodies, trying to ameliorate loneliness and suffering, and documenting in journalism or verse the profundity of his encounters. He saw "hospitals as navigating a borderland between the familiar, physical world of the body and the afterlife of the soul." Whitman described the hospital as "a new world . . . full of its separate action, play, suggestiveness—surely a medium world, advanced between our well-known practiced one of body and of mind."[49]

Released from the hospital with their new identity as veterans, these ex-soldiers altered their ideals of manhood to recognize and display their "honorable scars." The comparison of Christ's Side Wound with the display of these honorable scars is bolstered by the Second Great Awakening and its evangelistic fervor popular throughout the armies. Through their suffering, veterans emulated Christ. Veterans also reckoned with unseen wounds, including phantom limbs and their associated proprioception (awareness of body movement) or manifestations of pain without an associated visible lesion, a kind of "fraudulent body language" that imparted an effeminate characteristic to the veteran's manhood.

Immediately after the war, popular culture depicted "limbed" veterans as shown in figure 1.3, "The Empty Sleeve." Artist Adelaide R. Sawyer depicted a Union veteran holding a child whose attention is captured by the soldier's empty sleeve. The veteran appears lost in thought as he looks into the distance. The pose of man and child and the interior setting with a large window affording a view of a rural, peaceful countryside evoke countless Madonna and Child images from the medieval period forward. That the adult is a man missing his right arm suggests emasculation, "feminine traits that supersede his military masculinity

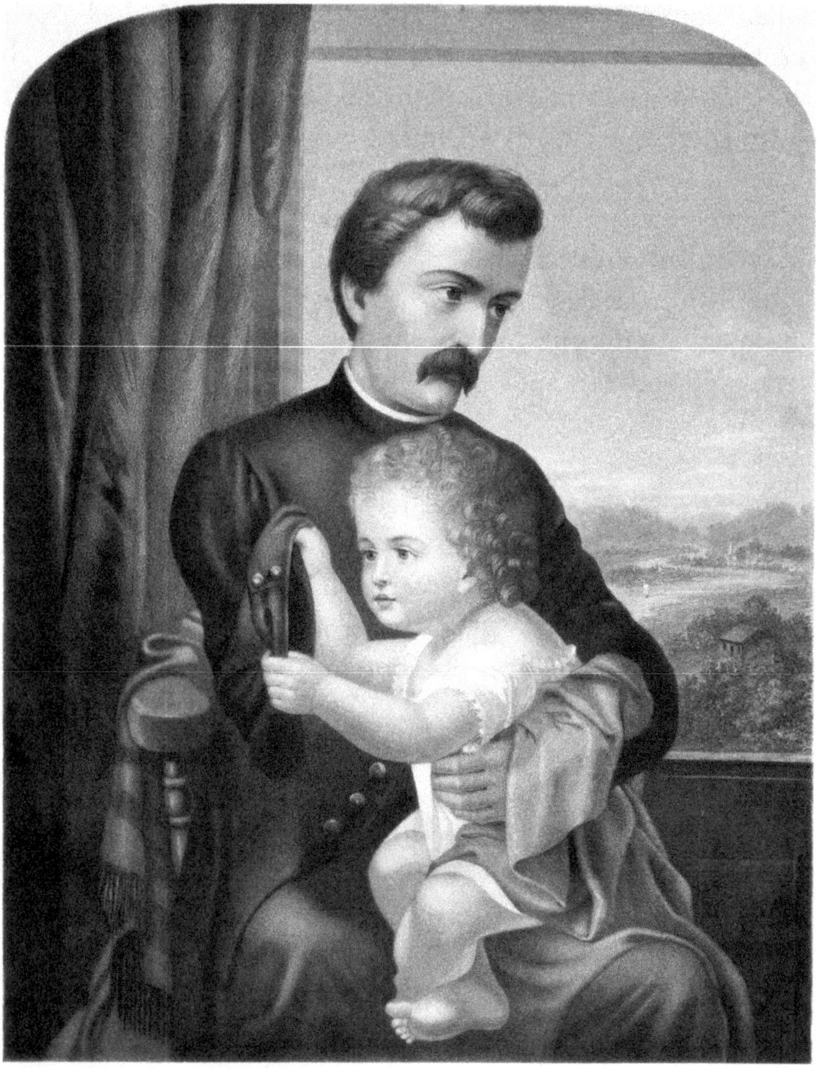

"The Empty Sleeve," a print published by J. C. Buttre, NY, 1866, based on a painting by Adelaide R. Sawyer. *Credit: Courtesy, American Antiquarian Society.*

and corporeal sacrifice." The setting of the image suggests domesticity, the home a place of caregiving to child and feminized veteran, an environment out of public view.[50]

The image also projects ambiguity. War wounds could be stigmata. Depictions and descriptions of wounds as disabling, limiting, or emasculating come from sources other than the veterans, just as medical terms used today to describe people with physical limitations come from physicians and insurers, not from people with those limitations. The maternal posture of the soldier in "The Empty Sleeve" suggests that his manhood has diminished by his embracing of feminine characteristics. Sawyer's soldier ponders future possibilities.

DISABILITY AND ITS REPRESENTATIONS

Today, disability has medical, legal, and social meanings, all of which are restricted by definition. The Americans with Disabilities Act (ADA) provides a legal definition: a person with a disability is one "who has a physical or mental impairment that substantially limits one or more major life activity." It can be challenging to determine what constitutes a disabled person in the context of the Civil War. Applying the ADA definition to Civil War disability is ahistorical, and perhaps applying the term at all is unnecessary. The war produced many documented examples of wounded or diseased soldiers who were unable to resume prewar occupations but found other pathways. *Disability* was a term used in the mid-nineteenth century to describe people with limited abilities or opportunities due to a physical malady. Veterans endured the views held by family and community that their disabilities occurred because of spiritual lapses, immorality, or characteristics of their ethnicity. Outside of employing the label in negotiating with pension authorities, veterans rarely used the term to describe themselves.[51]

Representations of Civil War disability, whether in text or images, reflected anxieties by onlookers, family members, or employers, and sometimes by veterans themselves. These anxieties derive from clinical reports, fiction and other popular writing, and popular imagery. These sources shaped society's responses to apparent disability. An amputee veteran might construct or alter his identity to anticipate people's responses or filter their gaze. The imagery of disability was suffused with cultural distress. The subject of physical disability "dominated the creative imagination, scientific understandings of the human body, and intellectual thought during and after the war."[52]

The veteran who bore the visible scars of war was a blank slate for evolving ideas about disability as the pension structure changed over time and public opinion about pensioned veterans drifted. The veteran's body remained "ideologically malleable." Some historians have written that amputations or vital operations meant a loss of autonomy for the soldier as the surgeon assumed greater power to reshape or modify his body. "The disabled body [was] a site where the authority of medicine subverted the individual's personhood." The case studies in this book argue for a different view. The soldier who has suffered a visible disability shared a dialogue and underwent therapies with one or more physicians, and together, they created a new body. Without the physician, veterans created their own pathways to respectability and independence. They exercised that malleability in revising their presentation of self as their wounds or illnesses from the war were reexamined and treated as medical therapies evolved. Medical intervention did not subvert identity: veterans absorbed therapies and forms of self-care, and the dialogue with surgeons helped them fashion their self-images. All the veterans studied here asserted agency in the world.[53]

An overlooked symbol that provides a clue to veterans' formation of postwar identities is the public statue. Severely wounded or amputee veterans became "readable bodies" to others, a public display the veteran could shape. All veterans who had experienced war damage recognized that their bodies were sites "where memories of the nation crystalize or fuse." The disabled or disfigured veteran supported the creation of monuments and statues depicting soldiers in attitudes of combat or vigilance, rarely in attitudes of suffering or death and never with gaping wounds or shattered arms or legs. The opposition between sculpted or cast soldier bodies and the living veterans required negotiation. Full-figure statues of soldiers did not appear in abundance on the national landscape until a generation had passed. Veterans, the main forces behind the movement to memorialize in stone or bronze, may have wanted to re-create in perpetuity the vigorous bodies of their youthful time of patriotic ardor. The obvious generalization proposes that veterans could own these stone or bronze bodies as emblems of the righteousness of their suffering and point to them whenever public attention was drawn elsewhere. Their sacrifice thus remained in the present tense.

Stone bodies also commemorated a state of mind. They show resolution, courage, vision, and dedication. They depict an American spirit and hold it in perpetuity to challenge future generations. These memorial bodies were under the public gaze. Onlookers scrutinized postures and attitudes and inferred emotions from stone faces. Subsequent generations made comparisons among the bronze or stone soldiers, the aging veterans, the public repository of photographic and other images of the war, and the ongoing discourse about vigilance against threats to national unity and purpose.[54]

Alongside statues at celebrations and dedicatory events, veterans may have projected their apparent disabilities as *improving,* not disabling. The disfigured body sometimes offended or startled others, but the disabled veteran might have perceived his body as having advantages over those of "normal" people, a category that lost meaning in a postwar landscape. The disfiguring wound or amputation stump, as stigma, "serve[d] to define . . . what it is to be fully human." The veteran's body challenged the long-held public perception of disability as indicative of fragility or decay.

Statues of determined and brave soldiers reminded citizens that no wound or disease that resulted from the pure motive of patriotism could possibly indicate an impure soul.[55]

PAIN

The soldiers portrayed in this book, consequent to their wartime maladies, endured pain, whether intermittent, chronic, sharp, dull, migrating throughout the body, or local. Pain defied and baffled the pension office, which had no way to quantify it. Veterans' lives attested to "the living wounded body" as "the final untellable legend."[56] Poet Emily Dickinson captured pain's uncharacterizable nature:

> Pain—has an Element of Blank—
> It cannot recollect
> When it begun—or if there were
> A time when it was not.[57]

Pain's strangeness relegated it to the category of medical anecdote. Mitchell's case notes on wounded soldiers and the many accounts of battle survivors confirm that a soldier struck by a minié ball may not have experienced pain at first. Some soldiers hit by bullets thought that a mischievous comrade from behind hit them with a ramrod and so turned to curse the suspected prankster. Another soldier might have collapsed in a faint. Another was excited to frantic and hysterical behavior. Another instantly felt numbness and lost the ability to hold a rifle or move fingers.

Common beliefs about pain during the Civil War can be glimpsed through assumptions about its moral value. Many people, including some physicians, opined that the use of anesthesia to dull pain came at a cost. Enduring pain or functioning as if pain were a minor impediment became virtuous behavior. Pain was a natural experience that was essential to being human. However, those who were unable to feel pain were deemed insensitive.

"Endurance involves strength and character; insensitivity can result from a moral or physiological defect." The nature of pain for Civil War soldiers posed confusion for these two categories. Mitchell's work identified pain so extreme that a soldier would plead to have the affected limb amputated. He was curious if this extreme pain could be endured. He wondered if the soldier who endured it was an exemplar of manliness or a sympathetic victim of a malady of as-yet unknown proportions. Possibly the soldier with clearly visible injuries or wounds who did not feel pain was a medical anomaly, one as deserving of study and sympathetic treatment as the pain-ridden man too weak to communicate the state of his body.[58]

Both doctors and patients coped with pain within a hierarchy of suffering and placed the soldiers' cases within it, filtered by race, class, and gender. White women occupied the top pain rung due to their innate delicacy, refinement, and clear evidence of a need for therapeutic intervention: They fainted, had headache spells, and were subject to temporary debility because of menstruation. Black women (and men, for that matter), occupied a much lower rung because of a common belief that African Americans had an innate insensitivity to pain that might otherwise subdue a white person. The effete white officer who graduated from Harvard might feel pain more exquisitely than a soldier who had been a teamster before the war. These distinctions were further nuanced by the ethnic backgrounds of the soldiers.[59]

The young men who became soldiers did not expect physicians to relieve their pain in every instance, nor did they seek pain medication for every malady. For their part, physicians were conservative in medicating pain. One reason not to anesthetize a patient before surgery was to preserve their ability to communicate verbally during the operation. Further, doctors relied on pain responses to ensure that the patient was recovering because they believed that pain signified vitality. "Bodily discomfort offered both patients and their doctors the reassurance that at least something was being done to alleviate symptoms, that symptoms were responding to a physician's intervention."[60]

Doctors conservatively used chemical forms of anesthesia to ease pain during surgery, both ether and chloroform governed by a considerable body of clinical literature. Because physicians believed that some pain was natural and promoted vitality, they also viewed anesthetics as potentially harmful, even lethal. Side effects included death from cardiac arrest and insanity. During the Civil War, however, the consensus of the medical profession was that more empirical data were needed on the effects of ether and chloroform. Their use might constitute experimentation on a patient. Even the fledgling American Medical Association did not yet endorse anesthesia. Veterans' manifestations of their pain and physicians' descriptions and analyses of that pain and their attempts to explore and treat it are complex and deeply entangled with how veterans managed bodily pain for the rest of their lives.[61]

Mitchell's therapies involving electricity elicited painful responses that required opiates to relieve. These treatments formed part of his investigation of the pain: its place within the body, how it travels throughout the body and under what stimuli, and the effectiveness of soldier self-care and physician-administered therapies. Mitchell's health questionnaire decades after the Civil War may have been mainly about pain, but the data he collected were somewhat confusing. For instance, respondents who had suffered amputations identified phantom limb pain that some of Mitchell's peers did not regard as a clinical reality. In trying to explicate pain incident to nerve damage, he struggled to trust the body's responses.[62]

CONCLUSION: CAN'T IMAGINE

Although it might be possible to construct a history of the Civil War veteran's body, there is one barrier most readers (and historians) cannot cross: the experience of combat. Veterans strove to make sense of it, as do all veterans of all wars. Mitchell's approach to evaluating war-torn bodies was to reenact the moment of injury or wounding: if possible, patients would demonstrate their movements preceding the moment the harm was inflicted. Similarly, they would demonstrate how in recovery their bodies had altered physical behavior. Mitchell's clinical writings incorporated soldiers' narratives of their suffering. Reading the case studies, one can imagine the larger environment of battlefield confusion, noise, and eviscerated men, but the reader cannot truly comprehend the scene. Mitchell later turned to fiction to capture this essence of destruction and death. Writer and critic Susan Sontag, in her masterful analysis of our photographic depictions of human suffering, also reached this ineffable barrier: "We can't imagine how dreadful, how terrifying war is; and how normal it becomes. Can't understand. Can't imagine."[63]

Poet Lindsay Tuggle wrote a meditation on an anthropodermic book—a book partially bound in human skin—found in the Historical Medical Library of the College of Physicians of Philadelphia. The skin, possibly from a Confederate soldier, bound a copy of Dr. Joseph Leidy's *An Elementary Treatise on Human Anatomy* (1861), owned by the author. Her poem concludes, "We are all flesh / toying architecturally with bone." Veterans and their physicians were all flesh, and in coping with injuries, wounds, and diseases, both participated in "toying" architecturally with bone, sinew, and blood to define new people. The next chapter explores how Dr. Mitchell toyed architecturally with soldiers' nervous systems to elucidate the nature of pain within bodies that were truly wounded for life.[64]

TWO

SILAS WEIR MITCHELL
(1829–1914)

SERGEANT MARKS AND DOCTOR MITCHELL

Sergeant Abraham D. Marks and the rest of Company C, Third Maryland Volunteers, marched forward through a field of felled trees, a cornfield visible to the right, and beyond it, Chancellor House. The men formed a line of battle and leveled their rifles at Confederate troops. On this day, May 3, 1863, when forty-three-year-old Marks raised his left arm to support his rifle as he aimed, a bullet entered his left armpit, passed through his pectoral muscle, struck the upper portion of his humerus, and exited his body through the coracoid process.[1] In glancing off the humerus, the bullet damaged Marks's brachial plexus, a nerve bundle descending along the arm from the brain. As he turned to leave the field, a bullet struck his back to the right of his eighth dorsal vertebra.[2] It traveled into the left side of his chest, where it remained. With this second wound, Marks fell to the ground.[3]

Confederates overran Marks's position and took him prisoner. He was taken to a field hospital and placed outside on the ground, exposed to the elements for some time. The hospital may have attended to his upper shoulder wound on the assumption that the humerus was fractured and immobilized the left arm with a pasteboard splint or adhesive strips to the shoulder. For either wound, a physician would have applied bandages to stop the bleeding. The bullet entry wounds were likely small and round and perhaps discolored from powder burns. The exit wound from the first bullet would have been "comparatively large, slit-like, everted, and free from color." Initially, Marks felt palsy in his left hand and little pain in his left arm from the first bullet. The second bullet, however, caused coughing and spitting blood, dysphagia,[4] and finally pleurisy[5] and a large amount of pus escaping as he breathed.[6]

During the first week after his wounding, Marks felt pain in his left arm, at first a "knife-like" pain that extended from the entry wound down the arm short of the wrist, later as "tingling and burning." Within the next few weeks, a prisoner exchange was arranged, and by June 10, Marks entered West Philadelphia Hospital in Philadelphia, where Dr. Silas Weir Mitchell examined him. By early July, the back wound closed, and the "lower half of the lung consolidated." Mitchell found Marks in a desperate state: "He lies on his back, anxious-looking, and pain-worn. The left arm rests on a pillow. It is cold, mottled, and swollen. The skin of the hand is thin, and dark-red, but presents no eruption. Tactility, nowhere absent, is dull on the dorsum [back] of the hand and fingers. . . . The whole arm and hand, except its back part, is, as he says, alive with burning pain . . . which cold and wetting ease considerably."[7]

Mitchell took on the case because other doctors either failed to recognize or had no resources or knowledge to treat injuries to nerves. The patients referred to Mitchell may have been considered hopeless because of the unlikelihood that they could ever return to duty. Mitchell's treatments began with applying ice to relieve swelling of the deltoid.[8] To encourage motion below the elbow with swollen joints and fingers partially flexed, he applied blisters[9] containing morphia (morphine) and administered hypodermic injections of morphia near the entry wound. The arm responded to the morphia, but the condition of the hand worsened. Mitchell abandoned the injections because the puncture sites developed erysipelas, a "superficial inflammation of the skin" now recognized as a bacterial infection.

When the infection cleared, injections resumed, first with conia (or conine, from poison hemlock). When that failed to relieve the pain, Mitchell tried atropia (a poisonous narcotic from deadly nightshade) that served only to relax the flexors of the fingers. He then resumed the morphia injections and turned to electricity, a novel technology in medicine, rare in American medical practice and nonexistent in army hospitals. The current could not activate the arm and forearm and induced pain. Both therapeutic and exploratory, electricity did not always yield consistent or predictable results. For Marks, electricity meant pain. Mitchell followed *electrization* (the contemporary term for applying electricity to the body) with more morphia injections. Mitchell dubbed the extreme pain "causalgia," and his clinical definition of the term thus acknowledged an extreme and almost unendurable pain occasioned by a poorly understood nervous system that had suffered trauma.[10]

By August, Marks's pain had not only diminished but seemed to increase. Marks now "moans and weeps incessantly." By September, Marks had received injections so "numerous that the part is dotted with punctures, and their irritation has aggravated [his] sufferings to such a degree that they have been presently laid aside for the internal use of narcotics." Mitchell turned to laudanum (alcohol and opium), "lead-water," vapor baths, douches of hot and cold water, "iodide of lead," "ointments of iodine," and various poultices and ice applications. He placed leeches on the wound scars followed by blisters, but "darting pains" continued to plague Marks's left arm. Nevertheless, "every motion or vibration caused pain." Most of these therapies failed to relieve pain or help Marks regain the use of his arm.[11]

By October, blistering applications appeared to be helping, particularly those saturated in morphia, ammonia, and cantharides.[12] These blisters remained in use until the pain ceased. Marks remained stable until December when he developed pneumonia of the right lung. That same month, Mitchell again tried electricity but stopped due to the pain it caused. Hospital nurses shampooed (massaged) Marks's hand and arm. Around the beginning of 1864, Marks could sit up and walk. He gained weight. Mitchell once again "electrized" Marks's body but failed to activate the muscles below the shoulder on the left side. He also took casts of the atrophying arm and hand for the Army Medical Museum. Eventually, the electrization stopped causing pain. Marks was able to move his fingers somewhat but not his thumb. The left hand was bandaged to manipulate the extensors,[13] which had been involuntarily contracting. By April, the hospital discharged Marks, who was pain-free but "having only three fourths of the fingers, without power to extend them. All other motions were improving.... Sensation perfect."[14]

Decades later, Mitchell teamed with his physician son, John Kearsley Mitchell, to survey the health of soldiers treated by his Philadelphia team of doctors, W. W. Keen and George Morehouse. This survey or questionnaire unites four of the soldiers discussed in this study.[15] The younger Mitchell extended his father's work to examine war veterans to update the condition of their wounds or injuries of the nerves. As an homage to his father's work, he published his analysis, *Remote Consequences of Injuries of Nerves, and Their Treatment.*

John K. Mitchell examined Marks in Philadelphia in 1890, a year before Marks's death from "dropsy from cardiac disease," apparently unrelated to his bullet wounds. Marks's pain had been unabated since 1863, although the second bullet had been removed in 1877 from an abscess that had formed around it. Marks did not continue the prescribed exercises for his arm and hand,

and thus his condition deteriorated after he was discharged from the hospital in 1864. He evidently recovered from the back wound with no problems, but his arm was another matter. At the time of his death, Marks's arm had been useless for decades, and "he suffered a good deal of pain." The 1890 examination consisted in part of John K. Mitchell using a needle to prick the skin along the arm to evaluate sensation. He also conducted an electrical test and found "quantitative reduction" to faradic and galvanic electrical stimulation (defined in the next chapter).[16]

This case study illustrates Mitchell's interest in nerve phenomena, his attempts to understand extreme pain—causalgia—which he named, and his treatments with the novel therapy of electricity. Marks's case is a prototypical one of nerve wound damage resulting in extreme pain and debility, and it illustrates the range of tests and therapies both Mitchells conducted thirty years apart. In exploring Marks's case long-term, both Mitchells developed an intimate partnership with their patient. Mitchell even replicated part of Marks's body in plaster for the Army Medical Museum. The 1890 examination reveals, too, how Marks stalled his 1863–1864 recovery under Mitchell's supervision by not continuing the exercises that might have improved his arm. He allowed the arm to deteriorate without contacting Mitchell to renew the helpful therapies. Mitchell effectively shaped Marks's recovery and, despite the deterioration of the arm, left Marks as a healing patient during 1863–1864, when both doctor and patient collaborated to build a postwar body. Marks's identity during the last decades of his life was shaped by that experience.

Mitchell's work was novel because his patients had been shifted from hospital to hospital when no physician had the time, patience, or expertise to observe and treat "phenomena which are rarely seen and which were naturally foreign to the observation of those surgeons whose experience was the most extensive and complete." Mitchell's unusual relationship with soldiers' bodies

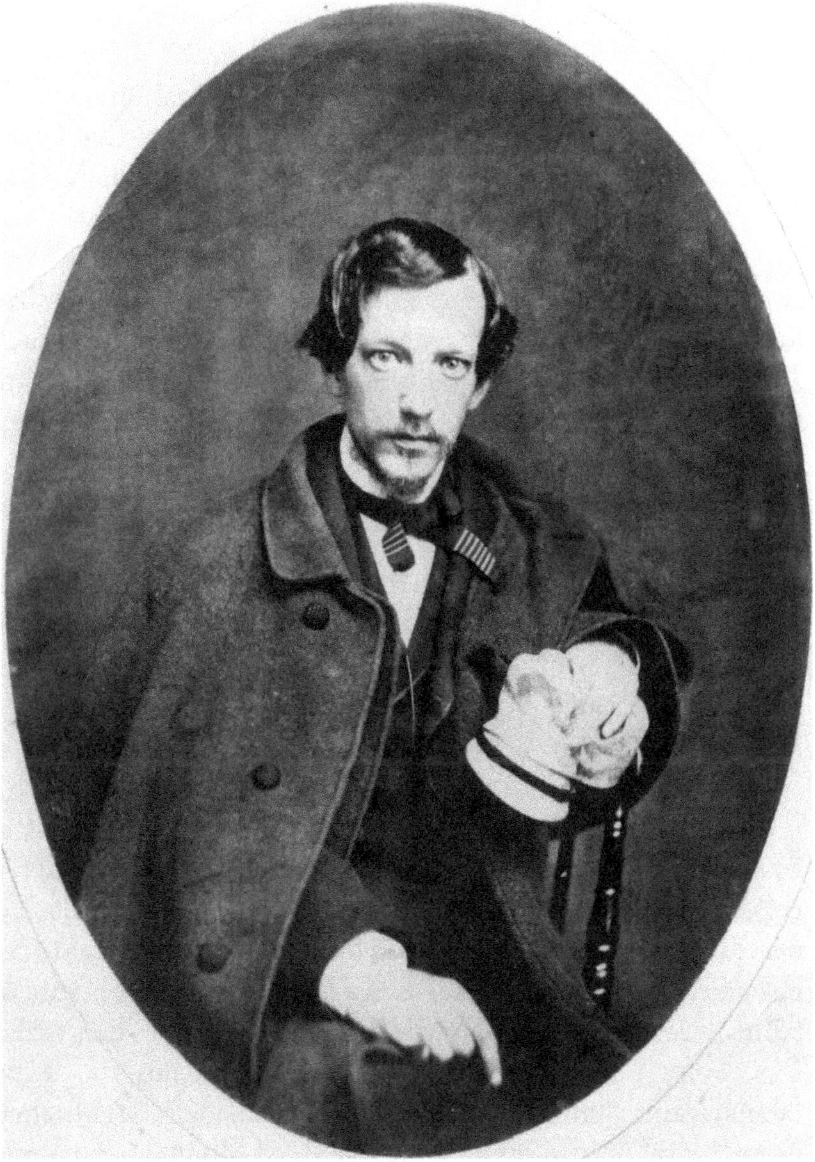

S. Weir Mitchell, MD, during the Civil War. *Credit: S. Weir Mitchell collection, Ms. Coll. 413, Kislak Center for Special Collections, Rare Books and Manuscripts, University of Pennsylvania.*

developed because the medical literature presented "wounds of nerves . . . as curiosities and as matter for despair."[17]

Mitchell's scrutiny of nerves through investigation into and manipulation of his patients' bodies was so atypical that he invented a language for the corpus of therapies he applied to soldiers' bodies. Mitchell's abundant clinical writings reveal a deep thinker whose works influenced medical practice well into the twentieth century. This chapter examines Mitchell's organization of a ward for treating soldiers suffering from injuries such as Marks's and his collaboration with two colleagues to create the medical discipline of neurology. Mitchell's work has been amply documented in other studies, so the focus here will be on his relationship with American men and the concept of manhood requisite for the type of doctor-patient partnership Mitchell found useful for treatment and recovery, a uniting of two bodies to produce a reconstructed one. My focus on Mitchell pertains to the physicality of interaction between him and his soldier-patients in treating peripheral nerve injuries and extreme pain.[18]

TURNER'S LANE

By the time Mitchell met Sergeant Abraham Marks, he and his colleagues had established a regimen for treating wounds and nerve injuries and had assembled a team for that purpose. Mitchell had rejected an offer to serve as a brigade surgeon because of family circumstances, so for the duration of the war, he worked as a contract assistant surgeon. In a makeshift hospital at the Pennsylvania State Arsenal building in Philadelphia, Mitchell began his investigations with George Reed Morehouse and was joined later by William Williams Keen. The three men were in their thirties and disposed to investigate phenomena through experimentation. Mitchell's leadership of the trio seemed obvious to all: "By breeding, instinct, and personality, Silas Weir Mitchell was the leader of this remarkable cast."[19]

At Mitchell's request, army surgeon General William A. Hammond, an investigator of nervous disorders, arranged for the transformation of Moyamensing Hall on Christian Street in Philadelphia into a hospital specializing in nerve cases. The "red tape" paperwork was assigned to others, leaving the physicians free for clinical work. Before the war, Hammond resided in Philadelphia and had collaborated with Mitchell and Morehouse, whom he had assigned to examine "the minute anatomy of the nerves and nerve-centers." Beginning in the summer of 1862, these physicians (they referred to themselves as "the Firm") began their investigations and arranged for all difficult cases involving wounded nerves to be brought to them. They traded non-nerve-related cases with cases they wanted from other hospitals and gradually developed their neurological ward at Christian Street. In late 1864, with a burgeoning caseload, they transferred to Turner's Lane Hospital, formerly a farm north of the city but converted into a hospital at the beginning of the war. At Turner's Lane, "for the first time, its capacity enabled us to classify in distinct wards the numerous cases which fell under our care. Never has such an opportunity for the study of nerve lesions and their results presented itself." Despite the opportunity, "In a kind of nightmarish substitution, human beings replaced the animals of his earlier experimentation—many of them very young men with torn flesh, shattered bones, burning pain, and phantom limbs."[20]

According to the hospital's division of labor, Mitchell examined damage to peripheral nerves, Morehouse studied patients with epileptic symptoms following head injuries, and Keen took on malingering, particularly the faking of neurological injuries. Incoming soldiers were washed, given clean clothes, and assigned beds. When the Firm began an examination, the doctors asked the soldier to describe or assume his body position at the time he was wounded and describe the larger environmental circumstances. And so the soldier's collaboration with Mitchell and colleagues began with a performance, the reenactment of the moment of wounding. In an almost forensic reconstruction of events, the Firm elicited a narrative of the wounding that enabled doctors to chronicle the path of the bullet through (and possibly out of) the body. The doctors appreciated and relied on their voluble, self-conscious patients who could deliver a chronology of actions, articulate bodily responses, and engage in dialogue about their treatments and recovery. The Firm took extensive notes while nonmedical assistants completed the administrative reports required by military regulations. "Recorded information included name, place of birth, general health, circumstances and initial reaction to injury, description of the wound, length of time before treatment, nature of treatment, and extent of recovery of sensation and motion."[21]

Mitchell's definition of the nervous system was conventional for the time. It identified the structures of the nerves without addressing the precise mechanism by which nerve impulses arise and are transmitted throughout the body. Most clinical descriptions of the nervous system did not reckon with wartime wounds to the nerves, much less clarify how pain manifested. Mitchell wrote that "the nervous system consists essentially of receptive or controlling ganglionic centres, and of the nerves which connect these with one another and with the skin, muscles, and viscera. Nerves are usually divided into those known as cerebro-spinal and those belonging to the great sympathetic system."[22]

When questioning a patient, Mitchell paid attention to any mention of numbness or lack of sensation, sure signs of nerve dysfunction. Mitchell probed the soldier's body with hands and a needle to ascertain "how great is the loss of sensibility, and by its limits, what nerves have been primarily affected." Once Mitchell had roughly gauged the extent and location of the nerve injury, he began a treatment regimen. One track included conventional remedies for pain, and another involved unconventional and experimental therapies. Conventional therapies included leeching, poultices, wet dressings, blistering, and various narcotics.

Unconventional therapies to reduce numbness and facilitate a return to sensation included shampooing (massage), morphia (hypodermically administered), and electrization. Time, bed rest, and nutrition were part of all treatments. Mitchell improvised other treatments, including the introduction of gymnastic classes, an early form of rehabilitative therapy. Other types of physiotherapy and hydrotherapy provided supplementary methods to revive bodies if the conventional ones were not effective. The unconventional therapies and most of the conventional ones required the surgeon to manipulate the soldier's body.[23]

PAIN THAT NEVER CEASED TO AMAZE THE THOUGHTFUL

Trauma is no simple pathology; rather, a wound "addresses us in the attempt to tell us of a reality or truth that is not otherwise available." Narratives of trauma, which Mitchell and his soldier-patients developed together, have an "endless impact on a life." Pain, however, confounds language and distorts perception and time, and for veterans who suffered pain throughout their lives, it became an indescribable experience around which the afflicted person created meaning. For all that Mitchell found baffling about pain, lifelong pain received little attention in the history of medicine. Pain, like the trauma that triggered it, remained a "narrative of a belated experience."[24]

By focusing on nerve injuries, Mitchell became familiar with a wide range of traumatic phenomena. Not every soldier struck by a bullet felt pain. Some went into shock, a life-threatening injury to nerves that causes the patient to become "cold, faint, and trembling; the pulse is small and fluttering." Some soldiers experienced incoherence or confusion regarding time, place, or circumstance; others vomited or defecated when shot. Some soldiers blamed comrades for playing a practical joke, while some thought that they had been hit with sticks or stones. "A clever sergeant, Canadian by birth, described his first pain as like that which is felt when a cricket-bat carelessly held is struck by a swift ball. The feeling of numbness, with tingling pain, is common in cases of slight nerve wounds or contusions." The diversity of responses to wounds and the degree of pain elicited when the body experienced violence or during later therapy intrigued Mitchell throughout his career.[25]

Owing to causalgia and the effects of electrization, Mitchell found Turner's Lane "a hell of pain." Believing that pain must have a physical location in the body, he searched unsuccessfully for a pain lesion. "Of the exact nature of the affection of nerve matter which produces pain we know but little," he wrote. He struggled to describe the varying degrees of pain. His inability to affix pain to a physical anchor corresponds with the challenge of language to express or discuss it. "Physical pain does not simply resist language but actively destroys it . . . [reverting] to the sounds and cries a human being makes before language is learned." For this reason, pain "resists objectification in language." Mitchell's two landmark treatises, *Gunshot Wounds* and *Injuries of Nerves*, have been characterized as trying "to reverse the de-objectifying work of pain."[26]

After the war, Mitchell came to understand that the pain he witnessed in recovering soldiers did not necessarily disappear but could come and go or remain chronic. Today, we might speculate that some recurrent pain may have been a reaction to trauma or the reexperience of catastrophic events, especially wartime violence. Mitchell and other astute physicians recognized symptoms of distress due to combat experiences and often labeled them melancholia. Those suffering from it exhibited lassitude and depression and a lack of ambition, desire, or interest in the world. Melancholia therefore militated against some of the characteristics of manhood, such as competition, achievement, and progress. In today's terms, melancholia means depression as a result of the "acting-out of trauma" that is unresolved. For Civil

War veterans, melancholia was joined with pain. By the late nineteenth century, Mitchell recognized concomitant phenomena to pain arising from inscrutable reservoirs of emotion. To him, intense emotions could contribute to lasting wounds of the mind. Even a dream "may occasion forms of temporary or lasting mental disorder, for which we have as yet no reasonable explanation. The largeness of the psychical and the smallness of the observable co-attendant pathological physical conditions never cease to amaze the thoughtful."[27]

Mitchell continuously explored the physical bases for emotional phenomena. He examined the nature of sleep and dreams and suspected that sleep involved "functionally actionless" nerve cells that are static during sleep. Using a military metaphor, he wrote, "When we begin, awaken, and the drowsied sentinels resume their posts," the nerves come to life. They close the day with a return to sleep. Mitchell described attendant hypnopompic hallucinations (those that occur when a person is half awake, half asleep, and dreaming) as "fairy country . . . a time for castle-building." He began taking mescal to heighten his sensitivity to these phenomena. Nonetheless, his observations and the experience of his narcotized body did not bring him closer to rationalizing the "co-attendant" pain and emotional highs and lows. In the end, he mathematized emotions by hypothesizing that everyone begins life with "a par of cheerfulness" that varies from person to person according to an innate "lifelong mood." Presumably, traumatic events permanently subtract hunks of cheerfulness—and a sense of time—from the body's storehouse.[28]

Mitchell's case study of Sergeant L. P. highlights the transitory nature of traumatic pain and the accompanying emotional changes with a significant diminution of that "par of cheerfulness." L. P. sustained a gunshot wound through the middle third of his thigh (Mitchell does not say which thigh) at Fredericksburg, Virginia, in 1862. L. P. immediately felt numbness and a loss of energy. Just over a week later, he experienced "sharp pain" at the wound site, alternating with aching and an "intense burning in the foot." The next day, he was delirious. "He begged at times to be killed, at others, to go home; while sometimes he would lie open-eyed, regarding ferociously the passers-by who shook his bed as they walked, every movement seeming to add to his torment." Gradually, the pain receded except for the burning foot, which took many months to subside. During the months of pain, L. P.'s emotional state transformed from his pain-free self.[29]

The persistent pain in the dorsum of L. P.'s foot coupled with the change in his personality indicated the presence of causalgia, the pain of pains. Indeed, causalgia "replac[ed] all other physical sensation and invad[ed] consciousness with a kind of nerve torture that shatters the body's discipline and coherence." Jos. H. Corliss, Company B, Fourteenth New York State Militia, was shot at the Second Battle of Manassas in 1862. He had emptied a powder cartridge down the muzzle of his rifle when a bullet entered his left arm. At first, Corliss "thought he was struck on the crazy-bone by some of the boys for a joke." Confederates took him prisoner and later exchanged him. Corliss was transferred to various hospitals in Washington, DC, before ending up in Mitchell's ward. Causalgia became the center of his life. "It is as if a rough bar of iron were thrust to and fro through the knuckles, a red-hot iron placed at the junction of the palm and the thenar eminence,[30] with a heavy weight on it, and the skin was being rasped off my finger-ends." In this statement, Corliss uses anatomical nomenclature to identify the pain center, revealing how the collaborative dialogue between doctor and patient affected his experience. Corliss underwent a personality change in "the presence of others from the fear of being hurt."[31]

Mitchell understood that pain was manifested through "the nerves of animal life" that somehow emerged from the spinal cord and extended throughout the body, but "of the exact nature of the affection of nerve matter which produces pain we know but little." To explain what he did know about the generation of pain, Mitchell used an analogy. "It is as if through a single tube were spoken various languages which could be only understood when, at its farther end, they reached the ear of the hearer native to each form of speech." Causalgia was "a form of suffering yet undescribed" that appeared following the sensation of burning pain, a pain that survived the initial wounding into later life. The Firm provided the first description of causalgia in print. Wet dressings seemed to be the most efficacious treatment, although their impact on nerves was very superficial until sympathectomy (surgical removal of nerves or associated ganglia that have been unduly stimulated) was developed in the 1930s.[32]

Striving for clinical precision to describe this pain, Mitchell used feminized language to explain how it debilitated manhood. He applied "hysteria" to the behavior of afflicted soldiers, a word he justified as "the only term which covers the facts." If the appearance and subsequent (possible) disappearance of causalgia remained a mystery, its related physical symptoms were unmistakable. The skin in the vicinity of the pain swelled and appeared stretched, glossy, and reddened. On the hands, the nails changed, "curving, thickening," and the patient endured hair loss near the site of the pain. Afflicted persons also exuded a peculiar odor described as "intensely acid," akin to vinegar. Sweat smelled like a bad drain. The associated pain, however, continually astonished onlooking physicians and presented as sheer torture. Indeed, sufferers "again and again [begged] to amputate the suffering limb."[33]

For example, Mitchell saw a thirty-year-old soldier, "a large, vigorous man, [who] was one of the leaders of the gallant storming party which took Fort Fisher." This soldier, who had "led the life of adventure and danger," had been shot by a bullet that pierced his lung and traveled into his right arm, injuring the median nerve. Causalgia developed and thus "reduced him in three months to a slightly covered skeleton, and transformed him morally into a peevish, timid child." Another soldier who had received a bullet to the right arm at Gettysburg experienced causalgia in the palm of his right hand, hyperesthesia so severe that "even to blow on it seemed to give pain." The soldier kept the hand wrapped in wet cloth that he rewetted by soaking the palm—pouring water only caused more pain. The pain worsened such that the distant noise of a band aggravated it: "His countenance at this time was worn, pinched, and anaemic, his temper irritable, and his manner so odd that some of the attendants believed him insane." Soon, "every strong moral emotion" just made matters worse, a disintegration of manhood. Still more unusual was causalgia's affliction of hands and feet while not appearing elsewhere in the body.[34]

Causalgic symptoms were so intense that they caused skepticism in onlookers, particularly other physicians with very conservative views about haunting pains not rooted in identifiable lesions. Mitchell wrote that some of his colleagues, on examining afflicted patients for the first time, "have been so surprised as to suspect that such extreme hyperaesthesia must be due, at least in some measure, to a desire on the part of the patient to magnify his pains." The boundary between the display of the symptoms of a disease and malingering, or faking symptoms, could be difficult to establish, yet in all contexts of treatment, physicians were conscious that their patients, even those with obvious wounds, might be deceiving their doctors. Dr. Keen, the Firm member charged with studying malingering, wrote, "*Pain* is not a feigned disease, but is the most easily feigned symptom, the most difficult and often most apparently cruel to gainsay or deny, and, at the same time, the most available stronghold to which the malingerer can resort." Sometimes the body cannot be trusted.[35]

The Firm used every analgesic that seemed promising to relieve the pain of causalgia. Of all the therapies they tried, hypodermic applications of morphia "alone in many instances seemed able to overcome the anguish of certain forms of neuralgic distress." Some soldiers received as many as twenty to thirty injections daily. Other drugs were tried—conia, datura, atropia—but only morphia reliably delivered consistent results. Repeated injections, however, and the corresponding puncture sites "produced a very unpleasant increase of sensitiveness in the part." Sometimes the injections resulted in abscesses or ulcers, requiring cessation of the therapy. Still, Mitchell decided where to inject the drug: at the site of the pain or elsewhere. As close as possible to the site of "burning neuralgia" seemed optimal for achieving the greatest relief, but eventually, first the soldiers and finally the reluctant physicians agreed that the injection site made little difference.[36]

To be more precise in his descriptions of causalgia and circumscribing its behavior and limits, Mitchell tried measuring it. Given the apparent increase in temperature at the locus of causalgia, calorification, the measurement of heat, seemed like a possible solution, but the apparatus proved troublesome. At first, Mitchell tried placing a bulb thermometer at the pain site, without success. Next, he tried "thermo-electric disks of M. Becquerel, in connection with a very delicate galvanometer. . . . The disks were applied on corresponding parts of the body, and the deflection of the needle of the galvanometer informed us which was the warmer."[37]

If one drew a cluster diagram of the therapies associated with nerve injuries at Turner's Lane Hospital, electricity would connect to every phase of the patient's treatment. Electricity was ubiquitous in Mitchell's work with peripheral nerve damage. "The use of electricity was more like actual exercise than massage, causing contractions of the muscles, increasing the absorption of oxygen, and changing the form and color of the red corpuscles." Electrization was a novel therapy absent from military hospitals except Turner's Lane and Christian Street. While it served as a form of exercise, it was also experimental and exploratory. Because of the pain it frequently elicited, Mitchell accompanied electrization with morphia injections: "hypodermic medication—at that time somewhat novel—was habitually resorted to, and its effects carefully studied." In some ways, electrization represented, short

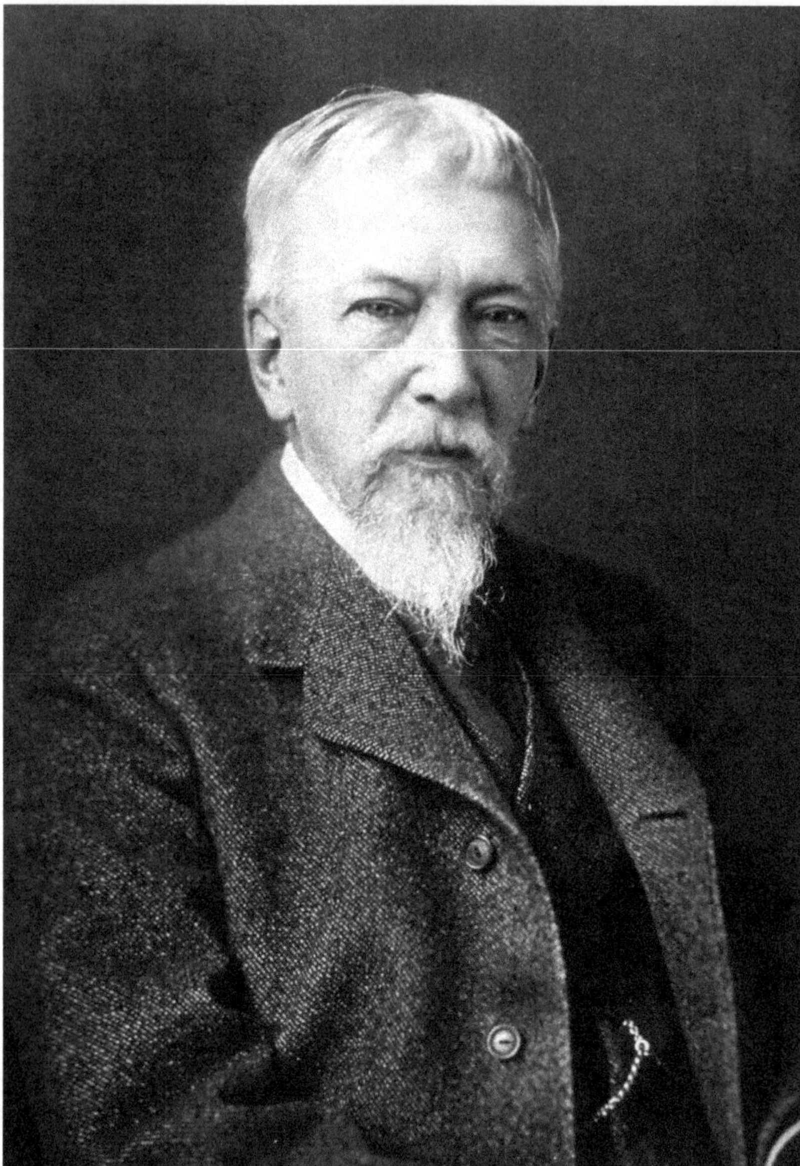

S. Weir Mitchell during the 1890s. *Credit: National Library of Medicine (ID B029404).*

of surgery, Mitchell's most penetrating therapy because it could send the patient within seconds into blinding pain. Electrization not only involved surface stimulation of skin; electrodes could also be inserted then electrified, thus placing soldiers' muscles in thrall to the machine. Electrization usually had an immediate effect of contracting muscles. While electrization helped Mitchell determine the nature of nerve damage, it also enabled him to estimate the possibility of recovery. Mitchell's faith in electricity strengthened, and he concluded, "Of this we are distinctly sure that there is no test of the restoration of nerve supply except the electric current."[38]

The use of electricity, for both Mitchell and patient, evoked associations grounded in professional and popular literature due to its inherent mystery and the widespread belief that the essence of the soul was electricity, simultaneously a material phenomenon and a spiritual essence. Michael Faraday's discovery of electromagnetism in the 1830s not only stimulated works of romantic art, philosophy, and literature; it also became the basis of a range of medical instruments manufactured in the 1850s and thereafter. Similarly, the advent of Samuel B. Morse's telegraph at about the same time had a profound cultural impact. The telegraph enabled people to be in two places at once, challenging "ideologies of the atomistic, isolated self." Mitchell's use of electricity as his dominant therapy to treat damaged peripheral nerves opened the soldier's compartment of a bounded self and allowed the physician to enter.[39]

TINCTURED WITH THE BLOOD OF THE CIVIL WAR

On a hot September afternoon, venetian blinds shutting out the harsh sunlight, Dr. Keen sat at a desk at Jefferson Medical College in Philadelphia with *Gray's Anatomy* open before him as he examined a human skull. He became aware that someone was watching him through the blinds, so he turned and caught a pair of eyes peering at him. A voice spoke: "Doctor, don't you want to help me in some experiments on snakes?" Thus began a lifelong friendship and collaboration between Keen and Mitchell. Keen regarded Mitchell with his eight years of seniority as the master, "a yeasty man" because his brain was fertile with ideas. Another colleague, Owen Wister, reminisced after Mitchell's death about how the good doctor was overwhelmed by the many soldiers he examined and treated. "Wounds, blood and agony were for him a daily sight . . . he conversed and argued with that past . . . every drop of ink is tinctured with the blood of the Civil War." These recollections speak to Mitchell's commitment to experimentation, his fertile mind and expansive curiosity, and his management of work. Then came the war. Mitchell fit uneasily within the military medical hierarchy. Without Hammond's interest and support, Mitchell's special ward devoted to wounded nerves would not have been established, and Mitchell would not have experienced a physical breakdown.[40]

While Mitchell excelled in meeting the military requirements, doing so came at a cost to his family, time, income, and professional stature. As a contracted acting assistant surgeon, Mitchell could avoid the strictly military attributes of the title (and, hence, identity) and concentrate on the work. Despite his military appointment, Mitchell remained susceptible to the draft and paid a substitute. Federal law permitted draftees to pay other men to serve in their stead. He retained a private practice in addition to his army work, making for an exhausting schedule. Mitchell's wife died of diphtheria in 1862, leaving to him the care of his children and widowed mother, so he required his private income to supplement government pay. He visited the hospital in the morning to "[dispose] of the routine work," then to his private practice, followed by a return to the hospital midafternoon where he would see patients and take notes until midnight or one o'clock the next morning. Then he and George Morehouse would walk back into town discussing cases and repeat the schedule the next day. Mitchell wrote to his sister on August 1, 1863, "I am tired of it and myself and am too busy to see my dear boys—Indeed it is a week since I saw them."[41]

Shortly after the death of Mitchell's wife, his cherished youngest brother Ned, a medical cadet in the Union army, also died of diphtheria. The death occurred in 1864 when Mitchell was seeing patients at Turner's Lane. Mitchell's memory of his brother revealed a feminization of character. Ned "was then a beautiful creature with so certain a rare spiritual look which troubled one to see . . . delicate masculine charm." Years later, Mitchell disclosed his anguish about Ned's death in a poem:

> Painfully
> He sickened, yearning for the strife of War
> That went its thunderous way unhelped of him;
> And then he died. A little duty done;
> A little love for many, much for me,
> And that was all beneath this earthly sun.[42]

By the time the war began, Mitchell had formed himself into the new physician, open to new technologies and techniques, determined to create a scientific foundation for his vocation. The war presented new opportunities for him. In the company of a circle of young colleagues, Mitchell reshaped medical practice as the war progressed. "Very simply the medicine of 1860 was vastly different from the medicine of 1863, and the medicine of 1866 was vastly different again." His professional trajectory had something to do with this rapid evolution. A graduate of Jefferson Medical College, Mitchell sojourned in Paris before the war with eminent physiologist Claude Bernard. Upon his return to Philadelphia, Mitchell embarked on a series of explorations ranging from the behavior of uric acid crystals in urine to the physiology of the chelonian to the toxicology of snakebites. As a contract surgeon during the war, Mitchell adhered to Hammond's Circular Number Two, which required Union doctors to "focus on specific organs, tissues, lesions, and specific disease conditions."[43]

To his patients, his fellow doctors, and himself, Mitchell presented a persona that mixed the civilian and the military. As a contract physician, he observed a chain of command and an administrative structure with its own rules. As a civilian doctor, he plied a solo practice "like his contemporaries in business and law, mixed work and sociability." Before the war, a doctor's chief clientele were pregnant women, and this fact might have influenced Mitchell's clinical observations, specifically the application of "hysteria" to men experiencing causalgia. As a military doctor, however, Mitchell would have responded to the increasing emphasis on scientific investigation. This trend characterized Mitchell's clinical work for the remainder of the century. "American medicine became firmly wedded to science." This orientation was strongly endorsed via military policy by the two wartime surgeons general, Hammond and Joseph K. Barnes.[44]

Under most circumstances, physicians in military services wrestled with their identities as officers. Doctors preferred the elite-sounding title of "surgeon" to that of their assigned military rank, which for Mitchell was the junior echelon of lieutenant but without the perquisites enjoyed by officers. While Mitchell followed his own path, other military doctors worked to create a corporate identity, a brand, a fellowship that promoted its own discourse, camaraderie, and esprit de corps. They nevertheless occupied a feminized niche: "The language associated with healing was feminized—nurturing, succoring, nursing—reflecting a gender differentiation between the two professions [military officer and physician]." After the war, Mitchell joined no veterans' organizations. Regarding his patients, Mitchell seemed to be both ward patriarch and comrade to articulate, intelligent, severely wounded soldiers. He constantly touched soldiers' bodies, medicating them with textbook remedies but also extending his touch, increasingly, with electricity.[45]

We assume that Civil War doctors treated soldier-patients while maintaining a clinical, professional distance. The surgeon's hands touch a patient who is not a friend but who implicitly consents to the doctor's ministrations. That understanding grants the doctor license to manipulate a patient's body in intimate, even violent ways. Mitchell's case notes and subsequent publications document his months-long relationships with many soldiers, attesting to an intimacy that soldiers would not have found with most other physicians. We rarely consider the picture of two bodies in an intimate healing partnership, that the physician's body may be joined to that of the patient through a surgical event or therapy. Mitchell's case notes reveal that "tincture of blood" in his own frustration to understand and cure injuries to nerves and thus enable a new veteran to resume his life.

Mitchell's clinical notes and publications reveal his "yeasty" mind and search for understanding and meaning in wounds. He has been cited for the clarity, narrative arc, style, and apparent completeness of his clinical writings. On the last point, one reads Mitchell's case studies as if the universe of possibilities is contained within each, as if no other phenomena or therapies are relevant, as if "their polish obscures the mechanics of the clinical encounter." Even when Mitchell writes searchingly about inconclusive cases, "the rhetorical appeal of [his] medical histories lies in their reconstruction of a clinical picture in which gaps have been filled and mysteries solved." The case studies, however, created narratives that embedded soldiers' own stories. For the rest of their lives, as soldiers were subjected to medical examinations by claims doctors (doctors assigned to examine pension claimants) or others, Mitchell's interventions remained affixed to their identities. His case studies may have pioneered an early understanding of the behavior of nerves and promoted a clinical conversation, but they also revealed a desire to find a way to come to terms with the war, a way to rationalize the suffering of his patients.[46]

Mitchell never experienced combat, but he arrived in Gettysburg the day after the 1863 battle ended. He saw corpses rotting in the July heat and hundreds of doctors at work on thousands of wounded soldiers in tents, homes, barns, and open fields. Although scarred for life by the sights, sounds, and smells, Mitchell remained politically neutral, even passive about the war. He would not "commit to the Northern cause," hated President Abraham Lincoln, and made pejorative and racist remarks about African American soldiers fighting for the Union, an attitude perhaps reflected in the lack of African American soldiers among his case studies. Regarding the rivalry between North and South, he wrote, "For my part I think all sides are insane—I have sympathy with something of all—entire sympathy with none." Mitchell's professed neutrality and detachment crashed against the clinical reality of the devastating cases he took on. To wounded soldiers, he offered his body as a healer who had undertaken a psychic journey of trauma and felt deep empathy toward the men in his care. He risked inflicting new wounds as he experimented, willing to take radical actions to ameliorate suffering even if his therapies caused further suffering that required treatment.[47]

Mitchell's presence at Gettysburg made an unforgettable imprint on his psyche. Three weeks after his arrival, in his additional role as a sanitary inspector, he visited the military prison in Fort Delaware, "that inferno of detained rebels," most of whom were taken prisoner at Gettysburg. Among the twelve thousand rebel prisoners there, he saw men dying of dysentery and measles, including medical comrades with whom he had trained in Philadelphia. Soon, Mitchell suffered exhaustion, depression, a breakdown, or all three: he took a leave of absence and traveled to Europe to recover. His body was shaken by war, personal circumstances, and an environment of endless suffering.[48]

VERY NATURAL CURIOSITY AND AMERICAN MANHOOD

Shortly after President Lincoln was assassinated at Ford's Theatre in Washington, DC, the building was converted into another kind of theater as the Army Medical Museum, a fulfillment of the army medical mandate to furnish specimens from the field, fresh from battlefields, graveyards, and hospitals to instruct physicians. The museum also "exemplifie[d] postbellum America's preservation compulsion . . . [the museum] enshrines the *sources* of trauma—extracted projectiles—alongside remains of the human bodies they shattered." Museum specimens were a "detached part of a specific body, preserved from decay and bearing no visibly discernible identifying markers." For poet Walt Whitman, however, these "human fragments" of bodies "epitomize[d] the enduring sublimity of the body." Self-described as a "hospital visitor," he found among the wounded and diseased soldiers a distinctly American manhood characterized by patient forbearance, generosity, and friendship. He wrote, "What I see, especially in the hospitals, convinces me that there is no other stock, for emergencies, but native American—no other name by which we can be saved."[49]

Mitchell's clinical notes on American manhood reflect his personal standards of presentation of self and conceptualization of identity. Indeed, he relied on discourse with suffering soldiers to describe symptoms and gauge the effect of therapies. Mitchell's observations about manhood parallel many of Whitman's character portraits, displaying similar interest, sympathy, and perhaps homoerotic sensibility. Mitchell, too, found sublimity in soldiers' bodies. In his 1864 treatise, *Gunshot Wounds,* he wrote, "The large mass of our patients being Americans, they were usually possessed of at least some education, and often of considerable intelligence and power of observation, which was certainly not dulled by the interest with which such men regarded their own cases." Mitchell, like Whitman, was intrigued and stimulated by the independence, free thought, native intelligence, generosity, and volunteerism of young American soldiers. These attributes crystallized in later decades as distinct characteristics of American nationalism: "'American' was a voluntary entity." In fact, the Grand Army of the Republic, the organization of Union veterans, espoused Americans' freely given service to the nation and volunteerism in war as the soldier's essential, indelible mantra of manhood, but it was silent about the commitment of draftees.[50]

In one case, Mitchell's dialogue with a soldier-patient informed his hypothesis that a body contains two distinct nerve centers, one for touch and the other for pain. Mitchell praised his patient for reliably articulating his symptoms, finding him to be "a very reliable and intelligent soldier, whose discharge was certain, and who could have no motive to deceive." Mitchell's dialogue with soldiers required "the utmost care . . . in ascertaining from the patient the state of [their bodily] functions." He was frequently rewarded by his young Americans' "very natural curiosity as to the condition of the wounded part, and are apt almost immediately to handle it, and to try to move it," anticipating the doctor's need to test damaged limbs. Before Mitchell prescribed a therapeutic regimen for his patients "at that time somewhat novel," including hypodermic injections and electrization, he discussed treatment and elicited patients' cooperation in a mutual exploration. He sought "intelligent sergeants of the invalid corps" to supervise treatments. Mitchell's intimate association with the wounded bodies of young men and their conversations about healing dissolved the social boundaries that would have separated them in civilian life. "The constant mingling of men of high medical culture with the less educated had also value, and the general influence of the war on our art was, in this and other ways, of great service."[51]

Mitchell's clinical studies also reveal when a patient's manhood failed to meet his expectations and Mitchell suspects that the patient's moral lack contributed to his lamentable outcome. This was the case for Chas. A. P., age forty-four, Company G, Eighty-Eighth Pennsylvania Volunteers. P. was not wounded but fell at the Battle of Cedar Mountain in 1862, injuring his elbow. Mitchell subjected him to periodic electrization to test the contractility of nerves and their sensitivity (called "sensibility" in the clinical report). The soldier responded poorly to treatment, but Mitchell noted that although he seemed bright and had received a good education, P. was an alcoholic who left the hospital prematurely. Expressing disdain, Mitchell wrote: "A sober man so situated would without doubt recover under the use of [electrization] for a length of time. P's case is utterly hopeless. Confinement injures his health, and every time he receives a pass it is used for the worst purposes."[52]

In the event of a language barrier—many soldiers were German—Mitchell's cultural lens provided a disparaging view of the patient and his prospect for healing. Swiss soldier Jacob Demuth, age twenty-one, Company D, 108th New York Volunteers, was marching into battle as an artillery shell burst nearby, sending a hunk of shrapnel into his right thigh. Demuth never adequately recovered after months of hospitalization and repeated treatments by Mitchell; he became "partially paraplegic." Mitchell did not describe Demuth with the attributes he prized in American soldiers. He described Demuth as exhibiting "lymphatic temperament," that "owing chiefly to the want of intelligence in the patient and to the fact that he spoke an impure German patois . . . made it no easy task to obtain from him a clear statement of his feelings."[53]

In other cases, where healing defied Mitchell's best regimen, he adopted a matter-of-fact assessment of a soldier's travail following wounding. He wrote clinical notes as though Providence had thrown some luckless soldier an excruciating wound that consequently disfigured his manhood. The previously mentioned case of Sergeant L. P. describes a soldier wounded in the thigh, losing sensation in the leg and foot that transformed in recovery to an intense, burning pain. He pleaded with others in the hospital to kill him. Mitchell described L. P. as "quite unmanned" and recorded how L. P. "shrieked with pain, and grew faint, pallid, and sick at the stomach." Although L. P. improved over time, the conventional attributes of manhood deserted him. "From being a man of gay and kindly temper, known in his company as a good-natured jester, he became morose and melancholy, and complained that reading gave him vertigo, and that his memory of recent events was bad."[54]

Sergeant L. P.'s case is contrasted with another patient who suffered a debilitating wound. This officer's soldierly mien of stoic resolve was insulted by his wound that induced spastic motions. He took an unusual step to restore his manhood. Conventional views of manhood required those with wounds to exercise self-control and perform their duties despite their failing and painful bodies. The officer had been shot in the heel and "was thrown instantly into a condition of the utmost trepidation, and behaved like an insane person." His men witnessed his wild, erratic gestures. In full view of the men he led, the officer felt ashamed of his behavior, which, while beyond his control, would be remembered by spectators as cowardly. The officer requested and was granted a court of inquiry to examine his conduct. As expected, the court "cleared him on the surgical evidence." Another officer, Colonel J. G. P., 139th Pennsylvania Volunteers, had a similar experience with a wound to the nerves but no public vindication of his character. Colonel J. G. P., "an officer of high character, in good health up to the date of wound," received a bullet through his right wrist, whereupon he "became at once singularly excited, and felt as if he were crazed. Under the sudden influence of these sensations, he ran along the line of his regiment, only half conscious, until he fell senseless, having gone about fifty feet." He was dismissed from the army because of an honorable wound that required amputation of the forearm.[55]

Mitchell characterized some of his patients as "exemplary sufferers" because of their response to pain. Mitchell believed that his wounded soldiers were inspired by the suffering of their comrades and may have felt that they were fulfilling divine will. In his clinical writings, Mitchell assessed his work in restoring activity to damaged nerves, thereby rehabilitating manhood: "We look back with unfeigned pleasure upon the great number who came to us, despairing cripples, and have left us eased of pain, and either entirely well or so far aided as to enable them to employ their limbs in useful occupations."[56]

When soldiers sacrifice their bodies as emblems of martyrdom, the inspiration of acolytes completes the Christian parallel. Many doctors, including Mitchell, did not allow women in hospitals. When women did work as paid and unpaid nurses, disapproving doctors, including Mitchell, frequently shunned them. He made an exception for the Catholic Sisters of Mercy whose vows of obedience corresponded to those of the patriarchal doctors. In Mitchell's wards, the nuns helped to uplift the morale of their wounded charges, treating soldiers as infantilized and feminized martyrs. Mitchell observed of this relationship "that good-looking, well-bred, low-voiced women exercised a wonderfully great control over our soldiers—a very American tribute with a physiologic basis." Whitman agreed with this sentiment about his hospital visits: "I never knew what American young men were till I have been in the hospitals. . . . O, how one gets to love them—often, particular cases, so suffering, so good, so manly and affectionate!" Mitchell may not have used that sort of language to describe his patients, but those soldiers whose manhood seemed to embody national ideals and a divinely inspired republic involved the most detailed and lengthy case notes.[57]

Mitchell's early research provides an idea of how he perceived manhood. Clearly fascinated by venomous snakes, his clinical notes suggest sexual interest in his admiration for their handling.

"Words explicitly associated with sexual organs and sexual intercourse become interchangeable with the anatomy and toxicology of the rattlesnake. The metaphors at play create a sense of penetration, ejaculation, and withdrawal and sustain ideas about the snake's phallic power." Mitchell's sexual language raises questions about homoeroticism in his case notes and perhaps homoerotic relationships with some of his patients. In the decades after the war, clinical literature on homosexuality was published by Carl von Westphal and Richard von Krafft-Ebbing, researchers who linked homosexuality (or "sexual inversion") to the nerves, particularly hysteria. In 1883, Mitchell's friend and patron Hammond published *Sexual Impotence in the Male* and was clearly interested in same-sex relationships.[58]

Mitchell's postwar literary career as a writer of fiction included novels that explored intimate relationships between men, such as *Roland Blake.* He was also Walt Whitman's personal physician decades after the war and hired a nurse to attend to the poet at a time when Whitman's sexual orientation had become known. Even when artist Thomas Eakins was, for a time, ostracized from society because of the nudity he promoted and participated in with his students, Mitchell stood by him. Mitchell either tolerated the sexuality of both men or was sympathetic, and in any case, he would have been interested in the science of nervous conditions as it related to sexuality. As he treated veterans in later years, Mitchell elicited their personal sexual histories.[59]

The army grouped men by company and regiment, inevitably spawning intimate relationships. Mitchell appeared tolerant of same-sex attraction among men, a relationship he explored in fiction. Public nudity in military camps and the hospital caused soldiers to take "on a new attractiveness for each other during the war." Mitchell was hardly immune to these perceptions and must have pondered the erotic component of male bonding through the wearing of military uniforms and participation in military rituals. Mitchell read Whitman and would have come across his Calamus poems with their sympathetic view of emotional bonds between men, “the manly love of comrades,” Whitman’s philosophy that may have informed Mitchell’s postwar “West cure” for men burdened with the weight of civilization and its rituals. This cure stressed the manly exploration of wild nature, men trying themselves physically—and together—in the wilderness, living off the land and in tents. Further, Mitchell was undoubtedly aware of the emerging literature on homosexuality as “androgyny of the soul.”[60]

MORAL INFIRMITIES

Despite Mitchell’s remarks about the manly qualities of several of his patients who underwent his innovative treatments for nerve injuries, several medical maladies without associated lesions or specific locations within the body could express symptoms deemed unmanly. Confusing for doctors, patients might have feigned their symptoms. Melancholia, for instance, could be identified through multiple symptoms, including lack of interest, motivation, or ambition. One aspect of the disease, nostalgia, particularly threatened discipline and the will to fight. In the parlance of the era, melancholic men reporting to sick call described their conditions in terms such as having the blues or being lonely or lonesome, nervous, discouraged, disheartened, used up, played out, rattled, worn down, sad, or homesick. Because Mitchell worked in a specialty hospital, he confronted nostalgia only when it manifested in patients with nerve disorders. Nostalgia, if unchecked, could undo healing or inhibit Mitchell’s therapies.[61]

Mitchell’s fellow doctors may have begun their day’s work with low expectations of the manhood of soldiers who reported for sick call. Roberts Bartholow’s *A Manual of Instructions for Enlisting and Discharging Soldiers* found “moral infirmities” difficult to spot because the “standard of qualification in respect to moral character is extremely low." In peacetime, "the ranks are filled up from the idle, the dissolute, and the unfortunate." A subcategory of melancholia, nostalgia could be especially pernicious because "the extreme mental depression and the unconquerable longing for home soon produce a state of cachexy,[62] loss of appetite, derangement of the assimilative functions, and, finally, disease of the abdominal viscera,—in fact, the objective phenomena of the typhoid state." These cases were worrisome because patients could progress to dementia, "the result of a diseased action supervening upon a healthy mental state." The only reliable remedy for nostalgia was to furlough the soldier so that he could visit his family and then return to duty recommitted to the cause. If this remedy did not help or was impossible to arrange, the physician may have looked for other contributing causes of a physical nature, such as heredity, fever, or triggering diseases. Absent somatic causes, the disintegration of manhood via nostalgia required a discharge from the army.[63]

Physicians who talked with soldier-patients about their mental states implicitly and sometimes explicitly criticized them for a lack of manhood. General nervousness was a malady both vague and articulable as the onset of infantile or feminine behavior. Mitchell characterized nervousness in terms of "its prominent peculiarity [that] lies in over-excitability. . . . The strong man becomes like the average woman, the woman like the unschooled child." To Mitchell, nervousness was uncommon in men because they had learned how to suppress feminine characteristics of emotional release: "The mass of men are naturally free from nervousness, and perhaps the hardening education which the man undergoes is a means of forcing him to repress emotion until restraint develops habit." Mitchell hypothesized a physical cause, anemia, and applied relevant drugs and tonics to ease the problem, but nervousness persisted because of "morbid habits" and therefore required substitutes to remedy a diminution of manhood, such as sports. Ultimately, though, dispelling nervousness required that men find a way to enhance their manhood. The physician labored to ensure that "the patient comprehend[ed] that he himself has some control over his symptoms, or, at least, that constantly to yield to them is to ensure defeat, and that constant struggle in a manly way is sure to bring nearer the day of perfect self-conquest." Despite an ignorance of the physical causes of nervousness, Mitchell placed his analysis within the domain of manhood. "When we come to ask ourselves what is the state of the nerve structures which give rise to the symptoms described, we are somewhat of a loss."[64]

Malingering or faking illness presented a manhood challenge to both physician and soldier-patient. Feigning pain or any number of maladies could be almost impossible to dispute. The soldier who fooled the doctor encouraged other soldiers to do the same. The doctor might never know that he was fooled, but if a malingering patient passed off fakery as a real malady, the doctor lost status, authority, and legitimacy. From a physician's perspective, every patient claiming pain or illness with no associated physical damage must be treated skeptically. "In peace and war, malingering was regarded as an evasion of man's duty to the state and to other men." The Civil War army medical establishment did not publish signs and symptoms to help physicians identify miscreants, but it embraced the view that other attributes of manhood required exercising to avoid the impulse to evade duty and "man up" to combat. Civil War physicians "reinforced the sentimental idea that courage came from character and that the body and mind, if properly disciplined, could withstand the hammer blows of war."[65]

Although Keen's report on the topic included the term *malingering,* the word was largely in British use. American parlance favored the terms *Abraham man* or *to sham Abraham* or *Abram.* Keen raised ethical questions for fellow doctors: How can they be sure of malingering? Not only were good order and discipline at stake; serial malingerers sought discharges to enlist in another regiment, claim the enlistment bounty, and repeat the process. Keen argued that all cases of suspected malingering called for detailed examination of the soldier's body, including the use of specialized tools and electrization:

> Always presume that the man can be returned to duty, absent catching the deception. In all cases, however, a thorough exam required . . . that the surgeon has faithfully used all the means of diagnosis at his command: that his physical exploration has been a careful one; that his inspection and examination have not been limited to the face, coat, pants, and pulse, but have been minute and bodily . . . that the special tests by ether, by galvanism [electrization], by the ophthalmoscope, the ear speculum, &c., have all been employed in vain; above all, that the doctor's eyes, ears, and brains have been active and observant.[66]

When careful examination of the soldier's body failed to expose malingerers, Keen recommended placing them under "a system of espionage" to spy on patients in and out of the hospital. Finally, if all means of detection failed, the physician could look at other areas of a soldier's life. "We should seek collateral evidence, such as the man's character, his willingness to work, the general tenor of his story of the origin of his malady, his conduct and gait away from the hospital, and when drunk, if it so be that he indulges thus." If recognizing these masculine traits and scientific evidence cannot identify the malingerer, the employment of feminine attributes might come to the rescue. Keen suggested that the doctor could rely on intuition where observation failed, thus allowing the doctor to "[fix] instantly upon a malingerer for no other than 'a woman's reason.'"[67]

Mitchell knew that soldiers throughout the chain of command viewed invalid soldiers languishing in hospitals in feminized terms. Throughout the war and after, Mitchell cited feminine traits and behavior in patients to distance himself professionally from them and to treat feminization as either an inherent defect of manhood within his patients or as one terminus in the range of pain phenomena. He shared with other experimentalist physicians the view of science as masculine because of its intellectual demands and discipline. "Reason itself came to be gendered as masculine, whereas emotion was evermore associated with the feminine." This entrenched view of masculine science—which persists today—led Mitchell to apply the term *hysteria* to the behavior of soldiers under the blinding pain of causalgia.[68]

Hysteria had been paired with shock when remote causes of nerve damage were listed; its symptoms included "fear of the place of the accident, sleeplessness, mental depression, loss of energy, stuttering, loss of sexual desire, contraction of the visual field, and sleep disturbances." To this list, John K. Mitchell added causalgia, a near-inexpressible pain. Resilience despite pain was an ideal of manhood. The so-called hysteria of men who suffered causalgia, however, presented a dilemma to Mitchell, who admitted that no other word seemed to fit the phenomenon. In other words, an extreme feminine reaction to pain, a disorganized, frantic, stereotypical wild and uncontrollable emotional outpouring characteristic of women due to a "wandering womb" was assigned to men. "The notion that men were as susceptible as women to hysterical pathology ran counter to prevailing patriarchal ideals and seemed to entail the need for a substantially revised understanding of masculine human nature." Mitchell did not provide that substantial revision. Likely, he applied a feminine term—hysteria—to manhood-threatening behavior and left open the question of how to embed descriptions of the pain within the masculine expressions of bodily phenomena.[69]

Among veterans who claimed to suffer extreme pain in the decades after the war, the expression of pain to pension physicians could evoke condescension, dismissal, or even contempt. During the late 1800s, many doctors "reconfigured [hysteria] as a kind of character flaw, the lamentable result of a lack of will power, a pathetic excess of emotionality, or constitutional degeneration." Mitchell's examinations of patients one, two, or more years following their wounding and nerve damage turned toward this judgmental direction. Mitchell pointed out that hysteria-ridden

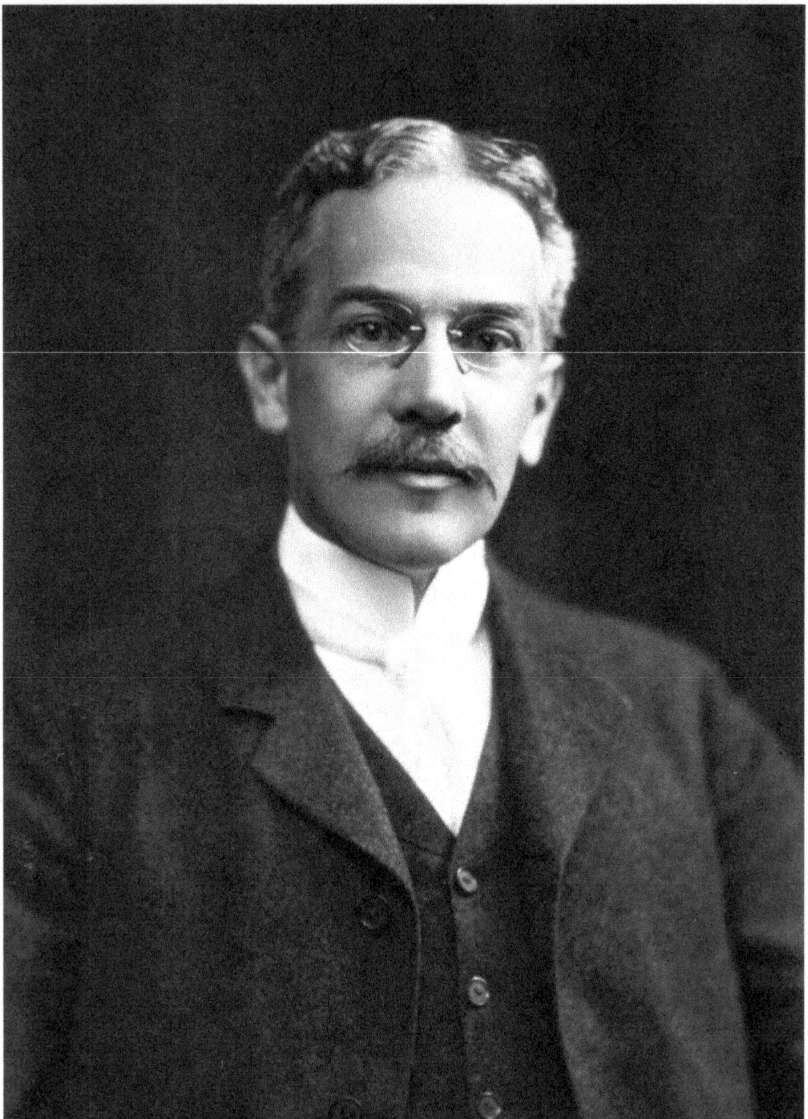

John Kearsley Mitchell, MD, about 1915. *Credit: National Library of Medicine (ID B019396).*

soldiers became "mind blind," a description of their failure to register what they saw, an obliviousness to people and the environment caused by pain: "The thing seen may be present to the man as an image is to a mirror, for the mirror has no memory, and cannot compare the present with the past." In a discussion of a patient with neuritis, an inflammation of the nerves that causes aberrant functioning, he wrote: "In fact, some of these cases become what in a woman we should call hysterical, and by turns bewail their condition, or pitifully apologize for their want of manly endurance."[70]

Three decades after the Civil War, hysteria in veterans still confounded Mitchell, who continued to resort to feminizing the sufferer. When discussing violent hysteria, Mitchell wrote, "Only once . . . have I seen a male exhibit all the acts in the long drama of hysteria precisely as we so often see them in the female." That "long drama" included nausea, "hiccoughs," regurgitation or vomiting, and spasms. In retrospection, Mitchell wrote that if the sufferer was a young man, he "should take him away, and with isolation, massage, and electricity treat him, and have hope." But in the 1890s, he did not support such a treatment, preferring to try hypnotism and hypodermically induced arsenic, a therapy recommended for anemia during the war. "I have used the label hysteria again and again. It is, and as yet must be, a word of somewhat loose employment." Later in the same work, he frankly admitted, "We do not know what hysteria is."[71]

WHAT POWERS HAVE YOU LOST AND REGAINED?

As part of his holistic approach to evaluating his patients, Mitchell believed that in diagnosing and treating cases of nervousness, the patient's life must be understood. This view may have inspired him and his son to circulate questionnaires about the current state of health among veterans who had suffered severe wounds, particularly those who had lost limbs. John K. Mitchell's *Remote*

Consequences of Injuries of Nerves embraced an analysis of the survey's results together with follow-up examinations of veterans still struggling at the end of the century to recover sensation and mobility and to rationalize why their pain had continued. His discussions and conclusions updated his father's ideas in some respects, notably in the evolution of language regarding electricity. By the 1890s, he was working at the same institution as his father, Philadelphia's Orthopaedic Hospital and Infirmary for Nervous Diseases, a hospital with an electrical department, where both saw veterans.[72]

What discussions preceded the dissemination of the health "circulars" is unknown. John K. Mitchell's studies date to 1890–1892 and revisit case studies from the Firm's 1864 and 1872 monographs to give the most comprehensive view of each veteran's health since the war, updated to include the younger Mitchell's examination of several former soldiers. Both Mitchells sought the assistance of the federal War Department to contact veterans on their behalf, and advertisements were placed in newspapers to encourage veterans to correspond. Mitchell sent a form letter dated October 1892 to veterans who had been treated at Turner's Lane or Christian Street Hospitals and asked them to respond to the following questions:

I. How are you as to the sensation of touch in the parts injured? How do you feel heat and cold? How strongly do you feel a touch and do you feel it as a pinch or a prick? Be as exact as possible, please.
II. How much movement have you in the part injured, and what powers have you lost and regained?
III. To what extent is the limb shrunken?
IV. What changes are there in the odor of the secretions from the injured part?
V. What changes are there in the character of the hair upon the injured part?

VI. What changes are there in the nails? Do they grow as fast as upon the other side?

VII. If the injury is upon the neck or face, what changes have taken place there?[73]

Mitchell's questions addressed the phenomena he observed in causalgia patients and others with painful peripheral nerve injuries, questions unlikely to be documented by pension examiners, much less asked at all. In September 1893, John K. Mitchell sent out a cover letter and accompanying questionnaire to veterans who had suffered amputations (appendix B). The letter states that he and colleagues "are very anxious, for scientific reasons, to make a study of the conditions of the men who have lost limbs some time since. The matter is one that has never been investigated, and the only extensive material that exists for its study is among those who were unfortunate enough to lose limbs in the service of the country." The letter acknowledged the help of the army surgeon general in endorsing the project and locating veterans and assured respondents of confidentiality. Recipients were urged to seek the help of their physicians in answering questions if they were unable to respond. Thus, perhaps the earliest longitudinal survey of Civil War veterans' health was begun. If both doctors could not touch and manipulate the bodies of these veterans, they could ask the veterans to do so for them.[74]

The Historical Medical Library of the College of Physicians of Philadelphia has fourteen completed questionnaires from amputee veterans and nine letters from other veterans. Of the subjects of this book, Henry Huidekoper and John Shields submitted letters (and Shields included a separate one from his physician). The former apparently did not respond to the published request for data; he wrote his letter in 1906 following a conversation with Mitchell. Three of the respondents had been wounded by minié balls—Huidekoper, Shields, and Henry Kircher (the latter completing a questionnaire)—and Richard Dunphy, who also

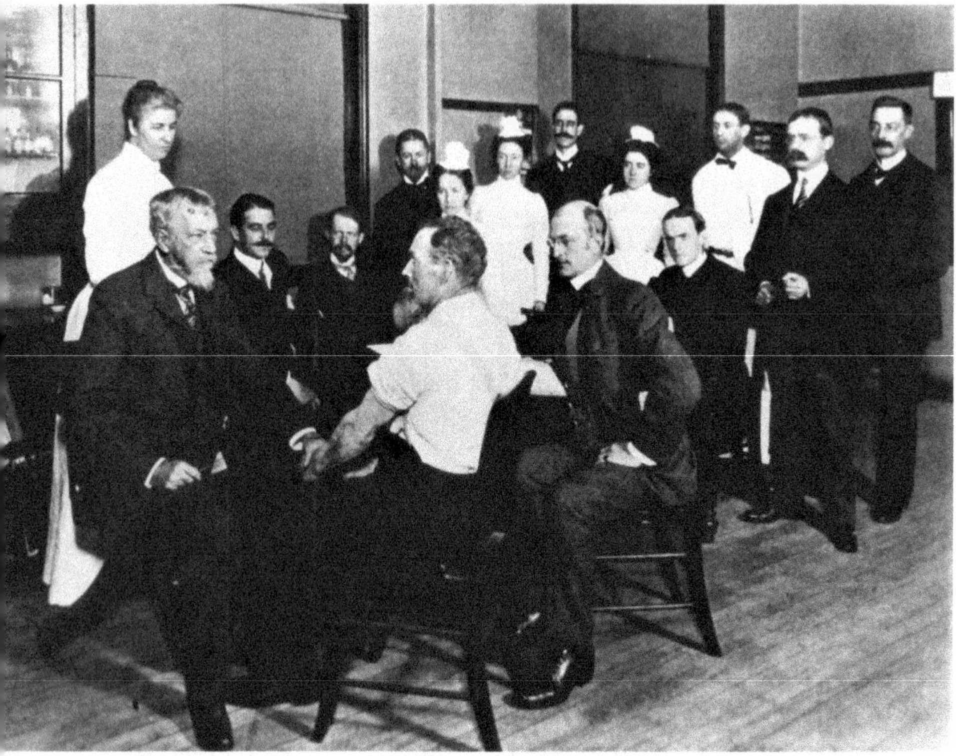

S. Weir Mitchell interviewing a Civil War veteran at his clinic in the Philadelphia Orthopedic Hospital and Infirmary for Nervous Diseases, 1902. *Credit: National Library of Medicine (ID B08398).*

completed a questionnaire, was wounded by cannon fire. He and Kircher were double amputees. The questionnaire focused on the nerve phenomena attendant with amputation, so the questions were pulled from Mitchell's Civil War publications to update and extend his data a generation on. On average, the respondents had survived about twenty-nine years since they were wounded.

When veterans received the letter and questionnaire, they likely thought of the meaning and implications of what they might say. Some recipients, apparently, did not complete the questionnaire and may have hesitated to reveal intimate information. John

K. Mitchell commented on the difficulty of eliciting responses: "I believe one cause . . . to have been the impossibility of convincing the men that many questions were not a device of the Pension Examiners, and that my anxiety to know various minute details of their condition was not prompted by a desire to reduce or take away their pay." Nevertheless, twenty men who had been treated at Christian Street or Turner's Lane contributed to John K. Mitchell's solicitation. Some veterans had tried to access Mitchell during those three decades to request his assessment of their continuing pain. Others approached the Army Medical Museum with written applications to Mitchell for help with their pain.[75]

In reading the questionnaires, one can imagine Mitchell sitting close to the veteran, asking questions while applying his hands to the veteran's body. Indeed, the questions seemed to follow the touching of the ex-soldier's body in roughly the order of a physical examination. A photograph (figure 2.4) shows Mitchell performing such an interview while physicians, students, and nurses look on. All the amputees reported continuing pain in nonexistent limbs (except Dunphy, whose intermittent pain seemed unrelated to phantom sensations), and several described a reduction of general health. Some noted behavioral changes such as loss of sleep and appetite, and many identified difficulties in maintaining physical and mental health. The veterans' responses revealed no challenges to manhood or anxiety about harboring conditions that might be deemed feminizing.

Both Mitchells doubtless agreed on diagnoses and prognoses most of the time. Although the son spoke to a generation of medical practitioners after his father, the elder Mitchell may have been more broadminded about identifying the site of pain owing to phantom sensations. While he departed from the imperative to identify a physical lesion in the nerves as the site of pain, John K. Mitchell had not abandoned that focus. When examining veterans, his first step was to locate and determine the extent of the neural lesion. His recommended therapy focused on treating a visible wound but allowing nature to exercise its healing power and then study the results. Taking a cue from his father's promotion of a rest cure for neurasthenia[76] in the late 1800s, the younger Mitchell opined: "Of the utmost consequence for the repair of wounded nerves is absolute rest of the part involved, which must be secured by position, by splints, and by strict injunctions to the patient." Ultimately, however, if the damaged nerve could be identified, and with advances in surgery after the Civil War because of antiseptic practices coupled with anesthetization, a nerve transplant became possible. John K. Mitchell recommended the use of sciatic nerve segments, for instance, taken from animals, particularly rabbits.[77]

CONCLUSION: YEASTY MEN

Dr. Keen's "yeasty man" led a team that "distinguishe[d] itself for its emphasis on research, experimentation, originality and clarity of expression." The Firm had no handbook for investigating nerve wounds, as none existed. Mitchell's therapies were exploratory as well as therapeutic. Sometimes the therapies did not work, but science requires analysis of failures as well as successes. The meticulous investigations of gunshot wounds required a full consideration of the soldier-patient's life; details of his behavior before, during, and after wounding; and an inquiry requiring empathy, an open mind, and an inquisitive nature. Mitchell necessarily became intimate with many soldiers: he massaged, probed, invaded, and reassured bodies. Equally important was his dialogue with soldier-patients: he needed to find a common communication based on white Americans' native intelligence, curiosity, and willingness to reconceptualize gender to find clinical truth in the body and ease pain. With these characteristics, Mitchell set an example for his colleagues Keen and Morehouse.

Of Mitchell, Keen wrote, "Never have I known so original, suggestive, and fertile a mind."[78]

The Firm's contributions included circumscribing the nature of causalgia, reflex paralysis, various palsies, epilepsy, the phantom limb phenomenon, and other afflictions of amputation stumps. The Firm took a methodical approach to gathering data exceeding the protocols commonly observed in Civil War hospitals. As Keen later reflected, "[Mitchell] taught me the important art of elucidating the case histories of patients; the importance of little hints which were often the insignificant surface outcroppings of a rich vein of facts; the importance and methods of cross-examination to ferret out the truth, and above all, the ability to interpret these assembled facts in making a diagnosis." Paying attention to those "insignificant surface-outcroppings" meant an intimate exploration of soldiers' bodies and the manipulation of their bodily responses to touch and pain. Doctors' hands are not only tools; they are conduits. As they apply their hands, doctors attach to the patient's body. They link the soldier's suffering to the physician's sensibility to motion, sound, touch, smell, and respiration, all mediated through dialogue. Mitchell, Keen, and Morehouse approached patients with their own bodily afflictions, impediments, stresses, and concepts of manhood and manly behavior.[79]

To a degree, however, the Firm selected bodies with wounds relevant to their study interests and experimental therapies. Their patients had ascended the healing ladder through field hospitals, regimental or brigade hospitals, rail or steam travel to distant cities, and ultimately special hospitals like Turner's Lane, where doctors had privileged access to senior medical authority and were spared the tedium of administrative work. Mitchell engaged with bodies that reacted with insensitivity to touch, pain that migrated and changed character over time, and sensations that did not appear grounded in identifiable, somatic causes. He later reflected, "The opportunity was indeed unique and we knew it. The cases were of amazing interest."[80]

The bodily essence of the afflictions among the Firm's patients was pain. Circumscribing pain in all of its evident permutations challenged Mitchell when he was writing his case studies. The burning, darting, piercing, stabbing, pricking pains were so overwhelming that they "replac[ed] all other physical sensation and invad[ed] consciousness with a kind of nerve torture that shatters the body's discipline and coherence." As Mitchell and patient linked, body to body, to plumb the depth of pain's misery, he was uncharacteristically at a loss for words. He reached for a feminine disorder and what he thought of as a woman's response to extreme pain in applying the term *hysteria* to young American men. "Hysteria" as a gloss for a reaction to pain, an emotional outburst, or other behavior deemed unmanly has never implied anything other than an attribute of the human female, despite ongoing professional efforts to desex the term. The word is wedded to its root meaning. Perhaps partly because of the clash between describing pain behavior and the male challenge of minimizing it, the Firm's work—and Mitchell's writing about it—explored the emotional impact of trauma to a degree not studied by other military or pension doctors.[81]

Mitchell and his son continued to study disorders of the nerves at the Philadelphia Orthopaedic Hospital and Infirmary for Nervous Diseases, the first such facility in the United States devoted to the emerging specialty of neurology. Mitchell made the rounds every Friday afternoon while his son examined veterans and took notes that became part of his treatise on nerve disorders. In reflecting on his work shortly before his death in 1914, Mitchell observed, "We hear little or nothing of the unequaled capacity with which we met the call on energy and intelligence, or of the extraordinary power of the trained American to deal with the unusual." The last clause speaks to the intellectual and emotional power to observe and comprehend pain and other phenomena of the nerves that challenge description, not only for empathetic doctors but also for the wounded American men struggling to regain manly vigor. In the process, they, in dialogue with the Firm, redefined their manhood.[82]

Arriving in Gettysburg on a hot July day in 1863, not even a day since the battle ended, the smell of human and animal rot entering his nostrils long before he saw the battlefield, Mitchell was seared by the experience. He never lost his depth of feeling for the damaged veteran or the young men now disappeared from life, including his younger brother. His subsequent writing, clinical and fictional, was tinctured with Civil War blood. One of Herman Melville's war poems likely spoke to Mitchell's sense of personal and collective loss and the transience of human life:

> Each bloomed and died an unabated Boy;
> Nor dreamed what death was—thought it mere
> Sliding into some vernal sphere.
> They knew the joy, but leaped the grief,
> Like plants that flower ere comes the leaf—
> Which storms lay low in kindly doom,
> And kill them in their flush of bloom.[83]

THREE

ELECTRIC AGONY

THE BODY ELECTRIC

On May 3, 1863, the second bloodiest day of the Civil War after the battle at Antietam, Maryland, former blacksmith Joseph S. Davis, twenty-eight, prepared for another assault by Confederate troops near the village of Chancellorsville, Virginia. His comrades of Company A, Twenty-Sixth Pennsylvania Volunteers, their faces and hands begrimed with sweat and black powder from days of fighting, huddled behind an embankment to await the inevitable attack. At the bend of the U-shaped Union line, Davis and his fellow soldiers expected to bear the brunt of the attack. Shortly, the rebels came, and Davis put his rifle to his right shoulder and aimed. At that instant, an enemy bullet entered his right shoulder several inches above the axilla (armpit), tore through flesh, and exited from his back just below the flange of the scapula. Davis immediately felt a shock through his arm and thought it might have been shot away. The pain was immediate: he felt a "stinging + burning pain from the shoulder to the finger."

Soldiers or medical orderlies removed Davis from the field. He traveled through several hospitals where his wounds were at least minimally treated until he arrived at S. Weir Mitchell's ward in

Philadelphia. Davis likely bore witness to his body's experience with pain and mobility with a mixture of horror and fascination. Although his entry and exit wounds were cleaned and bandaged, his arm, hand, and fingers defied his reliance on their expected behavior. At first, his right forearm and hand seemed painfully paralyzed, but over time, he was able to bend his arm at the elbow. Other motions returned except for the ability to flex his fingers. The hand appeared swollen and red with a burning pain, but the fingers refused to flex and experience full sensation. Mitchell ordered the limb douched (bathed with a jet of water) and electrized with galvanic current. After months and persistent electrization, sensation gradually returned and, by late fall, was restored in the hand except for the little finger. Swelling and burning sensations gradually abated. Electrization also stimulated pain, thus requiring intervals between applications. In November, Davis left the hospital but returned a week later. By February 1864, Mitchell could not release him to combat duty but arranged for him to work in the hospital as a medical orderly.[1]

Mitchell may have been the only army physician who administered electricity—electrization—to soldier-patients during the war. Electricity enabled Mitchell to engage with Davis's nerves directly, both to stimulate a return of sensation and movement and to learn how nerves function when traumatized. To electrize a patient, conductors (electrodes) were applied to parts of the body to communicate with local nerves, effectively placing the physician's hands within the body. To both patient and physician, however, electricity was a celebrity, a curiosity, an entertainment, a promising medical tool, and a cosmic mystery. People encountered allusions to electricity in poetry, fiction, science reporting, and popular discourse. Electricity "seem[ed] to refer to some intensified level of consciousness connected to the insights of poetic genius. . . . But metaphors of aesthetic electricity . . . were outgrowths of residual and emergent literary, popular, and scientific understandings of electricity."[2]

To advance his medical education, Mitchell traveled to Europe before the Civil War. There, he studied in Paris with Claude Bernard, a renowned experimenter who championed the application of science to medicine. In addition, Mitchell probably became familiar with the work of Guillaume-Benjamin-Amand Duchenne de Boulogne, a pioneering neurologist who photographed himself with patients, male and female, and on whose bodies he applied electrical stimuli. Many of these photographs show Duchenne's intimate manipulation of clothed and unclothed patients' bodies as he applied conductors or other electrical appurtenances. Mitchell would have studied Duchenne's clinical photographs, apparatuses, and conduction tests of nerves. His creation of a standard electrical examination was based on Duchenne's work.[3]

Mitchell considered electricity "as sensual and registered on the body, as shocks, or as a fluid moving through the material body" and tried to locate and trace its influence despite the frequent lack of an associated lesion. His Civil War work highlighted the necessity of determining how electricity might be measured and quantified. Scholars who have written about Mitchell acknowledge his use of electricity but have not situated it as an intellectual challenge rooted in the deep manipulation of the bodies of his soldier-patients. The electrical apparatus he brought to the hospital must have mystified both patients and hospital staff, yet in subsequent years, electrical tools became abundant and varied. Years after the war, as Mitchell treated veterans, he could rely on the resources of the hospital's electricity department.[4]

This chapter examines the relationship of two bodies, soldier and physician, trauma patient and arbiter of health, on a mutual journey of healing via a medium with unknown spiritual and physical consequences. Mitchell's practice of electrization during the Civil War can be appreciated for its significance to the professionalization of medicine, the education of physicians, and the promotion of a scientific viewpoint in medical practice.

Mitchell's replication of Duchenne's techniques in military hospitals validated the body electric as a new dimension of American manhood.

IMAGINING ELECTRICITY

Mitchell was doubtless aware of the debate within medical circles about the utility of electricity. The rapid growth of telegraphy promised more substantial applications of electricity in the future. Indeed, Mitchell lived to see radio, compact batteries, electrical power stations, and electric lighting. During the Civil War era, the telegraph reshaped identity "as individuals in modernizing U.S. society became more firmly entrenched in networks of commerce, information, and power." For veterans, that entrenchment impacted their futures as pension laws and public attitudes toward veterans changed in an increasingly industrial and urban society. The impact of cultural change also placed new boundaries around the veteran's body.[5]

Electricity was an omnipresent topic in household conversation, literature, and print, and the subject gradually permeated all forms of expression. Walt Whitman famously incorporated electricity in his creation of the spiritually democratic, independent American through his poetry. He was no stranger to science. To his mother, he declared his belief in the utility of electrotherapy, and he underwent it himself. In Section 27 of *Song of Myself*, which addresses touch, Whitman describes the effect of touch on the skin as electrical receptors:

> I have instant conductors all over me whether I pass or stop,
> They seize every object and lead it harmlessly through me.[6]

Whitman participated in a community conversation about electricity as a natural phenomenon, a medium of inspiration and energy, and he absorbed its abundant metaphors. So did other people of letters, including transcendentalist poet William Ellery

Channing, who was related to electrical experimenter William F. Channing. English poet Chauncy Hare Townshend spoke for many literary minds by invoking "the electric light of poetry," which "for one inestimable moment solves the universe for [the] doubting heart." In Townshend's poetry, electricity mediated his emotions ("And the fierce lightning through me flash'd / Electric agony") and drove his mind:

> The livelong eve in converse bright
> Had thought's electric flashes play'd.[7]

In employing electricity, Mitchell faced two challenges: first, locate apparatuses suitable to his ideas about nerves, and second, find an appropriate language for his use of electricity and the evaluation of its application. Establishing the language of electrization proved a challenge given the lack of standards for quantifying, measuring, or even discussing electricity. The conundrum of electrical language intensified with the arrival of telegraphy. An anonymous 1848 publication on telegraphy's impact on literature observed that the language of this invention "has been slowly yet certainly approaching the standard of perfection." The essay offered a view that telegraphy, because of its nature, required a style of writing that was "terse, condensed, expressive, sparing of expletives and utterly ignorant of synonyms"[8]—in short, a language called "telegraphic style."

Telegraphic technology required human operators to express "the greatest amount of intelligence . . . in the fewest words." The machine challenged language because it operated with the speed of thought. Ahead of humankind in the evolution of technology, "before us rise like exhalations from the western wave the islands of the blessed—the isle of engines, where the human race are to live by machinery, and *flash* from point to point in polar magnetic chariots." Clearly not expressed in the telegraphic style, this 1848 essay anticipated the proliferation of technological inventions that would close the distance between populations and increase the speed and urgency of work. Telegraphy would "constitute the nervous system of organized societies . . . its functions are analogous to the sensitive nerves of the animal system."[9]

Aesthetic electricity, the metaphoric language of poets, promised to transform the world. The telegraphic style was not limited to those tapping Morse code. All writing, clinical and romantic, was "a form of exploration and experimentation, and inseparable from the . . . period's forms of knowledge." Because of electricity's diverse audiences, for everyone trying to find a way to express its influence, effects, promise, metaphoric value, and clinical purposes, its meaning remained in flux. "Electricity had to be imagined in order to be understood or represented, making fictionality an embedded feature of its perception and conceptualization." The influence of popular writing on clinical descriptions of electrical phenomena is difficult to quantify, but some of the broader claims that electricity had a transforming power are implicit in Mitchell's clinical notes, attesting to its indispensability for recovery.[10]

When applying electricity, Mitchell concentrated on its therapeutic effects yet addressed or eliminated underlying assumptions about this force of nature. If telegraphy posed new demands on communication, perhaps the body's vital energy—electricity—was itself a medium of communication. Maybe the properties of electricity paralleled those of the nerves, hence the metaphor regarding "sensitive nerves of the animal system." Many people believed that the medium of spiritual contact with the dead was a kind of electricity and therefore a scientific endeavor. Scientific electricity somehow linked living and dead people in communication, "prompting the popular appellation of 'the spiritual telegraph' for séances."[11]

In searching for an appropriate clinical language, Mitchell balanced competing scientific theories about the nature and efficacy of electrical treatment. Michael Faraday posited a connection between the nervous system and electricity: "So, perhaps, in these organs, where nature has provided the apparatus by means of which the animal can exert and convert nervous into electric force, we may be able . . . to reconvert the electric into the nervous force." Physician and inventor William F. Channing, who quoted Faraday in his book on medical electricity, remained skeptical about nervous impulses being electrical, but he nevertheless opined that whatever may constitute "the physical agent" that passes along the nerves and within tissues, it "bears a remarkable analogy to electricity in its three principal characteristics,—the exertion of attractive force, the control of chemical affinity, and the rapid transmission of impulses."[12]

Other medical texts of Mitchell's era encouraged skepticism, cautioning that the metaphor of electricity should not confuse clinical practice. Several writers on medical electricity argued for more research and experimentation to ascertain electricity's application to health and healing. Physician Alfred C. Garratt, who invented a compact battery to be worn on the body for constant electrical current, asked, "Is Medical Electricity an art as well as a science? Is it a tangible remedy, that in certain cases and conditions can work a lasting, permanent cure?" While he pointed out that anyone could hold conductors to parts of a person's body, we ought to consider "medical electricity [as] *both*—a science and an art. A good medical battery, with its various electrodes, may be compared to a surgeon's case of instruments." For the instruments to be effective, however, the physician must be knowledgeable and skilled.[13]

The prevalent American and British views promoted caution. Physician and electrical experimenter Julius Althaus warned of "enthusiastic panegyrists" who "contend still, that it is a therapeutic agent superior to all hitherto discovered," while most physicians "entertain serious doubts as to the reality of the remarkable successes which are now and then recorded by medical galvanists [experimenters]." Pioneering neurologist and Mitchell's contemporary George M. Beard, who felt forced to address spiritualism to separate it from the legitimate medical use of electricity, bluntly stated, "At the present time electricity is the city of refuge to which all forms of delusion run."[14]

Public perceptions of electricity may have influenced some physicians to express beliefs that electricity's properties taught some lesson about consciousness, the hereafter, or otherwise furnished some organizing or unifying principle for all observable phenomena in the universe. Channing cautioned that if the life force "should be a form of electricity, we are at present wholly ignorant of the nature of its modification, and any control which we may succeed in exercising over it must still be the work of experiment." Mitchell's writings concluded that skepticism was well founded and that while "certain electrical phenomena exist in connection with all nerves and in the presence of all nerve action," his research showed that nerve impulses themselves were *not* electrical. He held, nonetheless, that in his work with soldiers, "there is no test of the restoration of nerve supply except the electric current."[15]

That test, of course, required instruments and the joint exploration and articulation of results between doctor and patient. Instruments, Mitchell wrote, "force us, by the time their uses exact, to learn, to be rapid, and at the same time accurate." His experimental machines reflected his own scientific manhood, enabling him to show patients that he could control a force of nature for their benefit. Even without a satisfactory scientific explanation of how his electrical tools worked, much less a solid grounding in the physics of electricity, Mitchell claimed that the clinical use of a battery or generator "exacts accuracy and teaches care; it creates a wholesome appetite for precision which, at last, becomes habitual. The microscope, the balance, the thermometer, the chronograph have given birth to new standards in observation, by which we live, scarce conscious of the change a generation has brought about." The clinical language demanded for expressing accuracy, for Mitchell, made no claims about the relationship between electricity and the soul or a life force. Mitchell's clinical language described the manhood of patients under electrical influence while also reflecting his standards of soldierly manhood.[16]

DIAGNOSTIC CURRENTS

Although electricity was used at Turner's Lane Hospital for only a short time, Mitchell integrated electrization into his treatment regimen for soldiers. He determined what measures were important, what tools to employ, and how to use those tools. As the nineteenth century opened, two sources of electricity were available for experimentation: static and direct. Both could be provided by an array of instruments from friction devices to early batteries. Electricity became a fixture in postwar hospitals despite lack of knowledge of precisely how electricity elicited healing effects. Other than the midcentury telegraph and the later advent of telephony, the greatest demand for electrical machines came from the medical and experimental science fields. As standards developed for measuring electricity—in voltages and amps, for example—it was possible to invent direct-reading tools to obtain data on what were, at Turner's Lane, unquantifiable electrocutions of wounded soldiers.[17]

What began as a "try this if nothing else works" electrical experiment at the Firm's ward became, through use, a template for assessment and initial examination: "The last and, perhaps, the best of all the means of exciting the tissues, and increasing the flow of blood through the part, is the judicious employment of electricity in some form." Electrical practitioner Channing explained why electricity applied to many bodily processes as it acted "directly upon the secreting organs, to effect the vital condition of the blood, to influence nutrition at its source, to produce structural change, in the nerve-centres and fibres themselves, as well as elsewhere, in fine, to act directly upon the life of the organized atoms." Said Channing, one only determined "the 'quantity' of the electricity employed" in relation to its intended effect. "Different parts of the body differ exceedingly in their sensibility to electricity." Despite Mitchell's experience with electrization, these two related issues—how much electricity to apply and for what specific purpose—remained unresolved during the war. The second issue, how and under what circumstances to apply it, was not resolved for purposes of standardization of measurement and treatment until late in the century.[18]

"If any one technic—diagnostic or therapeutic—can be said to have characterized early American neurology, it was the medical use of electricity. No other was either as closely connected to the field or as omnipresent in its practice." Mitchell's case notes highlight a spectrum of applications of electricity, from prophylactic faradization (application of alternating current) to topical galvanization (application of direct current) of nerves coupled with other therapies from drugs (such as morphia to alleviate pain caused by electrization) to massage ("shampooing"). Mitchell was sensitive to sensory phenomena stimulated by or concomitant with electrization: "Under favorable circumstances, the electrized limb flushes and gets warm, the muscles grow, and the atrophy disappears." Mitchell shared the process with his patients by pressing, palpating, pinching, or stroking the skin over nerves. He invited others to share in the experience, noting that repeated treatments could be performed by medical orderlies, friends, or even the patients themselves.[19]

Mitchell's use of electricity for both diagnosis and prognosis began with consideration of the nature of the apparent wound or injury to nerves. The symptoms could include loss of sensation or volitional control and lack of pain (sensibility). Faradization was employed initially, muscle by muscle, to map the damage, testing nerves for contractility and sensibility. If the soldier had suffered loss of contractility only, the prognosis was hopeful, but if the patient lost both, there was little chance of recovery. Generally, routine, daily faradization with a fifteen-minute session was prescribed. These methods are derived entirely from Duchenne's practice. The patient expected a long recovery, months or perhaps years if full restoration of nerves occurred. Occasionally, the final steps of treatment might have involved surgery or the fitting of a prosthesis to mimic muscular action.[20]

For example, J. S. L. Scott, age thirty-one, Company F, 121st New York Volunteers, was wounded by a bullet on May 3, 1863, at Chancellorsville. The ball passed through his right leg, narrowly missing his fibula and tibia, and passed out of his body. Upon being wounded, Scott lost the motion below his right knee. Substantial pain was not felt until the next day and was followed by inflammation. He did not enter Mitchell's ward until September. By then, Scott walked with a crutch, his right leg useless. A cast of the foot and ankle was prepared and submitted to the Army Medical Museum. At first, treatment consisted of hot and cold douches and faradization. By late October, there was some improvement, but "sensibility to pain [was] much impaired below the knee, but lost at the outer head of the gastrocnemius[21] and on the outside of the foot."[22]

Next, Mitchell tested for *electric contractility* muscle by muscle in the lower leg, but the electricity did not stimulate movement. Mitchell then tried an electric brush, which did not cause pain. Scott felt some response to electricity by late December, and by January 1864, electro-muscular contractility returned. Later in the month, contractility appeared "well marked." By February, Scott could walk with a cane, his lower right leg encased tightly in a gaiter. Based on his improvement, Scott was released from the hospital the same month, and Mitchell and colleagues felt "sure of ultimate cure with the aid of electricity."[23]

Induced, or faradic, current was "the greatest scientific achievement of the nineteenth century." It was invented by Michael Faraday and supported by his theoretical explanation of how it worked. The introduction of induced currents expanded

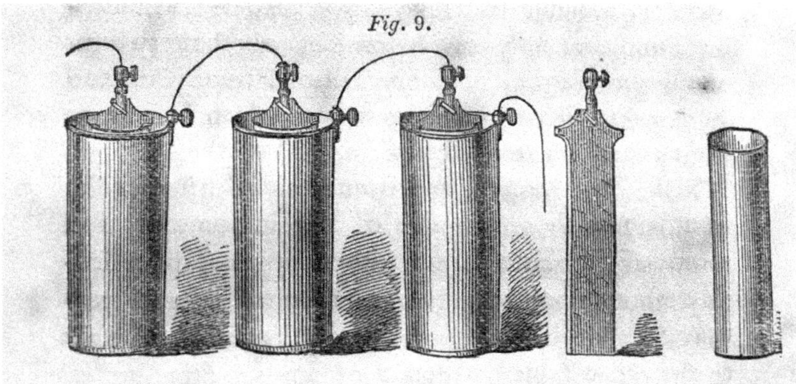

Illustration of a battery manufactured by Thomas Hall of Boston. Designed for "electro-medicine," this "constant battery" delivers a continuous supply of galvanic electricity. Each cell consists of an outer copper cylinder (*far right*) enclosing a porous cell and a zinc plate (*second from right*). To activate the battery, the operator adds "crushed crystals of blue vitriol" (copper sulfate) and water. Cells can be grouped from fifteen pairs to as many as fifty. Credit: William F. Channing, *The Medical Application of Electricity*. 5th ed. Boston: Thomas Hall, 1859.

medical interest beyond popular electrical entertainment to thoughtful medical applications. The essence of the technology consisted of two coils of copper wire (separated by insulation) wound around a soft iron core. Current from a separate source passing through the first coil, when interrupted, induced a current of higher voltage in the second, which delivered the interrupted or alternating current. Later, a magnet was added to the assembly, thus obviating the need for an external source of electricity. Magneto-electric generators were manufactured in small wooden boxes containing horseshoe magnets, rotating cylinders of spooled thin copper wire around iron bars, and a hand crank. Turning the crank rotated two identical cylinders that sequentially passed the poles of the magnet and created a current that entered the patient via two wired conductors. These machines became popular and were easy to apply to the body. The faradic

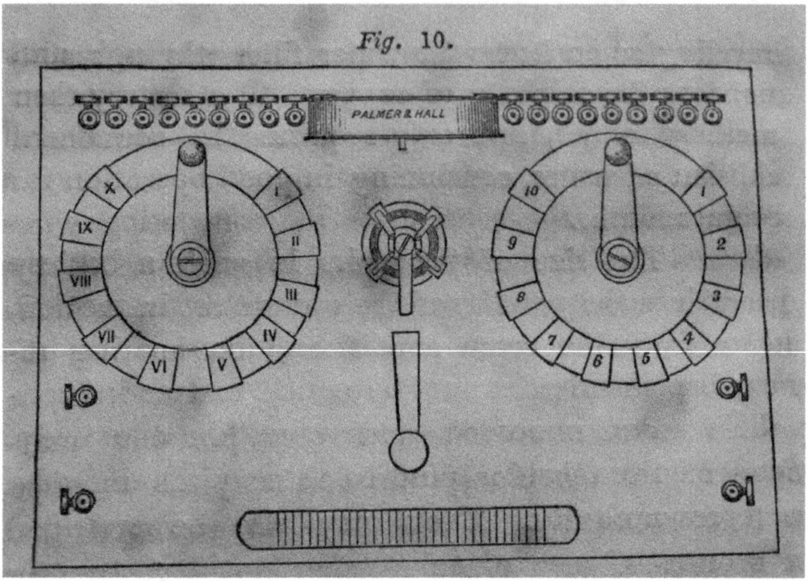

Schematic for a "switch- and key-board," or control panel for the batteries shown in figure 3.1. Also made by Thomas Hall, a manufacturer of electric devices, it allows the operator to control up to one hundred batteries in groups of ten, connected by wires to the panel. Should an interrupted current be required, the panel includes an electrotome "which, when wound up, causes a pendulum . . . to vibrate between two little metallic pillars, making and breaking the circuit with rapidity." By using a telegraph key, the current can be interrupted at the discretion of the operator. *Credit: William F. Channing,* The Medical Application of Electricity. *5th ed. Boston: Thomas Hall, 1859.*

current—faradization—could deliver a severe shock or a steady flow.[24]

Direct current, commonly known as galvanic (named for eighteenth-century physician Luigi Galvani) came from batteries. The process was known as galvanization. Users first partly assembled the batteries. A wooden box contained several glass bottles or waterproof cells connected to one another. Inside the bottles were alternating copper and zinc plates, strips, or disks. The user added brine, vinegar, or blue vitriol (or cupric sulfate, which is

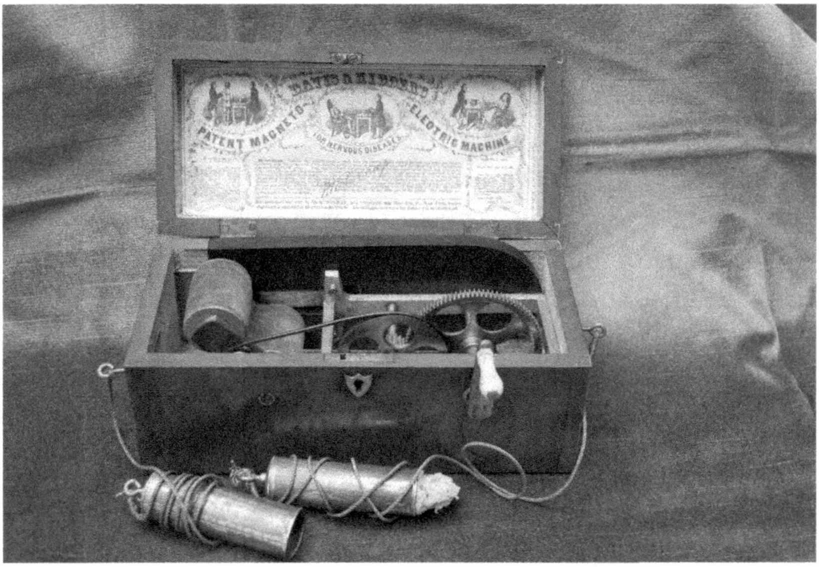

Portable magneto-electric generator made by Davis & Kidder, Lowell, MA, and New York City, c. 1855–1865. The machine generates its own electricity and requires no chemicals. The operator turns the hand crank, which rotates two velvet-covered cylinders. Each cylinder conceals a soft iron bar encircled by tightly wrapped copper wire. As the cylinders rotate against the poles of a horseshoe magnet, an electrical current is induced (faradic) and passes to the patient by two metal conductors connected by wires to the device. These machines were cheaper and more portable than those requiring many fluid-charged batteries. *Credit: Author's collection.*

still used today as a battery electrolyte) to put these substances into electrical communication. The chemical interaction of the substances produced electricity in a stable, direct current. The Civil War era stimulated expanding markets for batteries, and by the end of the century, batteries were commercially popular and delivered consistent, reliable results.[25]

Conductors of galvanic or faradic current varied. Manufacturers furnished several attachments for various purposes, some were contoured to be applied in specific ways to parts of the body, from eyes to genitals. For his purposes, Mitchell "buffered the metal conductor [with] wet buckskin, cloth, or sponge, over the bellies of the muscles."[26] The part of the instrument in direct contact with the body was the conductor, often a hollow metal tube attached by wire to the machine. The electrical discharge was mediated through various materials embedded within the tubes. Channing promoted the use of a sponge that "may be moistened with water, spirit, or a saline, or other appropriate solution, and it then constitutes the mildest and most grateful form of application."[27]

Occasionally, electro-puncture was employed. As the name implies, conducting needles were inserted into the skin and muscle and then electrized. Galvanic and faradic currents were not interchangeable. While galvanic current traveled in one direction from its source, the alternating nature of faradization meant constant reverses. The practical effect was that faradization was useful for eliciting muscle contractions, while galvanic current brought chemical changes to the tissue. "To effect nervous stimulation, the electro-magnetic current is generally sufficient; but to effect any organic change in the nervous tissue,[28] as well as in the other organs, the battery must be resorted to."[29]

Before or after electrization, a soldier's limb was "well shampooed [kneaded or massaged] twice a day, for not over ten minutes." Nausea could result from excessive electrization, which was eased by hot and cold douches and occasional blisters. Mitchell employed Duchenne's use of an electric brush as a conductor, "a bundle of thin wires." The skin must be prepared; it must be dry "and powdered with flour" before the brush is applied. "This is the most intense and painful local excitement known to medicine, while yet it has no power to injure the part it thus violently irritates." Channing described a method by which the practitioner applied electricity while continuing to touch the patient through massage or to localize painful phenomena. To do this, the physician held one conductor, thus introducing electricity into his own body, and then discharged the electricity through the other hand into the patient's body while simultaneously massaging or otherwise manipulating it. The bodies of both patient and physician experienced the treatment together.[30]

CONTRACTILITY AND SENSIBILITY

As the example of J. S. L. Scott shows, incoming patients at Turner's Lane received electric examinations that involved two distinct tests, both named and first applied by Duchenne. The first, electro-muscular contractility, evoked a stimulus response. When faradic current "of some power" was applied to a muscle, "contraction ensues and a deep pain is felt." This process was not limited to the muscle: electrization was accomplished "directly or through the nerves." Because of the hypersensitive ("hyperaesthetic" to Mitchell) responses of many soldiers to touch, Mitchell generally avoided using batteries for examination and favored faradization. "The amount of contractility present in a muscle under faradization, as compared to that of the healthy corresponding organ, is a good test of its condition." The healthier the response, the better the chance of the soldier's achieving "future volitional control."[31]

The second test, electro-muscular sensitivity, probed pain under faradization or, under some circumstances, galvanization. The latter had the advantage of "flushing and heating the skin" over induced currents. Batteries came into play to supply direct current to those paralyzed limbs that may have defied faradization. Channing cited battery-supplied galvanic current as "the most powerful electrical agency which can be brought to bear on the human system." To Channing, the battery was no mere stimulant, but its current acted as "more of a re-agent with the vital powers."[32]

Electricity may have been essential to the soldier's recovery of volitional movement. By the time Mitchell saw a patient at

Turner's Lane, the nerve wound may have healed, but the limb might still be paralyzed. Without the test for contractility, the limb "may lie dead as to motion, for years or for life; and it is here that electrical diagnosis becomes invaluable." A single instance of electrization could revitalize a limb, or repeated sessions over weeks or months might have been required. In sum, however, Mitchell "most earnestly repeat[ed] that without its use no limb, however palsied, should be abandoned by the physician as hopelessly injured."[33]

Mitchell expected, perhaps unreasonably, that the patient could respond verbally to the pain by distinguishing mild cramps caused by involuntary muscle contraction from the "deep muscle pain" of interest to him. Although doctor and patient may have shared the language of electrical treatment, the patient might not have been able to articulate the nature of his pain response, whether superficial or muscular. Further, because the conductor's contact with the skin was mediated by wet materials to limit pain, the patient may have had difficulty distinguishing the degrees of sensation so important to the Firm. The language challenge focused on what Mitchell called localization, "the power which the patient possesses of telling where exactly he has been touched."[34]

COPPER, ZINC, AND VINEGAR

In addition to using electrization to ascertain nerve damage and to improve nerve responses, Mitchell tried to measure skin temperature (calorification) in causalgia cases. At first, he applied a common bulb thermometer to the damaged skin, but he could not obtain useful measurements. The army did not supply electrical tools, so Dr. B. Howard Rand of Philadelphia's Central High School loaned Mitchell "thermo-electric disks of M. Becquerel, in connection with a very delicate galvanometer [that measures current]." Evidently, the disks were successful when applied "on corresponding parts of the body, and the deflection of the needle of the galvanometer informed us which was the warmer of the two localities." "M. Becquerel," the inventor, was Antoine César Becquerel, who pioneered thermoelectric investigation. The thermoelectric effect drove the thermopile, the instrument Mitchell was likely citing. Early versions contained two disks or plates of unrelated materials that, when heated or cooled, generated electrical current. Mitchell had reason to be confident: a thermopile invented in the 1830s could measure the heat emanating from a human hand from up to a meter away.

A similar apparatus was described in an annual publication that listed and described new inventions. In 1867, a "self-registering Electric Thermometer" appeared that incorporated Becquerel's "thermo-electric pile." The instrument included "thirty rods of iron and maillechort[35] ranged in parallel grooves" around a wooden cylinder. The ends of the rods were soldered together in pairs. One extremity was kept at a constant temperature while the other was adjusted to the desired temperature, thus generating a current that deflected a needle, marking a paper.[36]

Mitchell's galvanometer is not described or illustrated anywhere. Several versions of the instrument existed at the time, all of which produced an electric current passed through a coiled wire, which created a magnetic field. The field deflected a needle, hence the measurement, but no direct reading of numerical data was possible. Experts were uncertain about what was being measured: the intensity of the current or the quantity of electricity. No standards existed for baseline measurements; ammeters and voltmeters did not appear until the 1880s. By the time John K. Mitchell continued the examinations of veterans initiated by Mitchell, benchmarks and standards had been or were being established. Mitchell's clinical writings do not state whether he had any experience with electrical machines before working at Christian Street and Turner's Lane Hospitals other than what he might have gathered in Paris or through private study. Rand probably gave Mitchell a quick course in using the electrical apparatus, but it was Mitchell who determined how and under what circumstances to apply electricity to the human body.[37]

Mitchell evidently learned fast and developed his own preferences for the types and manufacture of the instruments he used. He also learned the pitfalls and cautions of applying electricity to soldiers. For instance, he evidently found batteries reliable enough to produce consistent currents. He mentioned using an "electro-magnetic battery" for faradization and cited a "large battery" of a Duchenne type that worked well but was too expensive. Under the direction of army surgeon general Hammond, a reliable portable battery was made "of copper wire gauze and perforated zinc, which is put into action by vinegar."[38]

Although Mitchell commonly employed "electro-magnetic interrupted currents," they often proved "too feeble" for diagnosis and prognosis. Mitchell cited a growing preference for "the rotating machines made by Neff & Sons, Philadelphia" and Thomas Hall of Boston. The rotating machines were probably hand-cranked magneto-electric devices. Channing believed that they almost superseded batteries and were generally useful for most instances that nerves required simulation: "Vital changes can therefore be effected by the practitioner . . . by cooperating with the nervous power." The current, however, depended on the speed of the hand cranking. Mitchell criticized the eventual deterioration or corrosion of wires and wished to see a clockwork mechanism operate these machines. Based on electromagnetism, sophisticated versions of these instruments were patented in 1854 but were not manufactured until after the war, primarily for hospitals, colleges, and schools.[39]

Duchenne's two relevant, pioneering works were *De l'electrisation localisée* (1855) and *Physiologie des mouvements* (1867). Mitchell must have thought his own work constituted vindication of Duchenne's exact mapping of the individual muscles and associated nerves to produce "a kind of living anatomy." Perhaps the soldiers on whose bodies Mitchell repeatedly applied conductors thought of themselves as blank maps with the nerves to be delineated, showing where features continued and proliferated or were cut off and nerve impulses stopped or detoured.

PAIN AND PERFECT SELF-CONQUEST

How and when soldiers communicated pain resulting from electrization was not straightforward. Despite Mitchell's praise for the analytical ability of American soldiers, interpreting the results of faradization presented a problem. How reliable was the patient's response in describing pain or identifying what part of the body was responding to electricity? Mitchell observed that people new to these treatments (which included all soldiers) may be "unaccustomed to these strange variations in the responsive power of the muscles [and therefore] may readily be misled." The language of treatment and the soldiers' intelligent and insightful observations were negotiated. Electrization required the patient to collaborate with the doctor and to share a vocabulary of treatment. Mitchell was clear about who among patients proved to be inadequate to the task: "In very sensitive persons, in hysterical women, in children, or in those of small intelligence, I have often found it difficult to make them discriminate between the pain in the skin, occasioned by powerful currents, and that which belongs to the muscular tissues."[40] Maybe the Firm tried not to select soldiers who seemed sensitive, hysterical, or "of small intelligence" to be patients at Turner's Lane. Apparently, African American soldiers were not considered for advanced treatment. Understanding white soldiers' spectrum of pain may have been the Firm's objective.

Mitchell's exploration of pain must have been challenged by blind alleys, inconsistent responses of relevant nerves, and the mysterious ways in which the body heals itself. Although Mitchell's most challenging form of pain was causalgia and its intense burning sensation, he was also interested in locating sources of aching and neuralgic pain. Remedies characteristic of other kinds of wounds and injuries were first applied, from blistering agents to various dressings and finally morphia and similar drugs. Electricity was applied sometimes simultaneously with other treatments or after other treatments either stabilized the malady or proved insufficient.

Physicians of Mitchell's generation did not believe that they could cure illnesses: at best, they could aid the body in summoning the natural processes of healing. A significant portion of Mitchell's therapy was dialogue with the recovering soldier, particularly when the latter was impatient to recover or despondent over his inability to do so. Given Mitchell's views about unreliable patient-narrators, he tried to convince the soldier "that he himself has some control over his symptoms, or, at least, that constantly to yield to them is to insure defeat, and that constant struggle in a manly way is sure to bring nearer the day of perfect self conquest." As a function of manhood, the patient accepted a painful therapy to remedy a larger pain.[41]

Both soldier and physician could see that any therapy's effects were transient and contingent on changing bodily phenomena. The electrization that prompted fingers to flex on one occasion might only induce pain on another. Pain relief was an ever-present need in cases of electrization. Mitchell and his colleagues depended on morphia, but by John K. Mitchell's era, cocaine had become as common and was administered hypodermically. He suggested that it be injected "as near the tender nerve as may safely be" and noted that joint application of both morphia and cocaine had no greater effect than either alone. Further, no better method of pain relief had yet been put forward.[42]

Occasionally, electrization-induced pain led some soldiers to reject treatment altogether. Chapter 2 recounted Mitchell's treatment of Chas. A. P., Eighty-Eighth Pennsylvania Volunteers, who left Turner's Lane but later returned for more treatment, perhaps narcotic pain relief. He was ultimately deemed incurable, but Mitchell's obvious disdain for the man's failure to exhibit the expected qualities of manhood might have played a role in his diagnosis. As Mitchell recalled, one measure of the harshness of electrization was that in one year, "over forty thousand injections of morphine were used." Most of these injections were intended to relieve pain due to electrization.[43]

Electricity could elicit strange and unexpected pain responses in the bodies of patients, inflicting pain, for instance, on nonexistent limbs. These unforeseen consequences may have intrigued Mitchell as much as those he and his colleagues anticipated based on experience. In amputees, electrization could trigger memories of motions or movements and the limbs that produced them. Even the attachment of a prosthetic to a stump could produce a similar result. In both cases, Mitchell wrote that "the limb is sometimes called back to sensory being with startling reality." In one case, Mitchell electrized a limb some inches above the amputation site on a soldier's arm. The amputation had been performed years earlier, and "the man had ceased to be conscious of the limb." When the current flowed into the soldier, the man felt excruciating pain and exclaimed, "Oh, the hand, the hand!" He tried to seize the nonexistent hand with his remaining one. As one confused soldier put it, "If . . . I should say, I am more sure of the leg which ain't than of the one that are, I guess I should be about correct."[44]

STIRRING MUSCLES

As John K. Mitchell matured into a neurological collaborator, medical applications of electricity evolved. The essential characteristics of Mitchell's electrical examinations and treatments remained the same, although the proliferating applications of electricity in American life had created new machines and standards of electrical power and its measurement. Just as Mitchell argued for the holistic appraisal of his patients' health before choosing the appropriate therapies, John K. Mitchell similarly proclaimed the need for a dynamic appraisal by scrupulous "observation of all the circumstances of the injury, the subsequent history, the electro-muscular contractility, the tactile and other sensibility of the patient."[45]

Similarly, he practiced faradization followed by galvanic current if the former proved ineffective, recommending that doctors "apply that current which will produce the most motion with the least pain." If both faradization and galvanization failed to elicit a muscular response, then the physician should repeat the regimen daily, as electro-muscular sensibility would likely return to the injured nerves. Just as his father embraced other therapies to be administered concurrently with electrization, the younger Mitchell focused on hot or cold douches and massage. The latter, according to Mitchell, should not consist of "mere rubbing" but should probe deep into the tissues of the injured or wounded area. Once the appropriate nerve responded, the physician should massage the locus of nerve damage vigorously despite the pain "it may cause to stiffened and disused joints and muscles."[46]

Hospitals acquired electrical equipment in recognition of the evolving importance of electrization even though its efficacy could not be explicated in most cases. Post–Civil War hospitals found, as current medical practices vindicate, that the electrical stimulation of arms, legs, hands, and feet can aid in recovery from trauma. Doubtless, many of Mitchell's soldier-patients were impressed by electrical technology and its effects and valued their partnership with him in exploring their bodies' capacity for healing. Even as they experienced pain in response to electrization, they had permitted Mitchell to stimulate the vital force as both bodies—the soldier's and Mitchell's—participated in the outcome. As both Mitchell and his son had learned, not only was the patient's trust required; his complicity and faith were also needed because success might "be dependent upon patient expectations, and . . . this may only happen if the patient believes there is an actual neuromodulatory effect."[47]

Electrotherapy departments in hospitals created suites of electrical apparatuses to suit both faradization and galvanization. At the Philadelphia Orthopedic Hospital and Infirmary for Nervous Diseases—successor to Turner's Lane and Mitchell's place of employment after the Civil War—a physician known as an "electrician" worked with electrotherapy. His function was not only to operate the electrical machines but also to deliver a current of reliable, consistent strength. By 1885, the hospital had installed "a galvanic battery with milliampere meter attached" that made it possible to deliver a consistent current. It remained in use as a "mainstay treatment" until about 1900. Machines became more reliable in generating galvanic and faradic currents. It became possible to quantify current: *volts* to measure force (in the 1870s), *amperes* (by the early 1880s) to measure current in terms of volts per *ohm* (by the late 1860s), a measure of resistance. During this time, the most widely read text on the burgeoning field of medical electricity was George M. Beard and Alphonso David Rockwell's *A Practical Treatise on the Medical and Surgical Uses of Electricity*, which was reprinted in many editions over decades. Mitchell's Civil War treatments and later applications can be found in this text, as they contributed to a professional standard.[48]

Over time, Mitchell learned about new techniques, tools, and medicines while continuing to use electrization. Even as the war ended and he anticipated a continuing need to treat Civil War veterans, he studied improvements and innovations. By the time he published his follow-up treatise to *Gunshot Wounds* (1864), *Injuries to Nerves* (1872), electricity was omnipresent among his cases, with consequent hypodermic injections of morphine and atropine, "their effects carefully studied." During the 1870s, Mitchell highlighted a different model of galvanometer from the one borrowed from Central High School, a "Thomson high-resistance galvanometer." This tool allowed for minute, "feeble currents" to be measured if they proved sufficient to "stir" muscles into activity. In addition, he took advantage of emerging antisepsis and refinements to anesthetization to expand ways of investigating nerve damage. John K. Mitchell cited nerve transplants including that of a sciatic nerve from a rabbit into a human.[49]

Over time, Mitchell found ways to share his electrical and associated therapies. Other professions besides doctors could apply electrization. Mitchell also realized that massage did not require doctors: the military personnel who worked as supernumeraries were trained to apply massage in a more sophisticated and effective fashion. Later, hospital orderlies and then nurses were trained to do it. After the war, he wrote that the Firm chose and "carefully trained several clever sergeants" to administer massage and conduct gymnastic classes. He noted that these "rubbers" or "manipulators" "must be not only tender and gentle, but also strong and enduring, because a treatment by massage extending over an hour, as it should do, will severely task the strength of most men." The intimate contact between patients and noncombatant soldiers who performed paramedical functions is not often mentioned in the medical histories of the Civil War, but they also participated in a bodily partnership with patients. Formerly ill or wounded soldiers thus jointly explored healing with soldier-patients, essentially camp and battlefield comrades. This mutual exploration reduced personal space, ignored civil decorum regarding the presentation of one's body, and created possibilities to redefine manhood through therapy, embracing feminine qualities.[50]

CONCLUSION: MAGUS OF THE MEDIUM

In imagining Mitchell's engagement with his patients while electrizing nerves, we can envisage intimate contact between doctor and soldier. Bodies in healing proximity share one another's touch, sweat, odors, heat, and breath. In *Gunshot Wounds*, for instance, Mitchell describes the glossy skin of causalgia sufferers, hair loss, eczema, and the odd phenomenon of the inactivity of nails in limbs due to nerve damage. Nails exhibited "curving, thickening" and became rough, hard, and discolored. Some conditions caused the skin to exude a vinegar-like odor that was "intensely acid." Mitchell writes of one case that "the odor of the sweat was disgustingly heavy, and resembled the smells from a bad drain." Mitchell's overworked body scrutinized, invaded, palpated, flexed, pressured, exercised, and managed patients' bodies to restore fractured, disabled, or useless nerves. To understand the behavior of nerves, he applied electricity with multiple instruments, perhaps the first diagnostic machines applied to bodies in hospitals.[51]

The pressure of private and army practice, the sounds, sights, smells, and incessant probing of soldiers' bodies undoubtedly contributed to Mitchell's breakdown while he worked at Christian Street and Turner's Lane. He must have experienced, either indirectly or by accident, moments of faradizing and galvanizing current. He must have imagined electricity's possibilities in a variety of bodily contexts. He must have wondered if electricity was the essence of the motive life force, perhaps in a cosmic sense a driving impulse of planets and stars. Channing's treatise on electro-medicine posited an "attractive force" in muscles and tissues that produces motion and "bears a close analogy to the attractive force so suddenly communicated to, and withdrawn from, the particles of magnetizable bodies by electricity." As the macrocosmos, so goes the microcosmos.[52]

Success with patients is measured by improvements in their health following treatment. Professional success is measured by how practice is articulated in print, demonstrated in the clinic, and evaluated by peers. The professional challenge is to "create a system of meaning with which the doctors and patients could interpret their illnesses and their respective roles in the rehabilitative process." Doctors and patients—and their bodies—are not easily separable or divisible: "Doctors are always patients as well, subject to the science that they practice."[53]

Mitchell's electrization, then, cannot be characterized as a mere transfer of electrical energy into a patient's body facilitated by the physician who controls the source apparatus. The rationale for electricity's medical use remained a matter of faith that some sort of positive outcome was likely, and if that outcome seemed elusive or nonexistent, then therapy would be continued to achieve a different outcome. The broad history of medical electricity confirms that its use has been propelled by innovations in technology. Since the eighteenth century, electricity has captured imaginations through parlor demonstrations and tricks, inevitably being applied to the human body to enhance life. From a twenty-first-century perspective, electricity has always found its way in, around, and out of human bodies following discovery, exploration, insight via hypothesis and test, theoretical debate, and restricted application, although why electricity is medically vital remains obscure.[54]

As electricity became legitimized over time, Mitchell stood out as a leader of the medium. His case notes incorporating electrization resemble the "humanitarian narrative," a late-nineteenth-century "expository technique that sought authenticity in large quantities of minute observation . . . about bodily pain and death in such a way as to engender an empathic response from readers, thereby blurring the boundaries between medicine and literature." Mitchell's style of writing case narratives blurs that boundary. That he blended observations on the "Americanness" of his soldier-patients with minute descriptions of their bodies under the influence of electric current does not present a neutral, "objective" clinical narrative. His case studies are widely read and cited today perhaps in part because of the empathetic response they engender. To describe the patients whose bodies have been invaded with pain-inducing electricity was to create a type of humanitarian narrative in which the physician calls down an elemental force and guides it to occasionally predictable results. The electrized body remained an inconclusive being. After the war, Mitchell concluded that among his instruments, "one of them, and the most efficient, is perhaps the most overrated and underrated of all the medical armamenta. Need we add that we refer to electricity?"[55]

FOUR

HENRY ADOLPH KIRCHER

(1841–1908)

RINGGOLD GAP

At the beginning of 1863, Henry Adolph Kircher prepared to lead his company in a charge across the challenging terrain outside of Vicksburg, Mississippi, against a fortified enemy, determined to break Confederate defenses. He awaited the command of "Forward!" and expected to die in the attack. He later recalled, "You can imagine that this was a painful half hour for many. I noticed many faces that almost visibly changed and got paler and paler. The eyes looked so hollow and as if they were fixed in the head. . . . Others looked terribly solemn and seemed impatient for the moment when they could sacrifice themselves." Despite Kircher's anticipation and mental preparation, the attack was called off. Perhaps some of the soldiers were disappointed that they could not face their mortality at that moment; they would have to revisit their apprehension later with the attendant physical symptoms, including trembling or shivering, nausea, vomiting, hot flashes, elevated heart rate, tightness or pain in the chest, or outright panic.[1]

Early on November 27, 1863, now-Captain Kircher and Company E, Twelfth Missouri, experienced those sensations again.

On that cold morning, Kircher and his regiment marched cautiously from Tennessee into Georgia following railroad tracks toward the narrow Ringgold Gap. Expecting to catch up with and defeat a retreating Confederate column, they were unaware of a substantial rebel deployment on the high ground. Kircher was ordered to turn the regiment east and proceed up the rocky slope of White Oak Mountain when gunfire erupted from atop the mountain and a grove of trees directly to the south. At the same time, from inside the gap, artillery was fired into Kircher's division. Rebel sharpshooters caused confusion. Kircher's and other regiments stalled for most of the five hours of the chaotic battle. Complicating things, gunfire ignited grass and forest debris, generating suffocating smoke and burning corpses.[2]

Kircher shouted orders and gestured commands to find cover and avoid retreat until reinforcements or artillery support could arrive. A bullet struck his upper-right arm, pulverized bone, and exited near his wrist, whereupon he collapsed. As he struggled into a seated position, another bullet struck his left thigh above the knee and passed downward and out, splitting bone. As he was being lifted and carried away from the action, a third bullet struck him in the left hip.

Kircher was taken to a temporary field hospital in a nearby house. He waited patiently to be inspected by a hospital steward or surgeon. There is no record of whether or to what degree Kircher felt pain at this point. Kircher did not lose consciousness and made every effort to present himself as stoically resolved to await his turn and not assert the privilege of rank. Surgeons were aware of the diversity of responses to bullet wounds: shock, then possibly spasms of pain, and then numbness. Given Kircher's copiously bleeding wounds, Surgeon Joseph Spiegelhalter feared that he would not survive. "I therefore hastened, after a slight examination, to remove the patient into a back room of the house, in which I had a fire built + a table ready," the surgeon later wrote in his order book. Kircher tried to stay conscious, to "keep [his] head level or [he] would have gone to—."[3]

Spiegelhalter and Kircher enjoyed a camaraderie not experienced in many regiments. They were both German Americans, as were most of the soldiers in the Twelfth Missouri. German was routinely spoken around camp. Both men were part of a division commanded by Peter Osterhaus, another German immigrant, who knew Kircher's family. Regardless of how Kircher's relationship with Spiegelhalter began, however, they remained friends until Kircher's death, not typical of most soldier-doctor relationships. Kircher likely turned to Spielgelhalter later to evaluate his wounds for applicable pensions.

Dr. Samuel D. Gross's manual for military surgeons states that a limb should not be saved "when, in addition to serious injury done to the integuments, muscles, or bones, its principal artery, vein, or nerve has been extensively lacerated, or violently contused, as the result will be likely to be gangrene, followed by death." Further, gunshot wounds that caused such injuries usually required amputation to save the victim's life. Kircher's apparent calmness and self-possession were vital to Spiegelhalter's decision to pursue surgery, without which he would certainly have died.[4]

Spiegelhalter cut away Kircher's clothing and wiped away his blood to get a better look. All three wounds were caused by minié balls (bullets fired from rifles). These .58-caliber, 1.5-ounce lead bullets made holes in the body the width of a finger and exit wounds the size of a fist. The soft lead bent, tore, or fragmented to obliterate bone, flesh, and sinew. Spiegelhalter noticed that Kircher "took it very easy" when he said to the doctor, "You will have to cut off my arm." The doctor responded, "I am going to put you under the influence of chloroform in order to examine your wounds closely. I have as much fear for your leg as for your arm. Do I have your permission to amputate your leg also, should it be necessary?" Kircher answered, "Do whatever you think best."

Other surgeons joined Spiegelhalter to consult on the decision to amputate. His assistant surgeon, Dr. Frederick Kohly, Dr. Charles Bruckner (Seventeenth Missouri), and a physician of the Thirty-First Missouri agreed on Kircher's treatment and likely participated in the surgery. Dr. Gross's manual advised caution in using anesthesia. It was not to be employed if "the vital powers are depressed and the mind is bewildered with shock, or loss of blood." One of the doctors administered the chloroform. This drug, a "distillation of chloride of lime with rectified spirit," was frequently chosen over ether because it was not flammable and smaller amounts could be used. It was nonetheless dangerous and could be fatal.

A funnel with a wad of cloth was placed over Kircher's mouth and nose. The attendant dripped chloroform through the funnel onto the cloth until Kircher became insensible. He was not necessarily unconscious; he may have been conscious but oblivious to pain. While the chemical took effect, his body may have exhibited involuntary spasms, so an attendant would have held his limbs steady. Spiegelhalter assigned a doctor or steward to monitor pulse, respiration, and pupil size while Kircher was under chloroform. If any problems developed—a change in breathing, pulse, or pupil size—the drug-soaked cloth would have been removed immediately. Being under anesthesia resulted in the disorganization of thought. Kircher was no longer able to reliably answer the surgeons' questions as they worked.[5]

Once Kircher was anesthetized, Spiegelhalter began a more thorough examination. As he inspected the arm, he noticed the entry wound about one inch below where the deltoid muscle attaches to the humerus. The bullet had progressed down the length of the upper arm to the joint, exiting through the "internal condyloid ridge," the bony bulge at the lower end of the humerus, "crushing the bone into small fragments."[6] That lower end also secured the muscles of the forearm. The arm was obviously beyond repair. Next, he inspected the leg wound. The bullet had fractured the internal condyle of the lower left femur,[7] traveled behind the patella through the knee joint, and split open the tibia such that the doctor could insert a finger deep between its fragments. This wound, too, was beyond repair. Finally, Spiegelhalter located the third wound, pronounced it minor, and dressed it. In all three wounds, the bullets passed out of the body.[8]

The surgeons all agreed that the immediate amputation of both limbs could save Kircher's life. Sawdust may have been scattered on the floor underneath the table, or an old blanket might have been put down to absorb fluids. Tools on hand included suturing material, most likely silk or cotton; needles; waxed silk ligatures (for tying off blood vessels); two tourniquets; various retractors or tenacula (long tools with a hook to separate tissues or blood vessels); "well-boiled sponges"; an assortment of knives from scalpels to near-foot-long catlins (heavy-duty, double-bladed cutting knives); a bone chisel; a director (used with a scalpel to direct the blade to the precise spot); a rongeur (bone cutter); and a bone saw.[9]

Spiegelhalter and his colleagues decided to use two amputation methods: flap on the leg and circular on the arm. The right arm was elevated, grasped above the injury, and massaged toward the shoulder "to empty it as much as possible of venous blood." The skin was pulled upward until taut, then the doctor quickly attached the cloth strap of the tourniquet around the arm several inches above the lacerated flesh and tightened it to stop arterial flow into the wound. He incised a circle about the arm, exchanged the scalpel for the catlin, and rotated it while deepening the cut to the bone. Assistants applied retractors to pull the flesh away from the bone so it could be cut without further injury to tissues and vessels.

Spiegelhalter exchanged his catlin for the bone saw and removed the lower arm. The protruding humerus end was scraped. Splinters were cut off with the rongeur so that as the arm healed and new flesh closed over the wound, sharp ends would not press

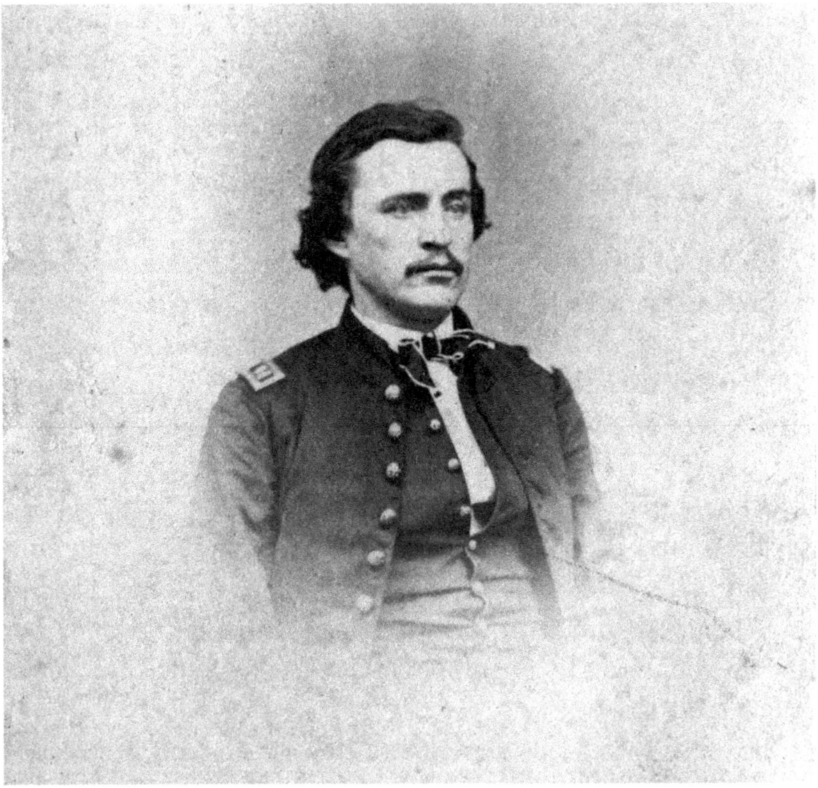

Carte de visite of Captain Henry A. Kircher in military uniform, 1863.
Credit: Abraham Lincoln Presidential Library and Museum.

inside the flesh and cause pain. An assistant sponged the wound, and Spiegelhalter tied off visible arteries with waxed silk thread or ligatures. The assistant slightly relaxed the grip of the tourniquet so the flow of blood could allow quick identification of other vessels to be ligatured. With the tension of the skin released, elasticity permitted the closing and suturing of the wound with a curved needle and silk thread.

Various ligatures were bundled or moved to the side. Distinctive knots at the thread ends protruding from the stump denoted which vessel was which. Kircher's arm was covered with reinforcing adhesive strips to hold all sutures and ligatures firmly in place. Before bandaging, a soft cloth or lint may have been set over the sutured wound "anointed with cerate" such as fresh lard or a cold-water-soaked dressing. Despite bandaging, the wound exuded liquid, including blood, for several days. As tissue was rebuilt, the ligatures stopped draining and fell off.[10]

The amputation of the leg was a different procedure. Instead of cutting a circle around the limb, Spiegelhalter cut two elongated flaps of cutaneous tissue (anterior and posterior flaps) that descended below the amputation line of the thigh. The flaps were drawn up and secured out of the way of the amputation saw by retractors. Following the amputation, the flaps were let down and folded over the new stump, thus providing an ample skin cushion for a prosthetic leg. The Union army favored circular amputations over the flap method because they seemed to heal more quickly and with less discharge. Kircher's circular arm stump suppurated[11] for nineteen days, whereas his leg healed much more slowly.[12]

The fact that Spiegelhalter used two different amputation methods may indicate that he and Kircher discussed prostheses beforehand. The choice of the circular method implied a decision not to wear a prosthetic limb because there was no skin cushion at the end of the stump. Indeed, Kircher never wore a prosthesis on his arm: "Never wore any on arm, stump too short. Leg has been worn constantly since July 1864," wrote Kircher in his questionnaire from Weir Mitchell many years later.

According to the federal accounting, the Union army experienced 1,761 cases of amputation at the forearm with 14.0 percent fatalities; 5,523 amputations of the leg with 33.2 percent fatalities; and 6,369 amputations at the thigh with 54.2 percent fatalities. The closer to the trunk the amputation was conducted, the higher the risk of death. Spiegelhalter realized these risks. Given the need for a double amputation—possibly the only one he had ever performed—he asked other surgeons for their advice. Further, he and his colleagues were aware that Kircher might succumb to shock, a point at which death was inevitable. Medical regulations at the time required that primary surgery (surgery before shock symptoms appear) occur within twenty-four hours if amputations at the hip were performed. Even so, primary surgery generally resulted in a 34 percent mortality rate, slightly less than that of immediate surgery, which led to a 35 percent mortality rate.[13]

One objective of amputation surgery is to minimize blood loss; evidently, Kircher did not bleed much during his surgery. Once he was bandaged, he was taken to another space for a brief recuperation before being evacuated from the battlefield. Spiegelhalter officially logged two successful amputations on one body: removal of the arm "in the upper third" and the leg at the thigh "in the lower third." The doctor recorded that Kircher "healed comfortably and was very encouraging." Between four and five hours elapsed between the wounding and the amputation. The day of his surgery and the next, Kircher "felt pretty cheap." The following day, Kircher was placed on a crowded railroad car and left there to spend the cold night. He "passed a hard day" on the twenty-ninth and arrived by ambulance at Chattanooga, Tennessee, where he was placed in a tent at Officers' Hospital, Fifteenth Army Corps. Kircher's godfather Henry Goedeking, representing the family in Belleville, Illinois, came to Chattanooga to visit and remained for several days to accompany Kircher home. The family planned his return. His father hired "a nigger . . . a nice mulatto who takes care of Heinrich [Henry]." For a time, his father pointed out, this arrangement "will be quite necessary, as Heinrich requires much care and lifting."[14]

As much as Kircher's family worried about his health and longed to have him home, his father wasted no time prodding his son to plan his future:

> The loss of the leg and arm is hard, but there remains nothing else to do but to adjust to what cannot be changed and to fit yourself into anything that will clearly lead to alleviate it. It must always be a great comfort to us

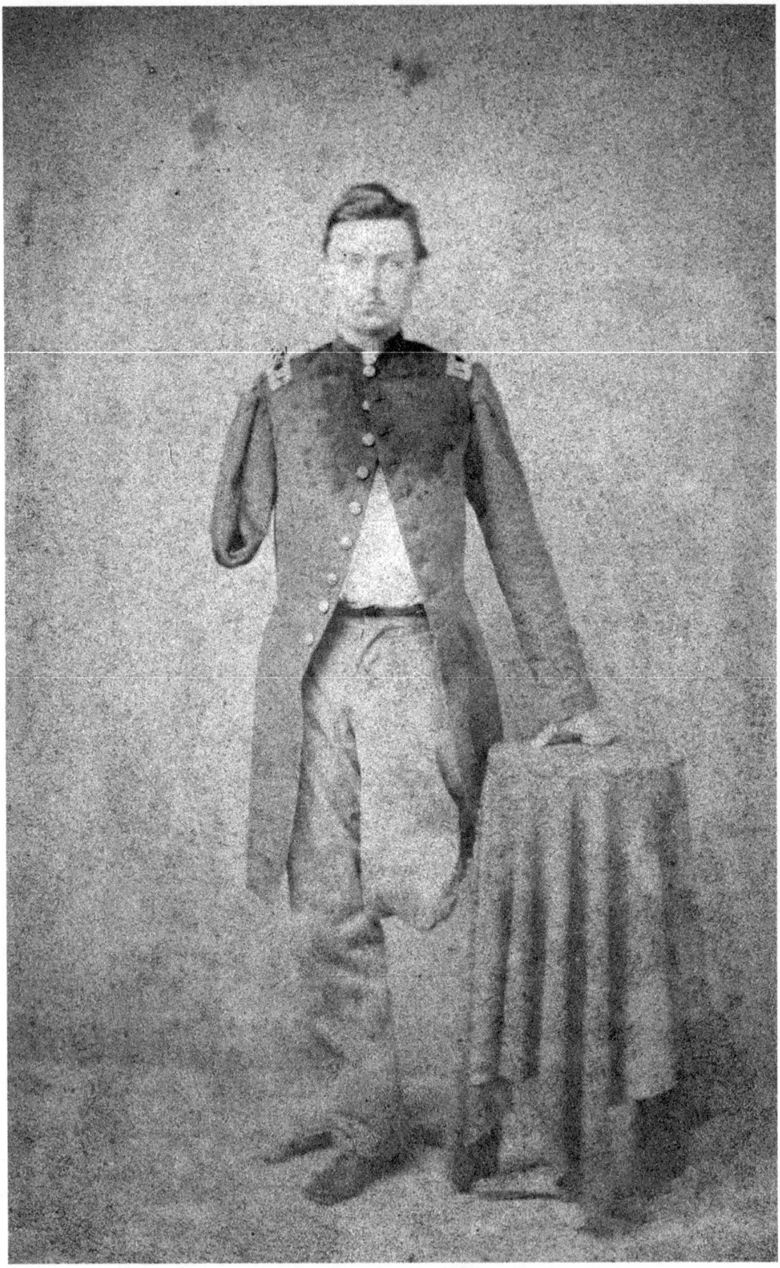

Carte de visite of Captain Henry Kircher, 1864, with campaign announcement "Henry A. Kircher, Candidate for Circuit Court Clerk." *Credit: Abraham Lincoln Presidential Library and Museum.*

> that it occurred for our country, which deserved to be remembered all the time . . . [the] amputation of the leg succeeded very well was reassuring, since that will increase the usefulness of the artificial leg so that in time you can walk without a crutch and cane. In a year, you will be able to write just as well with the left hand as you were able to do; and as you know, it is rare that somebody amasses a fortune by working with his hands. It is chiefly one's head, intellectual work, which brings it to light. In time, you will find the suitable activity in which you can gain a considerable fortune by thrift and industry.[15]

Later, after the Twelfth Missouri returned to Chattanooga, Kircher continued to recuperate as he watched his regiment march off to another campaign. By December 20, Kircher was ready to leave and, with his helper, traveled home to Belleville, arriving at two o'clock in the morning, Christmas Day.

The following year, Henry Adolph Kircher achieved the clerkship of his county's circuit court.

MANHOOD AND AMPUTEES

Walt Whitman described the postbattle landscape of the dead and the helpless living into which Kircher had entered: "Of all the harrowing experiences, none is greater than that of the days following a heavy battle. Scores, hundreds, of the noblest young men on earth, uncomplaining, lie helpless, mangled, faint, alone, and so bleed to death, or die from exhaustion, either actually untouched at all, or with merely the laying of them down and leaving them, when there ought to be means provided to save them."[16]

Doubtless, Kircher's thoughts ran among concern for self, comrades, and his family, and very likely his near future. The definition of manhood informed every aspect of Kircher's treatment: his beliefs and behavior before, during, and after he was wounded; his physicians' notions of their manhood and how these beliefs affected their surgical work; and the values and expectations of everyone in the medical universe of the Civil War.

Kircher had every reason to believe that his manhood was beyond reproach based on his conduct as an officer on November 27 and the lasting visible evidence of his wounds. At this time, he thought about being a veteran. The army kept him on sick leave for almost another year before discharging him into civilian life and the new territory of pensions and the comradeship of other veterans.

Before he was wounded, Kircher, in common with other soldiers, adjusted his sense of identity to conform to the circumstances of military service. As an officer, he supervised and directed soldiers and exercised an authority peculiar to the military. Through his correspondence to his family, he described difficult judgments about military tactics and strategy, thus placing himself as both actor and critic within a vast system engaged in a national crusade. His father's encouraging letter focused on stimulating thoughts of future accomplishments. The learned assertiveness and habit of command doubtless informed Kircher's future choices. His sense of manhood required anticipation for the future, active plans to achieve it, and creating a new identity as a veteran. "In becoming veterans, Civil War soldiers understood that they needed to find ways to trust in themselves, to reach their own judgments, and to pursue their own course of action without losing their religion or running afoul of the military establishment."[17]

Despite being characterized as reckless "sawbones" during the war, Union doctors were committed to saving limbs and preserving manhood, even when the preserved limb may have been functionally useless. To preserve patients' manhood, surgeons sometimes identified with soldiers who refused amputation altogether even if survival would have been impossible. In such cases, prizing their manhood at the expense of their life may have been the only course for some. Surgeons also related to amputees because of their wish to preserve manly ideals in the face of anticipated mixed public reactions. Spiegelhalter and Kircher agreed on the importance of teamwork in maintaining manhood in a medical environment.[18]

Integral to any physician's administration of therapy were his professional networks, ethnicity, and social class. When assigning therapies, military doctors of this era holistically appraised their patients' bodies, personal histories, and moral qualities. In Kircher's case, this shared intimacy with Spiegelhalter was no threat or problem. Unlike most doctor-patient relationships, Kircher enjoyed an intellectual reciprocity with Spiegelhalter. He deferred his body's care to the doctor's judgment because both men were social equals of common ethnicity and comparable "German-American-ness" and doubtless shared a common worldview about health.[19]

During Kircher's stay in a Chattanooga hospital, the hospital staff most likely did not talk with Kircher about the impact on his psyche of the recent battle. There is no record of any intimate interaction between Kircher and hospital staff or fellow patients. There was no doctor like Mitchell to question Kircher about the sensations of his nerves. He evidently never discussed phantom pain or other nerve sensations until he completed the 1893 questionnaire that he returned to Mitchell. Kircher was likely alone with his thoughts most of the time. In accepting that his military service was permanently over, Kircher redefined his life trajectory to consider how his bodily limitations might correspondingly limit his options. He obviously saw that these same limitations also created opportunities.[20]

While convalescing, Kircher's thoughts about soldiers' bodies may have become more critical regarding himself and those around him. His letters and diary reveal a sense of German bodily superiority over American and Irish soldiers. He believed—as did some doctors—that German soldiers were healthier and better able to withstand the rigors of campaigning because they practiced better personal hygiene and had healthier diets. This belief might have implications for pension awards, but Kircher would likely never know whether his German origin played a role in those decisions. In an analysis of Civil War pensions, researchers found that both German- and Irish-born soldiers were statistically less likely to become very ill from disease than native-born Americans and were therefore less likely to endure periods of hospitalization in military service.[21]

In the hospital, Kircher encountered far fewer German bodies and interacted more with native-born white Americans. He likely revisited the view he had formed in his first regiment, the Ninth Illinois, which included a tense mix of the two backgrounds. In a letter to his father in 1861, he complained, "You have to be much meaner than the average German to gain his respect. . . . Even if they gripe in a friendly way, however, you have to tell them dirty jokes and jestures. . . . Besides that, you have to tell them nice things and not forget to *treat* them." Kircher's recuperation in the hospital may have reinforced his views of the physical and cultural superiority of his body.[22]

One attribute of manhood is how to respond to pain. Kircher, like many others of the time, probably thought that men and women and white people and black people experienced pain differently. If this were true, then responses to pain under anesthesia might differ as well. According to the medical belief at the time, white people, particularly educated, socially refined ones, exhibited higher sensitivity to pain than uneducated manual laborers, especially African Americans who might therefore receive little or no anesthesia. This hierarchy of pain had wider cultural implications, "play[ing] an important, previously unrecognized role in such diverse areas as feminism, imperialism, abolition, penology, pedagogy, and poetry." Even for white men, stoically enduring pain was viewed as manly behavior, a view held by doctors who, during the first decades following the surgical introduction of ether, still conducted many surgeries without anesthesia.[23]

Kircher's thoughts about African American bodies may also have intensified while he was in the hospital awaiting his future.

He rarely noted the presence of any black people in his surroundings, such as the formerly enslaved Louis, who had served as his valet in 1862. Early in 1863, when his regiment fought in the siege of Vicksburg, Mississippi, he saw African American soldiers and wrote in a letter to his mother that he did not "like the idea of fighting side-by-side with a Negro. . . . If the colored and others do government work, I don't have anything against it. But to see him fighting with weapons in hand at my better side, hey now, no sirree bob." In a later letter, he clarified his stand: "You mustn't get me wrong when I say I wouldn't like to fight with a black. But that I am only saying that I wouldn't like to be a slave boss, a slave driver, and fight at his side, my blood with his, perhaps wounded by the same bullet that first traffics with a Negro and then pays me a visit. I am not far enough advanced in civilization that I don't know the difference between white and black anymore." In other words, black soldiers had their usefulness, but proximity on the battlefield increased the danger that blood oozing from a black body might affect his own.[24]

When Kircher was ready to leave the hospital, his stumps had not healed sufficiently for him to use a prosthetic limb on his leg; he had already decided against using one on his arm. People with amputations were seen on every street in the country, a feature of "new landscapes" that the war had created. Features of these landscapes were the tent camps of the armies, demolished towns, and the "new technologies that attempt[ed] to rebuild or replace what has been lost, such as the prosthetics that made veteran amputees whole again." Kircher had been living and fighting in an environment altered by war, and his journey home must have taken him through places of violent upheaval. Already emasculated by his two amputations, he came home to "the healing power and domination of women." We know little of the courtship that led to Kircher's marriage many years later, but perhaps Bertha Engelmann valued her fiancé's patriotic sacrifice in agreeing to the betrothal.[25]

The mere presence of a body with two stumps in public could elicit negative responses, Kircher must have reasoned, so what would he conceal, what would he display? His society had little tolerance for anomalous bodies. Social acceptance of wartime disfigurement was mercurial: people may have cheered and politicians supported ex-soldiers without limbs, but the public was fickle. Throughout the latter part of the nineteenth century, "ugly laws" emerged in many locales that banned people from public areas if their appearance might be deemed disquieting, if not disgusting. "People with disabilities were to be made invisible." Even an army guide for surgeons who examined prospective recruits cautioned about "the importance of disqualifying not only those men who were physically incapable of military duty" but also those who were "so disgusting in character as to render them repulsive and uncompanionable."[26]

Thus Kircher returned home for Christmas and planned for the new year. To him—and to scholars today—"the consequences of amputation on Civil War soldiers and civilians, both during and after the war, have remained largely unexplored." He presented himself as an exemplary citizen and simultaneously balanced his obvious bodily restrictions with the self-command expected of a community leader. In the interval between surgery and returning home, he reevaluated how he viewed his body, its utility, its value as a symbol and a badge of integrity, and its sexual being. Some people might have considered him a medical celebrity: double amputees who survived were rare. In fact, records of both armies reference only sixty-eight double amputees, not all of whom survived the war.[27]

Kircher's subsequent life constituted a ladder of accomplishments that cemented middle-class respectability with patriotic ardor. This ardor was fueled by a canny adaptation to the evolving paradigm of manhood via leadership in commerce and civic affairs. He was aware that many people were uncomfortable in the presence of an amputee because of class worries—a perception that the scarred or amputee veteran must be lower class. For the rest of his life, Kircher sought superlatives: he became the owner of the family business, served on boards of civic organizations and prominent local businesses, and frequently held offices from bank president to mayor. Perhaps these achievements reflected a desire not to be relegated to lower social status upon sight and to prove that the subtraction of body parts did not reflect a diminution of intelligence or ability.[28]

PENSION NO. 36,243

In the new year following his return, Kircher aggressively stepped into his future. He was not strong enough to wear a leg prosthesis until summer; nevertheless, he consulted with family and business associates to enter politics. At the same time, he began corresponding with the pension office in a campaign to have his specific wounds recognized and missing limbs compensated. To the government, Kircher was an invalid officer, 5 feet, 8 inches tall with dark hair, hazel eyes, and a fair complexion, assigned to the Twelfth Missouri Volunteer Infantry. The official record assigned him incorrectly to Company A, a mistake that was carried through almost all subsequent pension forms and correspondence.[29]

By the spring of 1864, with the help of his godfather and family business associate, Henry Goedeking, Kircher eyed the November election for the position of clerk of the county circuit court. The men conceived of an odd partnership: if Kircher won, Goedeking would function as the prime mover behind the throne. They planned a campaign that appealed to voters' sympathy for one of their own who had returned from war damaged and gave public notice of their proposed partnership. In a newspaper column, Kircher professed humility and promised to consult and be guided by Goedeking: "My youth, inexperience, and my almost helpless condition, would render me unable to attend to the duties of an office requiring such labor; neither could I make myself personally acquainted with my constituents throughout the county; hence I am induced to accept the offer of my kind and generous friend." Along with Kircher's announcement, Goedeking provided a kind of sworn statement: "I shall, if elected, superintend the office with him, so that his youth, and inexperience need create no apprehension. He shall however have the emoluments of the office, even if his corporal disability shall prevent him from attending to the duties of the same. . . . For his benefit, I hope to receive the cordial support of the voters of our county, who can thereby show their acknowledgement of the merits of a soldier wounded and crippled in their cause."[30]

Kircher would later call himself a "cripple," although this description was usually tinged with sarcasm. At this point in his recovery, he must have needed help with routine life functions and may have wondered if his body was up to this new challenge. Perhaps his "nice mulatto" was still supplying a second body to enable Kircher to manage his. But in July, he received his prosthetic leg, and he wore it for the rest of his life.

Many images of amputee veterans were published in newspapers, works of fiction, photographs, and other media. These images generally catered to a common public presentation of the amputated self, the pinned-up sleeve or the peg leg, the latter an ostentatious display of loss and, owing to its rude appearance, a clear indication that standing and walking in any "normal" way were not achievable. These images conveyed the message that the body could not be made whole, that the amputee was a being deprived of his manhood, a permanent living monument to wartime horror. A study of photographs made between 1861 and 1932 of 151 amputee men shows two primary types of clothing: first, no modification and, second, the use of fastenings. Interestingly, none of the photographs showed men wearing prostheses on their arms. The researchers found that most amputees pinned or otherwise fastened the sleeves of pants legs over the missing limbs. The researchers observed that such fastenings did less to conceal than to advertise the missing limbs. During the war and immediately thereafter, with the pall of misery suffusing all public life, veterans were more likely to conceal missing limbs than a generation later, when public opinion supported older veterans' maimed bodies for their sacrifices.[31]

The prosthetics industry had been burgeoning since the war began. The first years of the war saw a 290 percent increase in the number of patents for prostheses throughout 1846–1860. The first applicable pension law that provided artificial limbs dated to 1862; thereafter, over the course of Kircher's lifetime, the government continued to pass legislation that widened eligibility and specifically identified circumstances and criteria for claiming pensions for veterans henceforth denoted "invalids."

The government tried to facilitate the process of obtaining and fitting prosthetic devices by relying on the army doctor to order and fit them. The approved physician certified that the need for a limb was war-related and that the veteran possessed discharge papers. The examining surgeon may have been the one to amputate the limb in the first place. This relationship suggests reciprocity, a negotiation between the patient and the surgeon to determine the nature and shape of the stump that corresponded with the new limb.[32]

Physicians' notes attest to their desire to convince amputees that lifelike limbs could endure and absorb bodily stresses and outside threats. Manufacturers advertised their wares as machines that were not only functional but also comfortable in their method of walking, reaching, standing, and sitting. Kircher probably studied the advertising literature and the innovations claimed by various manufacturers, such as specially treated paper that simulated skin, the use of India rubber components to reduce noise and corrosion, or materials that boasted the sheer beauty of the craftsmanship. Still, no prosthetic was perfect: clothing may have been damaged or ruined, or the limb may have proved too difficult or painful to wear.[33]

As comfortable and reliable as a prosthetic leg might have been for Kircher, he would always have been conscious of the artificiality of a portion of his body. In concealing an amputated leg, he might avoid stares or impolite curiosity, but other social behavior might have reminded him of what he did not have. Prostheses "provoke[ed] anxieties about what was real and what was counterfeit in American society." Many people recognized that some men among them might have been physically less than they appeared to be. Kircher doubtless sensed this each time a stranger looked at his body. Mindful that war casualties were seen as people from the lower strata of society, "were Civil War amputees who they appeared to be?"[34]

Kircher's decades-long correspondence with the government began during the fall of 1864, when he was formally discharged from the army and applied for his pension. In making his case to a parade of pension officials, he used the terms *disabled, invalid,* and *cripple.* Nowhere does the military record reflect his civilian achievements and honors; he did not want to risk his pension claims by describing a body that did not fit the rating criteria.

Each communication with the federal pension office began with Kircher rehearsing the chronology of November 27 at Ringgold and his subsequent amputations. He carefully cited each applicable pension law in requesting his monthly allowance. Through the family business, Kircher had sufficient means for an upper-middle-class existence and did not require a pension to survive. Nonetheless, he wanted the government to acknowledge his sacrifice, see his body as extremely damaged, and force attention to his claimed disability as an invalid. He appeared before the clerk of the county court to make a sworn statement recounting his wounds and amputations, gave his occupation as a machinist (conspicuously manual labor), and stated that "this declaration is made for the purpose of being placed on the Invalid Pension roll of the United States," witnessed by Henry Goedeking.[35]

In November 1864, Kircher was elected to the office of circuit court clerk with almost twice the votes as his opponent. By the end of December, Kircher completed a "Claim for an Invalid Pension" form that included the army adjutant general's certification that he should receive a monthly pension of twenty dollars in recognition of "Total Disability + permanent—Disabled by loss of right arm + left leg by amputation." A handstamp on this form, added on October 12, 1872, states that the pension increased to twenty-four dollars[36] per legislation enacted the same year.[37]

DR. BLY'S LEG

Kircher decided not to accept a government-issued leg and instead opted for one that the government considered too expensive to pay for. Kircher received the cash the government would have paid, added his own money, and purchased Dr. Douglas Bly's artificial leg. The pension office recognized the leg's superiority. It relied on the use of rubber cords as tendons attached through the calf compartment to the foot. The foot's innovation was a ball-and-socket arrangement. An ivory ball supporting the leg was encased in a rubber socket, which resulted in a better imitation of the motions of a human foot. With enviable modesty, Dr. Bly endorsed his product, saying, "I do not want every awkward, big-footed, or gambreled shanked person, who always strided or shuffled along in a slouching manner with both his natural legs, to think that one of these must necessarily transform him or his movements into specimens of symmetry, neatness and beauty.... They are just what I recommend them to be—neither more nor less." Dr. Bly thus defined the standard of manly appearance and behavior to be shown by the wearer of his leg.[38]

Bly's 1862 promotional pamphlet claimed that his invention "embod[ies] the principles of the natural leg in an artificial one and in giving it later or side motion at the ankle." Bly highlighted the lightness of the leg, which used "rubber springs or artificial muscles" rather than metal connections to control the ball-and-socket joint. In his sales pamphlet, Bly described how the muscles of the legs and lower back conducted walking and analyzed a normal gait in detail. So "when walking, if one side of the foot happens to be placed on a stone or elevation, or into a hole, *the mobility of the ankle joint allows the foot to yield just ENOUGH to accommodate itself to the inequality, and thereby PREVENT stumbling or falling*" (italics and uppercase words in the original). Kircher valued these features possibly because he was afraid he might fall with only one hand and arm to support himself. Bly's leg minimized that risk.[39]

Kircher's new leg was designed in 1864. The federal government convened a meeting in New York City that included illustrious surgeons Samuel Gross, Valentine Mott, Joseph Pancoast, and Benjamin Franklin Bache, army medical personnel, and the surgeon general to determine what kind of limbs would be appropriate for the anticipated need and to solicit proposals from manufacturers. The committee named several manufacturers including Douglas Bly. Prices were set for "standard" prostheses, and contractors secured manufacturing orders. The committee continued to meet throughout the war. Their discussion, reflected in manufacturers' sales literature, reveals a growing expertise in the physiology of motion and the challenges of invalids' bodies. Later committee meetings were held in conjunction with modifications of pension law, which helps to explain Kircher's persistence with the pension office. For instance, in 1872, Congress approved funding for transportation of the veteran to places for fittings. By 1891, Congress allowed payments for limb replacements every three (as opposed to five) years and paid an allowance for annual repairs.[40]

A new limb to replace an amputated part had obvious advantages. It also had disadvantages. To a skin-covered structure of sinew, muscle, and bone, one fitted a machine of wood, leather, India rubber, silk, buckskin, steel, brass, catgut, and even cork and whalebone. Each material was matched with a specific function in the limb. The body sometimes rebelled against its new dependence on machines. Kircher experienced excessive perspiration. He and other wearers were self-conscious of the sounds and odors emanating from their artificial limbs, particularly due to the gradual absorption of sweat by wood and leather. Embarrassing metal noises or failures of parts necessitated the amputee to hurry into a hardware store and request an oil can and a private space.[41]

THE CIVIC BODY IS BORN

Kircher took office in March 1865 to serve a four-year term. Mindful that he promised the community, with Goedeking's endorsement, that his youthful and invalided self would be guided by the elder godparent to perform the job, Kircher was unable to follow through on this, as Goedeking died only six months later. Meanwhile, the family business renamed itself Kircher & Son to recognize Henry's promise to follow his father.[42]

Evidently, Kircher performed competently and did not appear to suffer from the lack of a mentor during his term as clerk. He seemed to regard the position, however, as a precursor to becoming a prominent local businessman of influence and status. The clerkship was first mooted as a possibility for Kircher when he was still recovering from wounds. Perhaps Goedeking and Kircher's father convinced him that the requirements of the clerkship would not be too demanding on a fragile body and would provide an ideal reentry into Belleville to create a public persona of trust and responsibility, attributes that could transfer to the hardware business and other pursuits.

During Kircher's first year home, he found an unusual opportunity to exhibit his damaged body in a way that enhanced his prestige and status. Looking for a transcript of a deed on property he owned, Major General William T. Sherman, under whom Kircher had served at Vicksburg, wrote to the St. Clair County recorder. Kircher was pleased and surprised to receive the letter, and he gave it his thorough attention. Following the correspondence, sometime in late 1865, the two met. Kircher doubtless regaled Sherman with his performance at Ringgold Gap, and his reduced body would have been on display. Sherman was grateful for Kircher's sacrifice and expressed "pleasure at knowing that Kircher's fellow citizens had rewarded him with a responsible civic position."[43]

By the end of his tenure, Kircher was examining his options and thought about visiting his family's community in Germany. In 1869, he applied for a passport. As the calendar turned to the next decade, the 1870 census listed twenty-six-year-old Henry as an invalid living with his family, including parents Joseph and Augusta, sisters Loulou (age thirty) and Hattie (seventeen), brother Willie (eighteen), and a servant, Mary Miller. There is no mention of the "nice mulatto" helper.[44]

In 1870, Kircher sent an application to the surgeon general requesting an "application for commutation for an artificial leg and artificial arm," meaning he would like the funds to buy another limb and not rely on a government-appointed doctor to do it for him. He acknowledged his use of the Bly limb for the past six years. The request was countersigned by the recipient with the note that Kircher was entitled to two prostheses, one for the arm and one for the leg. Perhaps his original Bly leg had been wearing out, or he wished to have a spare.[45]

The next year, Kircher used his passport to board a ship to Germany to visit his father's family in the town of Fulda, where he remained until the fall of 1872. Whatever Kircher's reason for visiting his family, upon his return, he was solicited for various positions in which he could guide civic improvement and influence the future of his community. Interestingly, between January and the summer of 1872, Kircher was elected in absentia to the board of directors of the Belleville Savings Bank, the Board of Education, and the Belleville Building and Loan Association, and as an incorporator for the new People's Gaslight & Coke Company (which had no board yet). These board positions required service for a year; each year, Kircher was reelected.

In September, Kircher left Hamburg for New York City and took a first-class cabin. He had earned the respect of his business community in only a few years, no doubt with help from the German community. We do not know if he traveled to Germany with his "nice mulatto" or worked in the hardware business with a helper nearby. By 1874, however, he began a complex negotiation with the pension office that lasted decades. First, he filed a "Declaration for the Increase of an Invalid Pension" in June. For submission to the pension office, he swore a notarized statement before the circuit court clerk "that he is disabled to such an extent as to require the regular aid and attendance of another person in assisting him in his daily duties of life; and he is permanently disabled in performing manual labor." This is the second glimpse we have about a shadow assistant who accompanied Kircher to help him. He used the same language in another document submitted in 1874, "Increase of Invalid Pension," in which he emphasized that he "can not perform arm manual labor and is more or less dependent upon assistance and aid of other [*sic*]. I have lost the two limbs named." The application was unsuccessful: an official stamped the form, "Reject: Not *helpless*—not under Pensions Act June 1874."[46]

THE TWO BODIES

Kircher had evolved into two separate bodies. The pensionable body remained in a perpetual state of disability, incompleteness, and disadvantage and required others to help with essential life tasks. This body existed outside of the universe of business, civic leadership, and broader dealings with the world. The other—civic—body was successful in business and family affairs, influential, confident, and apparently self-sufficient despite the constant public display of patriotic sacrifice. Of the two bodies, the latter was the more successful. The former body remained in suspension while Kircher repeatedly told the story of his wounds and amputations to assert control of the narrative to pension authorities. Given the rejection of the pension increase claim earlier, the government insisted on its own version of Kircher's struggles. While Kircher tried to wrest more consideration from the pension office, community members continued to seek out his other body for counsel. In July 1874, he was reelected to various boards; in December, the "ladies association of Belleville" issued stock to fund a kindergarten school, and Kircher became a trustee for the funds. The following year, he was elected treasurer of a local militia, Company A, Bellville Guards, which required him to wear a special uniform.[47]

In 1877, Kircher was still negotiating with the government to secure an increase in his pension. In January, he was elected mayor of Belleville and served two year-long terms. As with the vote for court clerkship in 1865, he received far more votes than his opponent, 732 to 397. His continuing work as an incorporator for the gas manufacturing company suggests Kircher's vision for Belleville's improving standard of living: the arrival of gas energy. Of the emerging utility company incorporated in July, he said: "Water-gas is said to be a prime agent for illuminating and heating purposes and can be manufactured and supplied to consumers at a cost which is merely nominal compared with coal gas."[48]

Immediately following the incorporation of the gas company, Mayor Kircher faced a public safety crisis. A railroad strike had led to an influx of striking workers in Belleville, and community citizens feared disorder, vandalism, and theft. He acted quickly, summoning a meeting of citizens to agree on a strategy and put it into motion. He organized citizens into "watch and ward" committees to police their neighborhoods and report suspicious activities. The strike ended, the tension passed, and plaudits followed Kircher's leadership.[49]

He returned to court to swear new statements of disability. In his October 1877 statement, he recounted his wounds and his twenty-four-dollar pension but also mentioned his third wound: "Also a flesh wound through the right thigh about half-way between the knee and the hip. That he is wholly incapacitated for the performance of manual labor." Kircher swore that he was "respectable and entitled to credit." The next month, the pension authorities appointed a physician to examine Kircher. The doctor's report described him as thirty-six, five-foot-six-inches tall, 149 pounds, dark complexion, respiration 18 1/2 p.m., pulse 78 beats. Spiegelhalter recorded Kircher's first wound in his arm and the second in his leg. For this new examination, the narrative changed to assert that the first wound was in the left leg, "which was totally shattered in neighborhood of the knee joint," and the second in the right arm, which featured "total destruction of the right elbow joint." The examiner concluded that Kircher "is totally disabled in performing his daily duties." The surgeon recommended a pension increase of thirty-six dollars[50] per month. Kircher received the new pension, effective beginning in February 1877.[51]

Why did the narrative change? The examiner recorded the facts of Kircher's wounding as he himself reported it. In 1863, Spiegelhalter would have recorded Kircher's narrative within hours after the wounds were inflicted. Perhaps one of the doctors made a mistake. Possibly, when Kircher was first examined, in pain and under the influence of morphine, he mixed the order when talking with Spiegelhalter. He also might have refashioned his story. There is evidence of Kircher—perhaps abetted by his family—altering the narrative later in other ways by the time of his death.

Meanwhile, Kircher's role as the business patriarch of Belleville continued. Based on his work for a women's fundraising drive, the Kindergarten Association appointed him as a trustee for another year. Belleville's expanding commercial interests led to the incorporation of a board of trade, and he was appointed as one of the directors.[52]

Congress continued to enact new pension laws, and Kircher was alert to any new provision that would justify a pension increase. In 1879, he filed a new application "for the arrears due me, under the act granting arrears of pension." His pension file number—listed in numerous places on official forms and correspondence, 36,243, to be exact—must have become as familiar to him as his birth date.[53]

CLAIMS AND MORE CLAIMS

In early 1880, Kircher ran for election to the school board. Controversy surrounded this election because one of the candidates opposed the teaching of German in public schools. The controversy reveals tensions between Belleville's mostly German older generation and the growing population. In this election, the three top candidates were a mere handful of votes apart. Kircher won by a single vote.[54]

On May 1, 1880, Kircher married Bertha Englemann, the daughter of a prosperous merchant and German immigrant. They married on the latter's farm in a ceremony attended by old army comrades. Dr. Spiegelhalter gave the couple "an elegantly bound vol. of Wm. Tell, handsomely illustrated." In the only surviving letter from Kircher to his betrothed that hints at romance, he bragged about helping the carpenter improve the newlyweds' house, Pine Grove. He proudly worked on a grape arbor and installed basement shelves. He seemed determined to prove to Bertha that his wounded body should not be perceived as a lack of manhood and that the new home plus the family alliance signified a civic body of stature and influence. In their sixteen years of marriage before Bertha's death, the couple had three sons: Harry Bertram, Joseph Casimir, and Theodore Engelmann. The 1880 census listed Kircher, age thirty-eight, as a hardware merchant and head of a household of two people, Henry and Bertha.[55]

Public opinion of impaired veterans became more tolerant throughout the 1880s; their visible wounds were viewed approvingly by the public as symbols of sacrifice. Union veterans had been attracting political attention through the Grand Army of the Republic (GAR). Although Kircher may have been a member, he does not appear to have been active as an organizer or leader. Maimed GAR veterans wore their identifying kepis (broad-brimmed hats), sported pins on lapels, or dressed in ways that called attention to their physical condition, as "fastening sleeves and pant legs [were] physically convenient and socially advantageous to men proud to show that they had given an arm or a leg in the war." Apparently, Kircher was not accompanied by a helper; family members may have acted in this capacity. Although he wore a prosthetic leg, his gait could not have been that of men with two natural legs. We do not know if he occasionally used a cane or a crutch.[56]

Kircher found new ways to use his physical condition to obtain an increased pension. In 1881, at age thirty-eight, he claimed that he was due fifty dollars monthly and requested a review of his case. Once again, the pension office assigned a doctor—the same one who saw Kircher in 1877—to perform another examination in support of the pension increase request. Kircher, thirty-nine, weighed 163 pounds; his other statistics were the same as in 1877. The examiner noted, "Claimant does not require the regular and continual personal aid and attendance of another person, only in the morning when dressing himself and evening when undressing." The doctor recommended a pension increase to forty-eight dollars per month. When the pension office rejected the request, Kircher, through a Chicago attorney, tried again, pointing out that he had been receiving thirty-six dollars[57] per month "for loss of a *hand* or *foot*—Can he receive more for loss of *arm above elbow + leg above knee*"?[58]

While always focused on receiving his due from the government, Kircher's civic persona branched out into new territory. Kircher once again served as an incorporator, this time for a new technology, the Belleville Elevator and Warehouse Company. He began service on the St. Clair County Agricultural Board. In 1884, however, although nominated, he declined to stand for election as a supervisor for Belleville Township: "I regret to state that I cannot accept the nomination, as present business relations and poor health would not permit me, if elected, to do justice to the trust—not to speak of the doubt of my ability to fill the office to the satisfaction of the citizens."[59]

This is the only recorded case of Kircher declining a civic post and the first time he had ever mentioned his worsening health. Months before, he may have been surprised to see a public convergence of his two bodies. Based on a published government report, the local newspaper listed all federal pensioners in St. Clair County. The majority were former soldiers. Kircher was listed as receiving thirty-six dollars monthly for the loss of his leg and arm, but his entry stands out because he had received more money from the government than any others listed. His closest rivals were two pensioners who were receiving twenty-four dollars monthly. Perhaps Kircher's reluctance to face the election was due to fear of public criticism that might arise regarding his pension. Or perhaps his health suffered in ways not recorded in Kircher's sworn statements or pension examinations.[60]

RESOLUTION, FINALLY

In 1886, Kircher underwent another examination, at which his statistics were as follows: age forty-five, five-foot-nine-inches tall, 163 pounds, pulse 80 p.m., respiration 20. The doctor described in detail Kircher's stumps: the leg stump terminated in a fold of "natural skin" with a "well-healed cicatrix" (scar). He noted Kircher's lack of an arm prosthetic but disagreed with his rationale not to wear one: "But while he claims not to be able to wear an artificial arm we see no good reason why he cannot do so. The stump is long enough and there is not sufficient tenderness about it to forbid the use of an artificial limb." The doctor nevertheless recommended an increase in pension, but the pension office kept the thirty-six dollar rate, which had been unchanged for the past nine years.[61]

Kircher's pension claims took on an increasingly legalistic dimension that must have required the pension office to circulate his thoughtful, dense, and thorough arguments for consideration by lawyers. In another sworn statement before the county court, he made (via a pension attorney) the following argument that he repeated in subsequent correspondence:

> He now amends his petition and claims a re-rating and advance to the first class on the ground that he has sustained a greater disability than is specified in the act of Feb 28, 1877; namely; the loss merely of one hand and one foot and avers that his disability therefrom is in all respects equivalent to the loss merely of both feet, and that he was at the times thereof and is now entitled to $25 per month from June 6, 1866 to $31.25 per month from June 4, 1872 to $50 per month from June 4, 1874 and to $72 per month from June 17, 1878 under the provisions of sections 4697 and 4698 Revised Statutes U.S. and the acts of Congress of June 18, 1874 and June 16, 1880 and now claims the difference between these ratings monthly and what has been allowed him.[62]

Each new pension law or amendment to an older one seemed to prompt a renewed argument for a higher monthly rate. Every morning when Kircher faced the day with his two stumps, he may have thought that another day demanded another acknowledgment by the nation that rebel gunfire took away about 22 percent of his body weight, roughly five pounds of arm and twenty-two (or so) pounds of leg. Every day, he reconciled his civic body with the loss beyond recovery. His implicit contract with the government required constant acknowledgment of that loss. The loss must be compensated.

Kircher may have known amputee veterans who did not have his persistence and knowledge of the pension system and therefore either did not receive pensions or lived with inadequate ones. As of 1888, the government had awarded pensions to approximately nine hundred amputee veterans, a number possibly about half or fewer of all amputee Union veterans. Some veterans were likely unaware of their eligibility for pensions. Some may not have wanted them.[63]

As Kircher privately engaged with the pension office, citizens sought him out for his business acumen. The St. Clair Nail Company, established during the spring of 1888, was soon to open and "operate the Western Mill." Kircher became the company's president. The following month, Henry's father, Joseph Kircher Sr., died. Shortly thereafter, Kircher approached the pension office again. He requested a review of his pension because of recent legislation noting that while pensions were set at fixed amounts for lost feet or hands, amputations of either the leg or arm that came too close to the hip or shoulder joints to permit prostheses could receive more pay. Kircher pleaded with the pension office: "Does it seem reasonable that the loss of arm or leg . . . above elbow or knee should be pensioned with thirty-six dollars for each, if loss has been sustained by two different persons or they then together receive seventy-two dollars while if one person alone loses both limbs (certainly a greater hardship for one than for two) should only receive one half as much for same disability." Kircher could not resist concluding sarcastically: "Your Honorable Predecessor once answered to above 'no person could draw two pensions' if that is the case, Uncle Sam should not allow his soldiers to be wounded more than once either."[64]

Dated a week later, the pension office filed an "Increase" form, signed by "Miss Desha," who was the latest bureaucrat to respond to Kircher. She reviewed his pension history and noted an authorized increase effective August 16, 1888, and added that "no further action will be had until he shall furnish [evidence] showing that he requires regular aid + attendance of another person." Kircher's sworn statements for the pension office did not argue for a helper, although the office appeared to be solicitous about that need and was willing to compensate accordingly. Kircher believed that his particular situation—not the mere subtraction from his body of a foot and a hand—the amputation site near the shoulder and that of the leg above the knee ought to place him in a more expansive category of pension. The nature of his amputations did not align with the government's chart of bodily losses and their monetary equivalents.[65]

In July 1889, Kircher's claim was adjudicated and a pension increase was granted on Miss Desha's recommendation. Backdated to 1878, Kircher received seventy-two dollars monthly. The conclusion of his years of claims appeared in an article in the *Milwaukee Sentinel* concerning rerated pensions. The *Belleville Weekly Advocate* quoted from it and cited Kircher, rehearsing his Civil War wounds and amputations and summarizing his pension history: "The report in his case says that when he was wounded, he was in front of his company in action. Kircher was pensioned at $20 a month on Sept 4, 1864; at $25 from June 6, 1866; at $31.25 from June 4, 1872, and at $50 from June 4, 1874. By the [new] ruling . . . he was given a rate of $72 a month from June 17, 1878, which gave him a total back pension of $6,341.72." The increases of 1866, 1872, and 1874 were authorized only at the time of the 1889 ruling, thus entitling Kircher to the large back pension award. Regardless of how Belleville citizens reacted when they read this information about their business leader, they were reminded of the courageous moment of unimpeachable integrity: Kircher was leading his men, facing the enemy. The government finally awarded Kircher his due following years of oversight.[66]

As the years passed from 1889 into the final decade of the nineteenth century, Kircher's civic body was enriched by additional appointments and elections. In early 1889, he incorporated the family business as Kircher & Son, dealers "in hardware and agricultural machinery." Another new local business was founded, the Security Fire Insurance Company of Belleville, promoted by Kircher. The Belleville Safe Deposit Company, also recently established, named Kircher to its board of directors.[67]

THE EXAMINED BODY

In 1893, Kircher received the questionnaire from S. Weir Mitchell and John K. Mitchell, completed it, and returned it. The form discussed matters not addressed in pension examinations and perhaps not discussed with physicians. While many doctors may have known about Mitchell's work with nerve injuries, they usually did not ask the veterans they saw many of the questions in the survey. Kircher's responses reveal his laconic and occasionally sarcastic self. When asked about the character of pain related to his amputation, his pen dug through the paper as he wrote, "Of course it hurts." In general, he maintained, "I enjoy good health can not say that loss of limbs made any changes in health." His "intellectual powers" remained intact, but he admitted to displaying a "quick temper." Some bodily functions had altered a bit. "My digestion is not as perfect as formerly, that is, certain articles do not agree with me as formerly," and although he stated that his habits remained "pretty regular," he could "eat and drink as my appetite dictates, avoiding such as I know does not agree—viz. pickels bananas—pork &c." Not surprisingly, he said that he needed "more sleep than formerly." He detected no "changes in the acuteness of the senses."

Had Kircher not been intimately associated with Spiegelhalter before his surgery, he might have resisted or subverted hospital treatments, a minor rebellion of manhood. Other soldiers—including some of Mitchell's patients—resisted or refused some therapies. Some of these refusals or other manifestations of resistance evolved from differing views of pain and soldiers' inability to secure pain relief that they thought they were due.[68]

The survey questions about Kircher's remaining limbs and stumps were more exacting. To the question about changes in strength or size of remaining limbs, he answered, "I think both remaining limbs are rather stronger than formerly but do not think changes in size much." Had his ability to use the remaining limbs increased? "Yes in so far as making more difficult use of same." What about the character of his stumps? Kircher answered that the skin of the stumps did not differ from other parts of the body. Skin texture, color, growth of hair, and temperature appeared to be unaffected in the remaining limbs, although the leg sweated more, as it was encased in a prosthesis.

Kircher allowed that his leg stump was "a little" sensitive, "mainly only in front of bone." He registered no identifiable sensitivity to extremes of heat and cold, but like other amputees, his stump had become a weather gauge: "Yes, storm—snow and other changes in weather I feel more sense in leg than arm." Living with a stump and wearing a prosthesis, had Kircher noticed any other changes over time? "Of course not being used the muscles have decreased and the constant pressure of artificial leg reduces the stump in wideness." On "some very hot days, when I take off the leg for convenience sake—I perspire very easily." Nevertheless, his leg "stump is sound and strong" but subject to some "involuntary twitching" or "spasmodic movements." He elaborated, "At times . . . nervous twitching caused sometimes by over exerting leg—walking standing too long or if I get the stump very cold." This has happened irregularly "ever since amputation," although it recurred with "no regularity." Chief causes were "overexertion, colds" accompanied by pain and "yes, nervous twitching, causes sleeplessness."

Several questions related specifically to the prosthesis. When asked "what artificial appliances [were] used," Kircher replied, "Dr. Bly pat. Wooden leg used up & now." Kircher seemed quite satisfied with his purchase of the more expensive limb, which evidently wore well over time. He could not resist some playful sarcasm when asked "Which [appliance] has been most satisfactory?" "My old bone + flesh leg." The most severe drawback to wearing the leg appeared to be the method of securing it to the stump: "Mainly the belt and strap for keeping leg in place." Kircher asserted that he had worn the Bly leg continuously: "I have not been without leg except at night since July 1864." He offered no details about what parts required replacement or necessary repairs over time.

While the two Mitchells found these responses useful, the questionnaire revealed a devastating insight: through the years, Kircher had experienced phantom limb pain, sometimes of an excruciating character. These symptoms are not discussed in the pension documents but may have been what Kircher meant when he claimed worsening health. The questionnaire asked if the respondent felt that the missing limb was shortened or fixed in one position. While Kircher felt that the missing limb (he seemed to answer these questions about the arm, not the leg) in its phantom state resembled the size of the missing arm, he could move his phantom fingers "but can not clinch [*sic*] them to make a fist nor straighten the fingers altogether—when I attempt these movements the muscles in the stump move." When asked if he continued to feel the lost part, Kircher said yes but that "at first [it was] more acute especially in arm." One infers that his responses about phantom sensations might have applied to both limbs, but the questionnaire only presumed one amputation event, just as the pension office had done.

The Mitchells probably found great significance in Kircher's answer to the question "How much of the limb do you feel now, and how does the feeling differ from what it would be if the member were present?" His response: "Mainly the hand and fingers similar sensation as holding a pretty hot iron." Here he revealed that for decades, he had suffered some degree of causalgia, the hyperesthesia of the hand, usually on the dorsal surface. This had been described by other veterans as clenched in a red-hot vise or rasped with a red-hot iron. As we have seen, some sufferers of this form of peripheral nerve damage, first described by Mitchell, found the pain so intolerable that they begged to have the afflicted limbs amputated. This awareness reflects on both Kircher's pension and civic bodies. His short temper and sarcastic nature, evident in his completed survey, may have been due to intermittent causalgia. He may have learned self-discipline in disregarding chronic pain. Apparently, he did not identify this pain to his pension examiners over the years. He may have thought the matter irrelevant to the government equation of a pension for specific lost limbs. Perhaps he failed to mention it because he suspected that the doctors would not be sympathetic to claims of pain in nonexistent limbs.

Unlike other respondents to the questionnaire, fifty-two-year-old Kircher wrote a note on the blank reverse side of the last page:

> Gentlemen: Should you really find any interest as to how we cripples get along can say that I think my general health has not suffered. . . . Still the inconvenience and being deprived of free bodily actions of course I constantly feel and therefore have to live accordingly. Should you want any particular description of my wounds would refer you to my former regimental Surgeon Dr. Joseph Spiegelhalter at St. Louis Missouri S.E. corner Lafayette + Missouri Avenue who at the time amputated both limbs for me, and thank him for his knowledge kind heart and my sound constitution all of which brought me through all right.

When Kircher completed Mitchell's survey, the law, per the 1890 Pension Act, no longer required veterans to prove that their injuries were caused by war. Veterans received bad press because of the perception that their incessant demands were draining the federal coffers. By this time, 42 percent of the federal budget was earmarked for pensions. It is little wonder that Kircher may have felt embarrassed or professionally vulnerable when his pension amount was published in the newspaper.[69]

Enough time had elapsed since the end of the war that local newspapers across the country published retrospective accounts by or about veterans and their challenges. In 1894, on the thirty-third anniversary of the date the first volunteer company left Belleville for war, the local newspaper listed the survivors still living in the community—thirty-two, including Kircher. Later, the paper published an account of "The Battle of Pea Ridge [Arkansas]," subtitled "Interesting Description of the Battle Written Thirty-four Years Ago." The account of the March 6–8, 1862, battle cited the behavior of Kircher's Twelfth Missouri, "a regiment that was largely made up of Belleville boys, and who in this battle experienced their first baptism of fire."[70]

On January 2, 1896, Bertha died at age forty-seven, leaving Kircher with three young sons, ages nine, eleven, and fourteen. The obituary recognized that Bertha "took great interest in all that pertained to the proper training and education of little children, and was an active member of the Kindergarten Association, of which society she was several times elected president." Soon thereafter, in 1900, Kircher's mother died at eighty-nine.[71]

At the turn of the twentieth century, the household, headed by fifty-eight-year-old Kircher, included sons Harry (eighteen), Joseph K. (fifteen), and Theodore E. (fourteen), housekeeper Emma Kribben (seventy-one), and a servant, Lulu Wehrle (twenty-five). Kircher clearly needed help in managing his family and home. He had become a local patriarch and successful businessman, and his Civil War exploits were occasionally recalled in public forums and newspaper reminiscences, all of which noted the diminishing numbers of veterans. Despite having dropped further pension claims since the 1880s, Kircher was contacted by the pension authorities again.[72]

In 1902, Kircher received a letter from attorneys in Washington, DC, explaining that due to accounting errors regarding the army's handling of pay and allowances, he and others might be due reimbursements. Although not a pension issue, the attorneys thoughtfully provided a form for him to sign authorizing the firm to represent him in litigation. Apparently, Kircher could not be bothered to get involved and communicated his impatience with, if not indifference to, further pension wrangling. Evidently, in response to a notice from the pension office, Kircher returned some forms or other papers with a letter:

> Enclosed papers belong to the waste basket—I do not think U.S. [cares for] anything else than my pension which I am getting regular and think I am fully entitled to for loss of arm + leg and want nothing to do with lawyers or Doctors if I can help it. Some years ago I saw a new pension act quoted in our local papers wherein numerous pension were increased, now whether my case comes under that law is not clear—since I lost 2 limbs had I lost either one, it seems clear there would be an increase but a double loss is not especially mentioned. Will please inform an old soldier and oblige.[73]

In other words, Kircher maintained: If I am due something, fine, but if not, don't bother me.

As the new century moved forward, Kircher's civic body remained on the ascendant. He had been a board member of the Belleville Savings Bank for years and was then elected vice president, then president. As reported in the local press, "Mr. Kircher is one of the oldest and most prominent citizens of Belleville, and has been interested in the savings bank probably longer than any other person at present holding stock in the bank. He is also one of Belleville's most successful business men and financiers, and the directors of the bank certainly did a wise thing in electing him as a successor to their late president."[74]

In 1905, a photographic paean to Belleville appeared in book form, a self-promotional tome that featured photographs of the homes of the local well-to-do and city patriarchs, including Kircher's Pine Grove: "One of the most delightful places in or about Belleville is the home and grounds of Henry A. Kircher on North Church Street." Among the local advertisements featured at the end of the book is one for Kircher & Son, "The Oldest and Most Reliable Hardware House in Southern Illinois." Kircher's successful dynastic family business was part of Belleville's upward trajectory as the book highlights the area's evolution since its 1813 founding as the county seat and coal-mining town to its

1905 identity as a manufacturing hub with foundries, breweries, boiler works, shoe factories, flour mills, and more—all of which happened in less than a century. By implication, Kircher and other families whose homes appeared in the book were the civic knights who ushered in a promising future.[75]

Henry Kircher died on May 1, 1908. Most Belleville citizens did not realize that he had been ailing for a week from a cold that became pneumonia, the cause of death. A brief news article about his life noted his training for a machinist's trade, followed by war service, election to court clerk and later mayor, his hardware business, civic achievements, and honors, particularly his twenty years as a director of the Belleville Savings Bank, where he became president.[76]

The official obituary was published the next day, May 2. While repeating much of what had been published on the day of Kircher's death, the brief recapitulation of his life presented a new account, romanticized and possibly secondhand, about his final Civil War battle:

> It was at the battle of Ringgold, Ga., while leading a charge that he was shot in the left leg. Unable to proceed, he took refuge behind a tree and continued to command his company. At this juncture Adjutant Fred. Kessler of this city rode up and ordered Mr. Kircher to drop back, and while delivering this command, was shot and killed. Mr. Kircher had reached out his right hand to remove Adjutant Kessler's ring from his finger to return it to his family at home, when a ball struck his arm. Later he was wounded in the hip, being wounded three times in less than thirty minutes, and as a result of the battle lost both arm and leg.[77]

This narrative, contrary to Spiegelhalter's notes, has Kircher receiving his first wound in the leg, as he apparently related to an examining pension doctor. The appearance and death of Frederick Kessler in this narrative highlight the closeness of the band of German brothers that constituted the Twelfth Missouri. Kircher's poignant gesture heightens his heroism: he lost his arm in trying to secure a memento for the slain soldier's family. The obituary presented the narrative of wounding that would be recalled and retold.

If Kircher's civic death took place on May 1, his pension death occurred on September 4, 1908. The last pension document in his file is a completed "Pensioner Dropped" form. His identifying details include "Class: Invalid," and again—and finally—erroneously listed his unit as Company A. The document reported the date and amount of the last pension payment Kircher received and his death date and requested that his payments henceforth cease.[78]

Given the prevalent view that disabling conditions feminized soldiers and that their subsequent care was conducted largely by women, there is some irony in the fact that Miss Desha handled the final pension communications between Kircher and government authority.

THERAPEUTIC LIMBS

Kircher willingly submitted to Surgeon Spiegelhalter's knife in 1863, and although the two men enjoyed a long friendship, Spiegelhalter's method of amputation involved explicit and implicit decisions about Kircher's future. Evidence of the former, the record of his amputation suggests a dialogue that may have led to the decision to employ the flap method of removing the leg and the circular method for the arm. Long after the original amputation, however, the amputating physician continued to exercise an influence on Kircher's body as a "legitimate arbitrator of normality," a description that applies to both Mitchells—father and son—in their work with veterans.[79]

Spiegelhalter's battlefield decisions influenced the rest of Kircher's life. Specifically, the amputations directly affected the body's ability to exert force or movement or carry weight. As prosthetic limbs became more sophisticated over time, manufacturers published treatises that both advertised wares but also provided detailed descriptions of the anatomical bases for the design of limbs. These descriptions reveal acute observations of how the body accomplishes various postures: standing, sitting, walking, running, or performing labor. The manufacturers may have had a command of physiology superior to most physicians. Spiegelhalter's abridgment of Kircher's body left it to others—manufacturers of limbs—to redesign.

Limb manufacturers became more critical of physicians. One of the leading manufacturers, A. A. Marks, argued that "the surgeon, therefore, can not be too careful in the choice of operation and the point of amputation, not only for the interest of his patient but as well for the protection of his reputation. . . . The surgeon should acquire some knowledge of artificial limbs. This is essential because the successful use of an artificial leg depends in a measure upon the character of the work he has done . . . [also] the surgeon is the first man the patient consults on the subject." For amputations at the thigh, Marks instructed the surgeon how to plan for the eventual prosthesis to bear the weight of the upper body, remain well fitted to the stump, and supply the necessary movements.[80]

On November 27, 1863, neither Spiegelhalter nor Kircher had the time or will to ponder the meaning of wearing a prosthesis. The primary goal was the restoration of leg function, not to convince the mind that the body remained whole, although a prosthesis that served as a simulacrum of a flesh-and-blood leg was doubtless intended to deceive onlookers and convince the wearer that it functioned as a substitute for the original. As twenty-first-century physicians and the designers and fabricators of customized limbs have evolved ways to integrate electronic or mechanical devices within bodies, from synthetic knees to heart pacemakers, Civil War limb manufacturers appear to have considered the possibilities of joining the organic to the mechanical. Increasingly throughout the latter nineteenth century, manufacturers applied anatomical names to mechanical components of limbs. As manufactured items, limbs and their components were changeable when they wore out, so the host body became a site for technological growth, an emblem of progress and innovation. As Kircher's civic body entered various spaces of urban improvement, from gasworks to banks, his body experienced a journey of therapeutic improvement. Over time, a limb wore out, necessitating a new limb of better appearance or increasing sophistication. Kircher applied more than once for compensation for a new limb: perhaps the "growth" of the mechanical limb over time was therapy. Perhaps he required a fresh limb as a form of therapeutic renewal of his identity.[81]

Manufacturers and those who wore limbs seemed to share the view that the artificial limb was a "natural replacement" for the lost one, but the discussion of limb-wearing (both in literature and scholarship) has focused on replacing what was lost, not the gain experienced by the wearer. That gain equated to the wearer developing insights into his body, his desires for his body, how he wanted to present his body in public, and learning new ways to combine the flesh body with the artificial. The presence of the artificial limb was therapeutic beyond the technical attachment of an appendage: it reassured its wearer that the body would not fail because of a lack of limb, it prompted the wearer to a deeper awareness of his body, it offered security, and it provided a clean, functional, responsive companion that "felt" what the body required. When it malfunctioned, the limb became an irritant or, at worst, a saboteur and required replacement with a new companion.[82]

Had Mitchell seen Kircher as a causalgia patient, both men would have explored the meaning of phantom sensations in a context of bodily integrity. Perhaps Kircher would have been subjected to electrization and other therapies not commonly practiced at the time. Mitchell seemed unconcerned with securing prostheses to restore lost functions. He was focused on how the fractured body reinvented identity. The view that the main contribution of prostheses to health is the restoration of lost bodily functions "maintains the very separation of mind and body that Mitchell argues against in his Civil War writing." His observations about phantom sensations and other phenomena of nerve injuries convinced him that human consciousness and measurable neurological and physiological phenomena are deeply integrated. The presence of artificial limbs cannot supply that sense of wholeness.[83]

Mitchell understood as few others did that wearing an artificial limb is a complex matter, combining the physical challenge of designing and fitting a limb and the mental challenges of manhood, identity, and social adaptability. His studies of stumps and the nerve injuries they concealed included periodic physical measurements of the circumference of limbs and stumps. Not only did the measurements change; so, too, did the phantom sensations of lost limbs. Over time, the phantom limb may shorten, or its sensation may increase or diminish. Mitchell wrote, "Eventually, the hand might be felt at the elbow, or the foot at the knee . . . such feelings as result in the notion of shortening are continually antagonized by the seeing of the foot in its position and by its fulfillment of function."[84]

CONCLUSION: THE LIGHT OF THE FUTURE

Kircher's personality emerges from his letters, diary, and newspaper articles as proud, forthright, forward-looking, socially adept, and smart. His presentation of self challenged anyone's dismissal of him as incomplete and perhaps unintelligent or limited in his capabilities. In short, no one caricatured or otherwise made fun of his double amputation, his very visible missing arm, or his cautious, limping gait with a leg prosthesis.

Physical or occupational therapy, counseling, and perhaps social work were not available to Civil War veterans. Kircher planned his life with no help but that of friends and family. The aperiodic appearance of a shadow helper suggests possibilities for his management of postwar life, but the evidence is too slim for conjecture. Kircher managed the pain and phantom sensations of the nerves in his stumps and rehearsed bodily movements to create a new presentation of civic self after the war. His experiences might have been invaluable to other veterans who were not as successful in finding their civic roles. Today we recognize the comprehensive whole of bodily sensations as kinesthesis, and that as part of "a broader system—proprioception—which includes the body's vestibular system[85] or balance mechanism as well." Kircher did not record in any detail his reconfiguring of his body or proprioception, nor did he write about or report to doctors his phantom sensations. Mitchell was the only one who asked him to do so.[86]

Kircher's insistence that it was impossible to wear an arm prosthesis was vindicated by the government. In 1892, the surgeon general of the United States declared that artificial arms were essentially useless and noted that most veterans preferred not to wear them. The empty sleeve became a universal trope to denote the amputee veteran and the implication of need and dependence. At his hardware store or board meetings, Kircher would have been ever conscious of the multiple meanings of his empty sleeve. On the one hand, citizens wanted to consign the war to the past and rid themselves of images of death and destruction. "The narrative of prosthesis redeemed the war by erasing all evidence of destruction from the body and history alike." However, Kircher would have enhanced his civic persona by asserting the exercise of leadership and counsel. His civic duties ran parallel to increasing national industrialization, mirrored in his community by the development of gas power, railway expansion, and labor disputes. He projected the image of a man who has adapted his body to meet the quotidian demands of life and who was physically competent to occupy important civic roles.[87]

We know little of Kircher's involvement in veterans' affairs. Perhaps his veteran's body, that which he would have shared and celebrated with fellow veterans, occupied a role secondary to his civic and pension bodies. No newspaper reports cite his involvement in the GAR. If he had been an officer or leader in the organization, the evidence should exist.

For a while, Belleville remembered Kircher as a business leader and war veteran, coidentities celebrated by his community. In 1914, Kircher & Son closed after sixty-six years, the business taken over by new owners. "In the last few years the entire business has been owned and managed by Harry Kircher, Joseph Kircher, Jr., and Theo. E. Kircher, who now retire from a business in which three generations of the family have been actively engaged." In 1916, local businessmen prepared to establish a local board of trade until someone reminded them that a board of trade had already been chartered in 1878, led by Henry Kircher. Today, Pine Grove still stands, now an apartment complex. The roadway that passes it is named Kircher Place.[88]

Had Kircher been a reader of literature, a stanza from Herman Melville's Civil War poems might have spoken to the ideals that informed his body's life experiences, from company captain to mayor to business owner:

> Catching the light in the future's skies,
> Instinct disowns each darkening prophecy:
> Faith in America never dies;
> Heaven shall the end ordained fulfill,
> We march with Providence cheery still.[89]

FIVE

RICHARD DOWNEY DUNPHY
(1841?–1904)

WITH SKILL AND COURAGE

At daybreak on August 5, 1864, a warm, cloudy day with a mild wind from the southwest, Coal Heaver Richard D. Dunphy,[1] begrimed with sweat and dust, worked quickly with the other sailors to feed coal into a hungry boiler to propel the Union flagship, USS *Hartford,* toward Mobile Bay to secure exclusive access for the Union navy. Dunphy's anxiety and anticipation must have peaked when he heard guns from Confederate Fort Morgan, soon to be mixed with gunfire from rebel gunboats as eighteen Union warships led by Rear Admiral David Glasgow Farragut's West Gulf Blockading Squadron steamed in parallel columns, wooden warships to seaward, a line of ironclads to landward, facing the brunt of cannon fire from the fort. Per the admiral's orders, the wooden ships suspended sheet chains over the exposed wooden outer hulls to minimize cannon damage and nets over the gun deck to trap splinters of wood smashed by rebel explosive shells and solid shots.

As the cannons roared to life above them, Dunphy and his fellow coal heavers shifted their duties to the shell whip, a dumbwaiter into which shells were placed and hoisted to the gun deck.

All manner of gunfire struck *Hartford*, including shell bursts in the vicinity of the whip and its exposed portal to the lower decks. Sailors manning the cannons were enveloped in smoke, debris, lethal splinters of wood, and fragments of iron. If Dunphy's boiler were hit by a shell or rifle shot, it could discharge steam sufficient to scald everyone in the vicinity to death. Other menaces lurked below: the enemy had surely placed torpedoes just below the water's surface that could detonate at any time. The word quickly spread that the armored monitor USS *Tecumseh* had struck a mine and sunk, losing nearly the entire crew.

When feeding the boiler, Dunphy lugged coal buckets that may have weighed over one hundred pounds. He repeated this process more than fifty times in a day. The work required raw strength and endurance, and the conditions even when not in battle were intolerable to most sailors: confined spaces in extreme heat and a combustible atmosphere of coal, dirt, and gunpowder. The concern that a shell could ignite the coal bunker and burst the boiler must have been set aside as Dunphy and his shipmates endeavored to provide ammunition to gunners and sufficiently power the ship's steam engine to maneuver in battle.

From about 7:00 a.m. to about 8:00 a.m., Confederate gunfire was at its most intense. After that, *Hartford* and its companion vessels cleared the fort and entered the bay, disabling the few attacking gunboats along the way. Sometime during that hour, an exploding shell near the whip sent shrapnel into Dunphy's body, lacerating his hands and forearms, shearing away flesh in jagged bits, and smashing bone. There is no record of whether Dunphy was on the gundeck or below placing shells in the hoist. The exposure of the coal heavers to explosive violence was not limited to Dunphy: during that same hour, Coal Heaver James R. Garrison may have been wounded in his foot, resulting in a severed toe, although he continued duty at the shell whip until he was disabled by a second, more severe wound. Coal Heaver Thomas O'Connell was a sick bay patient who nevertheless went to his duty station and assisted at the whip. An exploding enemy shell severed his right hand.

Shipmates hustled Dunphy below to the sick bay where Surgeon P. Lansdale examined him. Within three or four hours after Dunphy was wounded, the surgeon administered chloroform and amputated both arms about seven inches below the shoulders. During this time, Dunphy endured "a burning sensation of the nerves and weakness and hardly any appetite." Dunphy was later satisfied with the flaps the surgeon fashioned to turn into stumps, but in recovery, he experienced "extraordinary pain [in the stumps] + burning sensation of the nerves" that lasted for three weeks. For several days, urination proved difficult. Over the next three months before his recovery seemed to be complete, Dunphy endured "a great quantity of pus" and about a dozen "pieces of bone or splinters" emerging through the sutures.[2]

While Dunphy was recovering aboard *Hartford* following surgery, the battle was not over. Farragut, directing his fleet from *Hartford*'s quarterdeck or poised in the ship's rigging, observed that the most significant enemy threat apart from Fort Morgan's guns was following the Union ships, preparing to attack. CSS *Tennessee*, a wooden ship with a weather deck almost flush with the waterline, was surmounted by a well-armored casemate to protect its powerful guns. The superstructure had slanted sides to deflect cannon balls and was impervious to exploding shells. Farragut directed his ships to approach the ironclad at full speed and ram it while firing guns. *Hartford* likewise came about and was the third vessel to attack *Tennessee* in this manner. The Union flagship collided with the rebel ram, but "the blow was a glancing one, and as she rasped along [*Hartford*'s] side we poured our whole port broadside of IX-inch solid shot within 10 feet of her casemate," according to Farragut's report. *Tennessee*, however, did not return fire up to her capitulation at about 10:00 a.m. Battered and disabled, *Tennessee* surrendered, surrounded by Union ironclads. The battle was over.[3]

Dunphy had been in the naval service only since the previous December. At his enlistment, he told the navy representative that he had no previous naval service and so was assigned the rating of coal heaver. He was healthy and able to handle the rigorous and exhausting duties in the boiler room. At Dunphy's enlistment, the navy made a record of his body and documented its essential statistics: twenty years old, five-feet, eight-and-a-half inches tall, blue eyes, black hair, and "ruddy complexion." The enlistment record includes the comment "Has had small pox."[4]

A hospital in Pensacola, Florida, admitted Dunphy on August 6. The hospital ticket recorded that his arms had been amputated due to "action with the enemy"; specifically, "Vulnus sclop[etarium]," the Latin phrase used by many physicians to denote gunshot wounds. The same description appeared on the ticket at the Naval Hospital, in Chelsea, Massachusetts, to which Dunphy was admitted on September 21. This ticket recorded that "at first there was some oozing of blood and patient's strength was low, but later he has gained vigor and the stumps are nearly healed." The Chelsea hospital discharged Dunphy on January 25, 1865, whereupon he returned home, possibly to relatives or another Irish immigrant community.[5]

Farragut wanted to honor the bravery of his crew and submitted recommendations for Medals of Honor. Of the dozen recipients aboard *Hartford* who were awarded the medal on December 31, 1864, three were coal heavers: Dunphy, Garrison, and O'Connell. The latter two men's official citations described the specific actions that resulted in their wounds. Dunphy's, by contrast, was more general in citing "extraordinary heroism": "With his ship under terrific enemy shellfire, Coal Heaver Dunphy performed his duties with skill and courage throughout this fierce engagement which resulted in the capture of the rebel ram *Tennessee*."[6]

Thus Dunphy was to be known as an "armless veteran" for the rest of his life. The epithet would precede his name in numerous official pension records and newspaper reports. This descriptor, in fact, was enough to render the mundane into the newsworthy because the country viewed him as a pitiable unfortunate, an anomaly or spectacle, a man shorn of his manhood, a feminized interloper with no place in the scheme of civil life. Unlike Henry Kircher, Dunphy was not supported by a community of relatives successful in business who welcomed his return. His status as an Irish immigrant relegated him to lower-class status in the eyes of most Americans. For the rest of Dunphy's life, his key occupation was that of armless veteran but one distinguished by the Medal of Honor. This honor did not have the social value it later acquired when Congress stipulated criteria for its award. Dunphy, however, did not even receive the medal and its accompanying citation in 1864; he waited for years while persistently requesting it from anyone in authority who might be able to deliver it. Dunphy regarded it as the chief honor of his adult life and proof of his manhood. His other chief achievement was fathering fourteen children, of whom ten reached adulthood.

As the precise facts were not recorded, it is impossible to give a detailed accounting of the circumstances of Dunphy's wounding. Later, popular reports of his moment of heroism, reinforced by Dunphy's account, offered a romantic view of a titanic struggle between two antagonists equal in strength and ability, a duel between *Hartford* and *Tennessee,* in which Dunphy sacrificed his arms to help ensure victory. Sea duels between USS *Monitor* and CSS *Virginia* (1862), USS *Kearsarge* and CSS *Alabama* (1864), and CSS *Hunley* and USS *Housatonic* (1864) received much press because the contests profiled agile and brave naval commanders directing the largest war machines in existence, the future of a republic at stake. *Hartford* and *Tennessee* did not fight such a duel. The Confederate ram did not return fire. In the early stage of the battle, as Farragut's fleet struggled to pass Fort Morgan, *Hartford* was fired on from multiple directions, the most severe fire coming from the fort. Dunphy may have wished to ascribe his mutilation to a specific, worthy assailant, but it is impossible to assign the shell that burst near him to a source. The preservation of manhood, however, required an identifiable, brutal but crafty foe, a worthy opponent. Indiscriminate gunfire from afar would not do.

MANHOOD AND PENSION CERTIFICATE NO. 845

Before his double amputation, even as he looked at the remains of his arms, Dunphy could not imagine a future without them. He possessed a strong body and was used to heavy manual labor. As a teenager, Dunphy arrived in New York City from Ireland in 1856, apparently alone, but he may have connected with relatives or family friends in New York where he worked at various unskilled jobs. He saw himself as self-reliant, confident in his strength and adaptability to confront almost anything. He chose an occupation requiring physical strength and stamina. He may have decided in late 1863 to enlist in the navy because Congress recently had instituted the draft and he wanted to avoid army service.[7]

During his time in Boston and Pensacola hospitals, Dunphy observed other severely wounded men and may have reflected on his own apparent loss of virility. Perhaps he exhibited extreme emotional responses to what had happened to his body. Most people made distinctions between men and women in their responses to pain. A mature man was presumed to have a rational mind and basic intelligence that would see him through most of life's vagaries, whereas women could be irrational regarding pain or bodily dysfunction. Dunphy's hospitalization and double amputation rendered him visibly emasculated to others—and perhaps to himself. Irrational "feminine" responses ensued.

In subsequent years as a veteran, Dunphy was conflicted about the degree of his apparent feminization because of the help he required for essential life tasks. Without someone like S. Weir Mitchell to analyze, guide, and record his healing, no other doctor in the pension system bothered to examine Dunphy's body: after simply observing his lack of arms—signifying

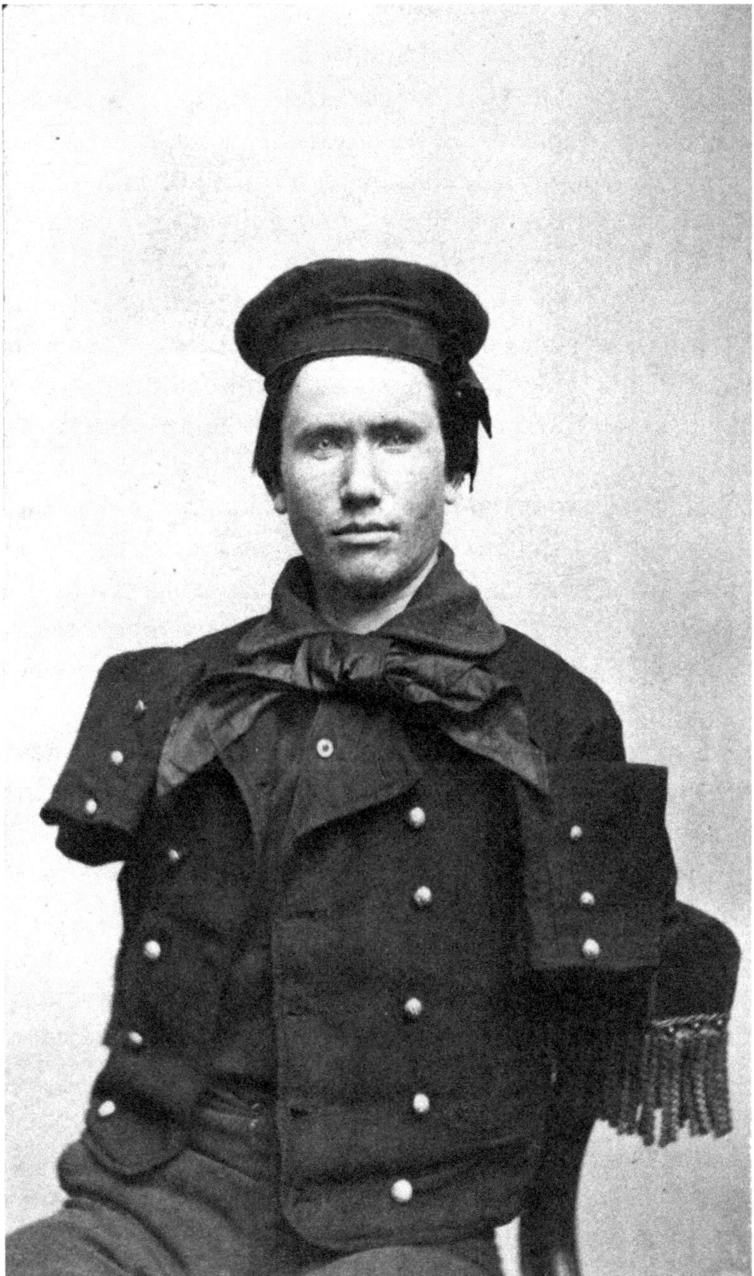

Richard D. Dunphy carte de visite showing him in naval uniform, c. 1864.
Credit: Library of Congress (LC-DIG-ppmsca-41740).

an obvious lack of manhood—they signed off on pension forms with no examination. His disability was thus rendered static for life. Unseen disabling wounds were viewed suspiciously by many: they could be fraudulent or exaggerated, thus requiring a doctor's testimony. Dunphy's double amputation, however, was incontrovertible and thus became a "powerful cultural touchstone" requiring no inspection.[8]

Many images of amputee veterans appeared in popular publications. These men were shown to be powerless, with a woman nearby to quietly apply her innate nurturing abilities to help with what the man could no longer do. For the rest of Dunphy's life, the medical world followed Mitchell's view that hysteria and other manifestations of female irrationality might characterize men, a clinical exploration that "risked uncovering the elements of mental and emotional 'femininity' in the 'male' psyche itself." To preclude gender ambiguity, Dunphy sat for many photographs in his naval uniform, looking confident and engaging the viewer's gaze directly. He sold these photographs to help support himself, a widespread practice. No photograph exists, however, showing Dunphy with his entire family. Such amputee images with family members proved that, despite the loss of a limb, a soldier's virility remained intact.[9]

Before Dunphy was discharged from the hospital, surgeons completed a "Form of Application for Navy Invalid Pension" and a "Report of Medical Survey." The former described Dunphy's line-of-duty injury and subsequent amputations and provided his New York City address. The surgeon completing the form confirmed that the Chelsea hospital admitted Dunphy "affected with vulnus sclopeticum." The latter report repeated much of the same data and recommended a pension for total disability. Dunphy thus entered the record as navy pension certificate number 845.

Following his release from the hospital, Dunphy had trouble supporting himself until his pension took effect. A letter to the pension authority from the Navy Department, Bureau of Medicine & Surgery stated that the veteran amputee was "utterly without means, + if a higher pension cannot be granted, he will be glad to know the decision of the Commissioner in any event." In January 1866, Dunphy filed a pension application, endorsed by a naval authority, which granted him a pension of twenty-five dollars[10] per month, retroactive to January 21, 1865.[11]

In every American city, men went about their business with obvious war injuries. Their bodies displayed scars, they sported folded trouser legs or sleeves, or they moved around with crutches or canes. The warscape was thus omnipresent even if the landscape was cleansed of evidence. Wounded veterans were constantly under public scrutiny. They "were seen through multiple lenses and exposed to critical commentary on their choices." While veterans faced an ambiguous future, both North and South strove to remove evidence of destruction, leaving veterans' bodies to recall it. As the years passed, veterans continued to embody the war's massive destruction despite the reshaping of the central narrative of why the war happened.[12]

Dunphy, however, resided first in New York and later in Milwaukee, Wisconsin, and San Francisco, California, places with no visible signs of the war's devastation. His public appearances in such places disturbed, startled, and frightened people. The first commemorations in stone or bronze at Civil War sites, largely erected in the decades since the war, gave veterans hitching posts to which they attached themselves, creating small areas of war remembrance that were distinctly theirs. How active was Dunphy in these veterans' activities? We do not know if or how he participated for many years until near his death, when other veterans held up Dunphy's stumps to define a small "echo of the ruin" that "reverberates forward" at Civil War sites, generating "nostalgia rather than a true understanding of the past." Dunphy may have struggled to maintain his sacrificial manhood by adhering to his tale of the great sea duel. He may also have allied himself with other veterans who struggled to maintain their vision of their manhood as the rest of society moved on.[13]

Although Dunphy received a pension backdated to January 1866, he remained in a precarious financial state with no practical vision of a future. The next month, he dictated a letter to Secretary of the Navy Gideon Welles and included a carte de visite of himself. He introduced himself as a *Hartford* crewmember who took pride in his body's badge of valor, his amputations: "I believe I stand to day the only one in the American Navy who lost both Arms in the late Rebellion." He pointed out that Farragut had told him he would receive a medal, but to this date, he had not. "I place a great value on it and I believe I am justly entitled to it." He also prodded the secretary to lobby for increased pensions: "The pension is low especially in my case where I have to pay a man to accompany me wherever I go. I cannot help myself to anything not even feed myself for my Arms are off above the elbow." In the enclosed carte de visite, Dunphy posed in uniform, sleeves pinned up, his face expressionless and gazing into the camera. The printed caption states that he "lost his arms by a shell, from the Rebel Ram TENNESSEE."[14]

Sometime in the late 1860s, Dunphy relocated to Milwaukee. He might have moved there because supportive relatives were willing to assist him. A local census in 1855 for Menomonee (now Menomonie) in Waukesha County lists a household head, Richard Dunphy (not the coal heaver), and spouse as living there. During his sojourn in Milwaukee, Dunphy married another Irish immigrant, Catherine M. Cooper, in 1866. Despite this happy event, Dunphy's financial woes followed him to Wisconsin. On his behalf, the state legislature sent a resolution to Congress in 1868 requesting an increase in pension. Citing the cause of Dunphy's wounds as being "struck by the fragment of a shell from the rebel ram, Tennessee," the document argued that he "has a wife, and one child . . . dependent on his labor to support; that he is entirely disabled and is the only person that served in the navy during the late war who lost both his arms and is living." As his pension record shows, this resolution had no effect. Federal pensions adhered only to the evolving standards set by Congress. Dunphy fathered his first son, James William, who was born in Milwaukee in 1868, and the city directory for 1869 lists him as a pensioner resident in the city. That same year, his second son was born, John Richard.[15]

During these first years living as a double amputee, Dunphy doubtless negotiated a new civic body. He did not earn a salary, his wife was unemployed, and his family was growing. The existence of a family may have implied stability and responsibility to pension authorities despite Dunphy's apparent disability. To other people, his growing family betokened Irish Catholic irresponsibility. During these years, too, he must have relied on many people to help him with the activities that required two hands. He decided to try prosthetic arms at war's end but gave them up. If his experience was similar to that of other amputees who recorded their challenges with prostheses, he must have occasionally felt pain, spasmodic twitching of his stumps, and even phantom sensations. The only evidence of these experiences comes from the completed health questionnaire that Dunphy sent to Mitchell. These phenomena constituted "fraudulent body language," precisely the body sensations attributed to hysterical women. Perhaps Dunphy's many carte de visite poses were intended to challenge the perception of himself as helpless, as an invalid relegated to the margins of life. In these poses, he appears ready to serve his country again at a moment's notice; he holds fast to his wartime identity. These images "became a form of coping" while remaining disturbing to viewers. "An almost grotesque tension results between the horrific wounds and the placid domestic settings in which they are displayed."[16]

SOLD BY A WOUNDED SOLDIER

When he lived in Milwaukee, Dunphy applied for new prosthetic arms or a commutation allowance to buy his own. Immediately after the war, the navy provided him with two arms made by the National Leg and Arm Company of New York, but either he could not adjust to them or they were impossible to wear. Most soldiers and sailors knew that amputations close to the shoulder might not support prosthetic arms and did not bother to apply for them. For several reasons, most amputees who obtained prostheses never had them fitted and soon discarded them. Within months of Dunphy's 1870 application, the Bureau of Medicine and Surgery (formerly the Surgeon General's Office) endorsed his request and confirmed that he had received two limbs on June 15, 1865. We learn through Mitchell's questionnaire that Dunphy tried various types of limbs, but all were unwearable.[17]

By the 1870 census, Dunphy and his growing family had moved west to Vallejo, California, just outside San Francisco and opposite the Mare Island Naval Shipyard, where he found employment as a messenger. Admiral Farragut might have arranged this appointment (as he soon commanded the yard), or the navy offered him this opportunity when he lived in Milwaukee. His pension plus "a little salary," as the newspapers put it, may have been sufficient to raise a middle-class family. The move must have been recent: according to the census, the family lived in a boarding house and owned no real estate.[18]

Meanwhile, Dunphy continued to distribute photographs of himself without arms or sell them to raise funds to support his family. These images, usually in the form of cartes de visite, bore fundraising captions such as "Sold by a Wounded Soldier." Importantly, these images communicated clear messages: here was a clean, neat, clearly disciplined, and morally centered young man whose uniform attested to military achievements and whose visage (or "countenance," to use the nineteenth-century term

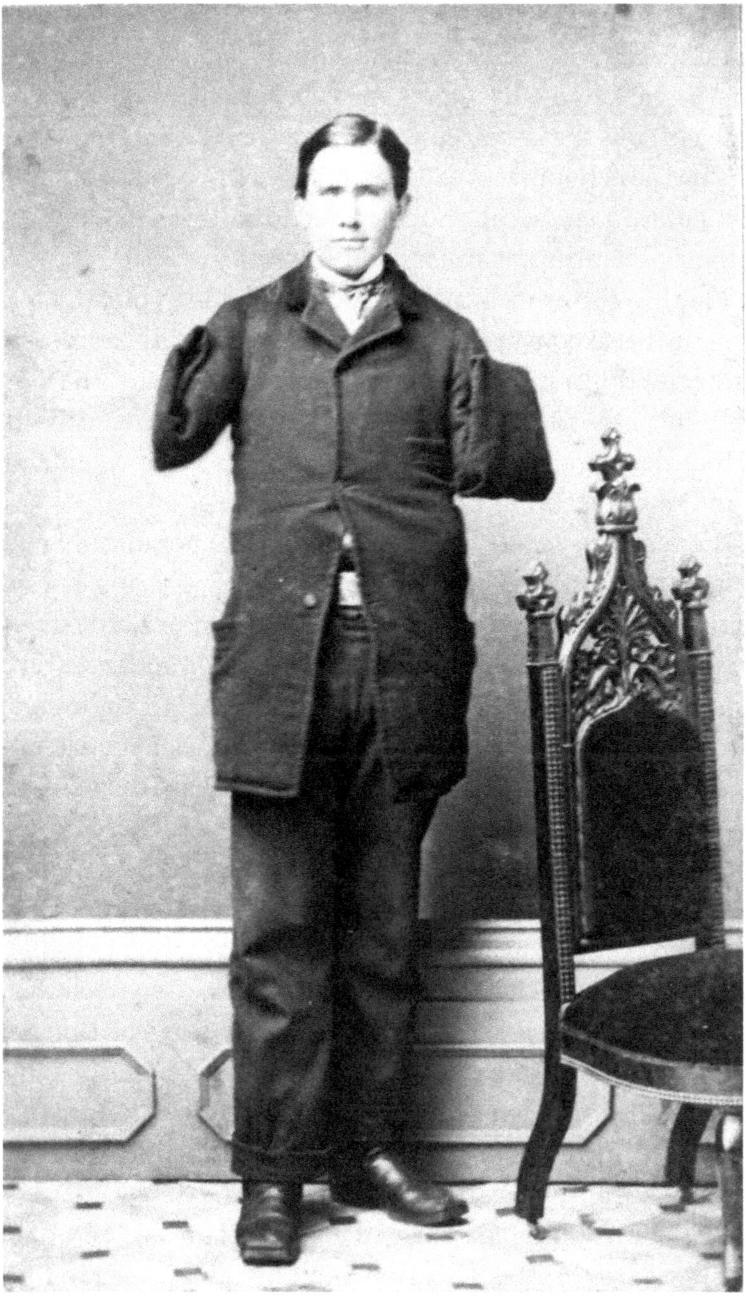

Richard D. Dunphy carte de visite showing him in civilian clothes, c. 1864. *Credit: Library of Congress (LC-DIG-ppmsca-41742).*

that encompassed class, education, intelligence, background, and lineage) showed resolution, high ideals of patriotism, and determination to build a life (and rebuild a nation). As such, the image "marks the impaired veteran's return to a paternal national fold via the economic assistance he solicits and receives." A Connecticut women's association decided to embrace Dunphy as one of their philanthropic causes and sold his images on his behalf. While this gesture was born of goodwill and sympathy for the veteran, it also conveyed a point about the body by "reinforc[ing] the perception among their potential customers that the viewers of the image were 'normal'; Dunphy physically 'suffered' for them so that their bodies would not have to do so and could emerge from the violent conflict 'healthy' and 'whole.'"[19]

The terms *disability* and *disabled* appear sporadically in pension documents and newspaper reporting. During Dunphy's lifetime, the terms were never elaborated on or defined within the pension system, but "disabilities are social and cultural constructs, rather than isolated medical events." He and other veterans—including Henry Kircher—sometimes negotiated with pension authorities from a disadvantaged position. First, the government always treated claims with skepticism to minimize fraud. Second, pension claims carried an implicit assumption of stasis. The veteran claimed that the state of the wounded body was fixed, its limiting features permanent. Disability certificates had been granted during the war with a date by which the disability must be reviewed in case the body had healed sufficiently for the veteran to gain employment. With amputees, of course, pension officers did not expect anything other than stasis. Third, any use of the terms *disabled* or *disability* was contingent on the larger cultural and legal circumstances of the time; hence Henry Kircher's and Dunphy's repeated pension claims when Congress tinkered with the law. "Defining disability, and determining who had the power over those definitions, was a central tension."[20]

The prevailing model of disability for Civil War veterans was a medical one, still a governing criterion today. Pension payments were made based on the extent to which veterans' bodies deviated from an imagined normality. In this view, the pension ethos presumed that the veteran recipient aspired to this normality but accepted a body that fell below the so-called normal standard. Each pension payment reminded the veteran that the government viewed him as a lesser being. Disability, then, was the inability to be normal.[21]

A relevant essay by Leonard Kriegel, an African American man who used a wheelchair, written at an intense cultural moment in the 1960s in the wake of federal civil rights legislation and the assassination of Martin Luther King Jr., compares the black man to the cripple (his word). Both black man and cripple are "still asked to accept definitions of what he is, and of what he should be, imposed on him from outside his experience." Further, the cripple is subject to incessant voyeurism in that "normal" people might pry into any circumstance of his life, no matter how intimate, without any reciprocity. In time, as Dunphy found himself retelling the story of his armlessness on demand, he would have been expected to behave in a supplicating manner due to his lack of normality. His daily interactions with the world required continual justification of self and an assertion of manly attributes that commanded respect, such as being a father, householder, and veteran.[22]

Assertions of manly swagger in saloons got Dunphy in trouble. He considered his pension and his Medal of Honor to be due payment for services rendered for the country and expected others to see him as a social equal. Like Kriegel's cripple, he was "a social fugitive, a prisoner of expectations molded by a society that he makes uncomfortable by his very presence." Also, since many people associated physical abnormalities with people of lower class and less intelligence, Dunphy was sometimes presumed to have a weak mind, possibly a mental illness as well as a physical disability, a further feminization of character. Dunphy's later drinking episodes, which invited pension office scrutiny and newspaper reporting, heightened this perception.[23]

During the 1870s, the Dunphy family settled into life in Vallejo and welcomed more children. Henry David was born in 1871, the first child to come into the world in California. George Patrick followed in 1873, Thomas Francis in 1875, Mary E. in 1876, and Bernard Stephen in 1879. Meanwhile, Dunphy's pension rose for the first time from $25 to $31.25 in 1872, then to $50[24] in 1874. He continued to apply for pension increases, arguing total invalidity. In a sworn statement made in 1874, George W. McGill attested that he was "well acquainted" with Dunphy, who was

> totally unable to help himself either in putting on clothes or attending to any call of nature. That [he] has no means whereby he could cook any food or eat or drink any food but by having the [food?] placed near to his mouth and cut up or fed by a spoon. That by consequence of his said inability to do any thing for himself he requires, wherever he is an attendant is necessary to clean him after stool and to lave [wash] the filth from his person and clothes when making water. That said Dunphy has a wife devoted to him and worthy to be compensated for her unpleasant position.

This statement reminds us that Dunphy was a public double: he required a shadow person to act as his hands, even for distasteful duties. At home, he may have relied on family members to perform these jobs. Whenever Catherine was mentioned in pension documents, including sworn statements, she was described as dutiful, clean, virtuous, patient, understanding, and competent in the management of home affairs. There are nevertheless suggestions that she found the handling of Richard's bodily necessities to be distasteful, although she received credit in these documents for his clean, neat presentation in public.[25]

McGill's statement parallels a document that was prepared a month later that argued for a pension increase (and was duly annotated to note that an increase to fifty dollars had been authorized), which acknowledged "that claimant requires the regular attendance of another person, and is totally unable to help himself either in putting on his clothes + etc." The week before McGill provided his statement, however, a Solano County sheriff's deputy escorted "Richard Dunphy, insane" to an asylum in Stockton, California. References to Dunphy's brief sojourn at an "insane asylum" occur sporadically in later pension correspondence. Whatever the circumstances, these references do not appear in official pension records, and pension authorities seem to have regarded this episode as outside their concern. No examining physician for the pension authorities asked about this mysterious interlude in Dunphy's life. Perhaps the pressures of raising a growing family on pension funds and the uncertainty of raises in allotments demanded an escape from world affairs for a brief time. It is also unknown how long Dunphy resided in Stockton or what brought about his release.[26]

In 1878, Dunphy made another sworn statement, noting that although he had been receiving fifty dollars per month, he needed more because he was "disabled in the following manner, to wit: Loss of both arms above the elbow, and other wounds on the right leg, and breast. Caused by the explosion of a shell from the Confederate ram Tennessee in Mobile Bay in 1864." For the first time, Dunphy claimed other bodily wounds, giving the impression of the fragility of his body beyond the loss of arms. The government responded by raising his pension to seventy-two dollars[27] per month. The early pension laws did not anticipate the necessity for periodic acts of Congress to remedy systemic problems. Pension doctors relied on a schedule of payments for the circumstances and extent of wounds or injuries. These policies amounted to the creation of "a hierarchy of abnormalities [that] acknowledged the symbolic logic of the medical model—the missing body part or function was the diminished veteran, and a standard monthly payment was the appropriate response once the condition (and its service origin) had been identified."[28]

WALKING TO WASHINGTON, DC

The 1880 census listed Richard (occupation "laborer") as head of the household, his wife, Catherine, shown as "keeping house," and six sons and one daughter. The sons ranged in age from five to thirteen, and daughter Mary was six. Four sons aged seven through thirteen were listed as students. In June 1880, another daughter was born, Theresa Catherine (Kitt). As was the case with Kircher, Dunphy's pension allotments were a matter of published record. Among pensioners living in Solano County in 1883, Dunphy was listed as receiving seventy-two dollars per month, the highest on the list. The publication of this information reinforced the paternalistic attitude of the government toward disabled veterans and ensured that Dunphy's private affairs were thereby public matters.[29]

Veterans unable to continue their former professions took whatever jobs were available to them, such as security guards or night watchmen. Amputees like Dunphy also endured the prejudices against former soldiers as lower class, shiftless, and untrustworthy. Many of these jobs contributed a meager income to supplement pension payments and provided only precarious employment. In 1887, Dunphy lost his job as a messenger at the navy yard due to political patronage. Appointed under a Republican president, he was moved aside for a Democrat. He wrote to the president to protest his firing but received no response. Perhaps courting press coverage, Dunphy called attention to his injustice by walking to Washington, DC—approximately 2,800 miles—to make his case. He wanted his body on display as exhibit A in his objection to this alleged injustice and to remind the nation that for wounded veterans, the war had not ended.[30]

The five-month journey attracted some notice, although the newspapers were cynical about its success. "Of course, it will do him no good. What are the claims of an armless veteran compared with those of an able-bodied Democrat who votes early and often?" Dunphy did not meet with the president, and he required a hospital stay due to the stress of the journey. In a naval hospital, seventy dollars was stolen from him. His tenacity attracted local attention in Vallejo and no small measure of support in his cause. By the end of the year, he got his job back. The "armless veteran"—the odd figure ambling along with a cape to conceal his stumps—was well known by this point in his hometown.[31]

Managing one's pension required constant vigilance regarding changes in federal and state laws, continuing competence in completing government forms, and some skill in negotiation. Dunphy must have long regarded pension laws as a mixture of mystery and calculation based on premises governed by foreign logic. Henry Kircher had disputed pension authorities over interpretations of the law that did not appear to recognize the loss of a leg and arm from the same body as being equal to the loss of two hands or two feet. Dunphy, similarly, ensured that government regulations acknowledging the loss of two hands also recognized the fact that the arms might also be missing. He argued to a pension agent in San Francisco that a raise to one hundred dollars per month was justified according to the "February 12, 1889 . . . Act of that date for loss of both hands." That year, the federal government increased Dunphy's pension to one hundred dollars,[32] where it would remain for the rest of his life.[33]

Although no pension doctor examined Dunphy's stumps or questioned him about them, this does not mean that he had nothing to say about his health. His pension applications do not mention pain or suffering beyond the inconvenience of not being able to feed, dress, or clean himself. Despite these inconveniences, he seemed to see himself as a healthy and virile man who presided over a large household. He may have viewed his pension—which was doubtless inadequate to sustain a growing family—as a form of salary, something that the government ought to pay him in compensation for what the war took from him.

TEMPERATE BUT CRANKY

The behavior surrounding traumatic injury—cardiac stress, what would become known as combat fatigue or a phenomenon of the nerves—had been under increasing medical scrutiny as the "second scientific revolution" in medicine began to develop at the close of the century. Hysteria, long associated with the "wandering womb" in women, came to be seen as a pathology not exclusive to women. Mitchell's later writings freely applied the term to men who experienced severe pain of the peripheral nerves. He and his contemporaries acknowledged "the existence of masculine nervous and mental illness among all social classes and in diverse guises." With the emergence of psychology and psychiatry, the professional dialogue about hysteria was no longer only about women but also a "blurring of demarcations between genres of commentary about the nervous distempers . . . and clinical case studies read like short stories."[34]

In *Lippincott's Magazine of Popular Literature and Science,* Mitchell highlighted the enigma of amputations by stating that there was no equivalent Latin term for an amputation "stump." Rather, a "stump is rarely a perfectly comfortable portion of the body" that can be easily injured. Stumps can create a "form of neuralgic torture" due to the "inflamed or hardened" nerves encased within them, which may require a second amputation. Stump pain may arise under many circumstances, from intense emotional reactions to changes in wind and weather. The most annoying, embarrassing, and unmanly phenomena associated with stumps were the "automatic gymnastics" whereby "the part thresh[es] about in a wild and meaningless fashion."[35]

In his 1872 treatise, Mitchell lamented the lack of research into the physiology of stumps (noting that only one study existed at the time) and based his observations on approximately ninety-one of his own cases. He described specific "nervous afflictions of stumps" as chorea ("irregular and involuntary motions of one or more limbs"), neuralgia ("a generic name for a number of diseases, the chief symptom of which is a very acute pain"), neuritis ("inflammation of a nerve"), and sclerosis ("any hardness or induration," especially concentrations of nerve endings and adjacent tissues).[36]

Dunphy responded to Mitchell's questionnaire in 1893 with help from an amanuensis, probably one of his children. Dunphy's responses reveal bodily circumstances that pension doctors had either not noticed or not asked about. He evidently never sought specialists who could have explained the reasons for some of his bodily phenomena over which he had little or no control, phenomena cited by Mitchell as early as 1872 in his treatise *Injuries to Nerves*.

Dunphy was fifty-two when he completed Mitchell's questionnaire. After describing the initial circumstances of the amputations and his recovery, he stated that following his recovery (complete healing in about three months) and discharge from the navy, his general health had been good with no changes in pulse or body temperature. He had followed "temperate" habits but admitted to a "cranky" disposition. His eating habits, sleeping schedule, and the acuity of his senses remained unchanged.[37]

Dunphy had plenty to say about his stumps, offering valuable data to both the elder and younger Mitchell and providing an intimate look at the ruins of his arms. The stump skin appeared "small and thin, no muscle." The stump ends remained red for almost three decades following amputation. No hair grew on the stumps, but their ends were susceptible to both winter cold and summer heat. They perspired less than other adjacent areas of the body. Sensation in the stumps, however, was challenging to describe. One question required a self-test: administering pinpricks in and around each stump. Some parts proved sensible to pinpricks, other parts insensible. The stumps were more sensitive to touch than other parts of the body; mere touching could elicit pain. Abrupt changes in weather caused "a jumping sensation of the nerves" that caused brief jabs of unpredictable, recurrent pain that continued until Dunphy's death. His stumps were not immobile appendages: he could raise them to the back of his ears.

Dunphy provided insights into his use of prosthetic arms. He first wore arms in 1866 but only sporadically after that. He cited three manufacturers, G. Monroe, Thomas Wrens, and B. F. Palmer, and said that the Wrens limb was most satisfactory. With these limbs, Dunphy "could do [his] own writing + feed [himself]." It is not clear how often or when Dunphy wore his prosthetics (or perhaps he only wore one), but if doing so enabled him to write, none of the documents bear his signature in the pension file, as he routinely signed with an X. Wearing prostheses was challenging: they made Dunphy "perspire more" and tired him, although they helped keep his stumps warm in winter.

Importantly, Dunphy still felt phantom arms in their entirety but shortened, fixed in one position despite any movement of the stumps. He felt each finger, but all remained folded around his thumbs. The phantom sensations were not painful. He discovered that moving his stumps backward could bring spasms or the "shakes very rapidly until I bring [them] forward." This action brought no pain either.

As if affirming Dunphy's phantom sensations, Mitchell found that amputations caused more sweating and a faster pulse and noted that stumps could change over time. They could shrink in atrophy or gain bulk. Tumors could appear where nerves were severed, hence the sclerosis cited in his 1872 treatise. Mitchell also described the variations in skin sensitivity to touch, from zero response to hyperesthesia, and variable responses based on weather changes. Twitching and chorea-like phenomena were more prevalent with arm stumps than legs. Many respondents complained of the nonwearability of prosthetics, especially during the summer heat. Mitchell noted that extreme temperatures could also induce chorea or "some [other] unpleasing sensation."[38]

Occasionally, Mitchell's observations coincided precisely with Dunphy's experience. Mitchell wrote that the "most common . . . referred sensations [pain during reflex actions]" included thigh-high pain during urination. As for phantom limbs, Mitchell said that "sensory hallucinations" were "so vivid, so strange, and so little dwelt upon by authors, as to be well worth study. . . . Nearly every man who loses a limb carries about with him a constant or inconstant phantom of the missing member, a sensory ghost of that much of himself, and sometimes a most inconvenient presence, faintly felt at times, but ready to be called up to his perception by a blow, a touch, or a change of wind." Mitchell emphasized that "the limb is rarely felt as a whole."[39]

Not surprisingly, when Mitchell applied faradic electricity to stumps, patients reacted with great sensitivity and "choreoid [spasmodic] movements" and pain. If the phantom sensations disappeared, the same current could reactivate them: "It is not easy to forget the astonishment with which some of these persons reawaken to a perception of the long-lost leg or arm." Electricity could also stimulate a persistently clenched phantom fist to open its fingers. Electricity exacerbated pain induced by a blow to the stump. The "pain is often unceasing" and "opiates in excess become at last the only comfort."[40]

It is not clear from the medical questionnaire whether Dunphy required a shadow helper, as he had asserted he needed in 1866 in his letter to the secretary of the navy. The 1873 pension law allowed government funding for a full-time medical attendant if required. A shadow's help may have extended beyond opening doors and toilet assistance; the shadow might have eased Dunphy's sporadic pain through massage or some other form of exercise. Pension laws, however, expanded and became more complex over time regarding what and how much help was required to aid a veteran. Pension law distinguished between a person in need of medical assistance, a veteran unable to perform *manual* labor (specifically, agricultural or industrial labor), and a veteran who could not perform *any* labor. Pension authorities were willing to compensate for lost arms, but if Dunphy was able to perform some paid work at the navy yard, doing so could limit his pension eligibility. If this was the case, the pension file says little about these distinctions. No official pension document acknowledges his work at the navy yard. The pension file does not show that Dunphy hired a shadow assistant. If he did, the person's name went unrecorded.[41]

AT THE MERCY OF EVERY MAN

Dunphy navigated the world with his dignity intact, despite the pitying looks he received. He supported a growing family, albeit on a pension, performed some work for the navy yard, and eventually acquired real estate. He also drank liquor with barflies at local saloons. Dunphy became estranged from Catherine, and the pension, according to her, was imperiled by Dunphy's heavy drinking. During 1899, Dunphy's pension file was filled with accusations and counteraccusations between husband and wife. In September, J. H. Shepard, whose law firm described itself as "attorneys and solicitors of government claims," wrote a letter to the pension agent in San Francisco, referring to a "distressing case" that had been brought before the pension office in 1880 and 1883, although to this date, no action had been taken. Representing Catherine, Shepard stated, "Now for the past several months the soldier (sailor) appears to be entirely without common sense, and will not yield to advice or do anything that seems reasonable to take care of his own person, his pension money, or his family." He argued that Dunphy "is at the mercy of every man who handles his money," cannot pay debts, and had once been committed to an asylum. Shepard repeated Catherine's desire to gain access to her husband's pension directly "to draw and dispense [it] for the benefit of his wife and minor children."[42]

Shepard enclosed various letters to support Catherine's claim, one from the local Catholic priest who asked Dunphy "to act like a man and care for and stop abusing his wife and children" and similar ones from senior navy officials at the shipyard that attested to "the dissapated [*sic*] habits and habits of the man." Despite a legal requirement that Dunphy receive his pension via US mail, the letter went on, he had arranged to receive mail directly "by express" to prevent his family from accessing the funds. He had announced, said Shepard, that he would give his wife 33 percent of his pension income and no more, and if she tried to get more control over the finances, he would give her nothing. Shepard's letter concluded, "Some time ago the priest of his church sent him a letter requesting him to stop drinking and treat his family better than he had been doing for some time past."

A month later, an official with the law division at the pension office referred this matter to the chief of the Special Examination Division with another forwarded letter from Shepard. Quoting from the Shepard letter, the pension official wrote "that the pensioner appears to be entirely without common sense, will not yield to advice or do anything that seems reasonable to take care of his person, his pension money or his family, and is at the mercy of every man who handles his money. That he fails to pay his debts except to saloons. That he has been committed to the insane asylum and would be there now but for the sympathy of his family and the county judge. That he has three children, one of whom is in the insane asylum on account of his brutal treatment."[43]

The pension officer who wrote the letter took the conservative view, asserting that "there is no evidence . . . that the pensioner is insane or incompetent to attend to his business affairs, nor does it appear that he has deserted his wife and family." The officer pointed out that the law did not permit diverting the pension to other family members. On the possibility that Shepard's claims could be true, the letter requested that a special examiner be assigned to visit the Dunphy family "for the purpose of determining whether the pensioner's mental condition is such as to require that he have a guardian" and take appropriate testimony. In October, E. G. Hursh, a special examiner with the San Francisco office, was appointed to visit the Dunphy family.[44]

While the Dunphy case progressed through the pension system, Congress continued to modify and expand pension laws. In earlier decades, the underlying premise of the medical pension examinations was to determine if the veteran had become self-sufficient enough to perform manual labor. In Dunphy's case, doctors waived examinations because his two stumps (and therefore his disability) were readily apparent, and Dunphy was therefore a priori incapable of work and lacked self-sufficiency. By the 1880s, however, the examining doctor was replaced by a three-person panel that scrutinized veterans for conditions that prohibited self-sufficiency; namely, "vicious habits" such as sexually transmitted diseases and alcoholism. In 1890, Congress created a new pension category that disregarded how a veteran was originally disabled and focused solely on self-sufficiency to earn a living. That same year, the federal Census Bureau conducted a special survey of Civil War veterans to determine the number of veterans in need of assistance and to forecast budget needs for pensions in the new century. By this time, pensions made up much of the federal budget.[45]

Before Special Examiner Hursh began conducting interviews, he reviewed other documents that accompanied Shepard's letters. Catherine detailed her family's dilemma in a sworn statement, describing her husband as existing "in a state of total helplessness." Because he could not physically handle money, he relied on strangers to reach into his pockets "at all times and places." Catherine wanted to accompany her husband on pension days to make the rounds of businesses to pay bills, but Dunphy refused. He always first paid his saloon debts, but he rarely received receipts and sometimes paid the same bill twice. She had tried earlier to have a guardian appointed but gave up when the effort proved unsuccessful. "But of late the pensioner has shown such a mental and physical change. That I cannot let the matter pass."[46]

The pension office also received a letter signed by various Vallejo merchants who affirmed Catherine's character as meritworthy and acknowledged that Dunphy was "helpless, and at the mercy of every man he meets. And especially . . . when he is in possession of the large amount of pension money. That he must depend upon others often strangers to help and attend to his wants. And especially when in possession of money." The merchants requested that a guardian be appointed.[47]

Shepard wrote a second letter to remind the San Francisco pension office that the commissioner of pensions requested a review of the Dunphy case and wanted to see all relevant documents. The office duly sent a letter to the commissioner with the statements from the merchants and Catherine and added a note that "nothing has been put in this petition about [Dunphy's] habits of drinking or what are the results of the same." Hursh, however, was already on the scene and taking statements. One deponent, the local druggist, could not resist mentioning Dunphy's drinking behavior as a wonder: "I have never seen him drunk, though I have seen him take up a glass of soda off the counter between his teeth and hold his head up and drink it down." All deponents extolled Catherine's virtues as wife, mother, and housekeeper. Neighbor Julia Borland, for instance, stated that Catherine "has taken good care of [her husband]. He is always clean. His clothing looks very well and seems to be always ready for him."[48]

Catherine repeated the statements she had made in the recent affidavit but intensified the observations of her husband's drinking and his behavior under the influence. "When under the influence of liquor he is really insane. . . . Whenever he has been drinking the day or night before the next morning he is perfectly crazy and does not seem to know what he is doing." Catherine and daughter Mary were the only family members whom Hursh interviewed. They are the only deponents who asserted mental illness. Catherine mentioned Dunphy's stay at an asylum in 1874 and implied a concern that the children might be similarly affected. In her deposition, Catherine referred to their "boy," Stephen Bernard Dunphy (or Bert) "who has been confined to the Insane Asylum at Napa, but now the boy is at home [for a] trial, he has not been discharged. He will be 21 years of age April 17, 1900, or next April." Although there are no details about Dunphy's treatment of his children, Catherine blamed him: "I believe it was his ill treatment, while intoxicated, of our boy Stephen Bernard that made him insane." To those close to the family, Dunphy's behavior regarding drink constituted insanity. Pension officials, however, required a much higher standard for applying this label; excessive drinking did not suffice.[49]

Daughter Mary, now twenty-two and described in the affidavit as "assistant housekeeper," reported her father's "crazy" behavior. She recounted how she accompanied him to pay saloon debts, and once he "tried to force" her to put twenty dollars in his pocket to pay a "breweryman," but she refused. "He tried to make me do it right on the street, and get me up against the fence, but I did not do it. He frequently becomes intoxicated. He is generally out all day, and seldom comes home after supper until late at night. He comes around for his supper, and then goes out again and don't get home until later."[50]

Hursh obtained affidavits from Vallejo citizens, some of whom had known the Dunphy family for decades, including merchants, a real estate agent, a druggist, a jeweler, a dentist, a justice of the peace, and a physician (although not one who treated Dunphy). The consensus was that he was "not insane, but gets cross and cranky at times." All claimed hearsay knowledge about the drunkenness and expenditure of pension funds in saloons but declined to comment on family dynamics or mental illness. All attributed the drinking to Dunphy's lack of arms and associated depression. All placed confidence in Catherine to act as a guardian if necessary.[51]

Dunphy also supplied a statement but not a deposition. He first asserted his bona fides as a man: he declared that he was a veteran, a pensioner, and a married man with six sons and four daughters and that two sons currently served in the navy. Dunphy stated that Bernard had been placed in an asylum without his consent, that the asylum officials discharged him because they found no evidence of mental illness, "and that affiant can not to this day understand the object of said action on the part of his wife." Dunphy claimed to be a good husband and had saved money to purchase a homestead valued at over $5,000. Contradicting Catherine's statements, Dunphy stated that *she* cashed his pension checks and dealt directly with creditors. He added that his wife's behavior humiliated him, and "when he respectfully asks of his wife to give him an account of how his Pension money has been expended, she says it is none of his business and abuses him."[52]

Dunphy affirmed his manhood. He ran a household, reared and educated his children, and owned substantial property, but he could not accept his wife's behavior, which emasculated and feminized him by challenging his manly prerogatives to handle family finances and make important decisions about his children. His response to Catherine placing their son Bernard in an asylum was also a reflection of his own experience: Who committed him in 1874 and why? Or did he commit himself?

Although Hursh did not depone Dunphy, he spent time talking with him and concluded in a report to the commissioner that "the pensioner uses intoxicant liquors at times, and then becomes cross and seems to act foolish." Hursh pointed out that most of the testimony he collected "is of the heresay [*sic*] character and is such as might be circulated about any one who cannot live amicably with his wife." Hursh added that he learned that Catherine and Dunphy "have not lived amicably together for a great many years and although they live in the same house they seldom speak to each other." In his conversations with Dunphy, Hursh decided that the original Shepard letter contained exaggerated claims and unfounded observations, and he found the veteran "of ordinary intelligence, possessed of as good common sence [*sic*] as one will generally find in persons of his class." Hursh's letter summarized his conversation with Dunphy, who denigrated Catherine's behavior, explaining to the commissioner "that his wife for years had done nothing for him and that he had been depending for personal help upon some of his children. I also learned that they had not shared the same room for a good many years."[53]

Hursh dismissed Catherine's claims as exaggerations. He pointed out that Dunphy's last pension was duly deposited in a bank and that Catherine had claimed a portion for household expenses, thus disproving her claims that Dunphy refused to support her. He interviewed the parish Catholic priest—possibly the one mentioned by Shepard as having intervened in the Dunphy family's affairs—but Father Dugan told him that he did not know about Dunphy's conduct, although he acknowledged that the couple were not cohabiting. Hursh could not reconcile Catherine's claimed penury with his view of their "nice home, comfortably furnished, even with the luxury of a piano for the use of his daughters who have been fairly well educated," so "Mr. Dunphy cannot be such a dreadful spendthrift and bereft of all common sence [*sic*] as Mr. Shepard's letter would indicate." Hursh also dismissed the allegation that an abusive father drove his son Bernard into an asylum because the son had been serving in the navy for the past few years.

Hursh's judgment of the Dunphy family dynamic may have been influenced by the common prejudice against Irish immigrants, that one ought to expect conflict between spouses, especially with a shrewish, miserly wife. While admitting that he had tried marriage counseling with the couple, Hursh concluded that although he did not condone Dunphy spending his money in saloons, "I do not think that the Pension office should humiliate an old veteran like him to the extent of appointing a guardian . . . against his will and without having first been adjudged incompetent by a proper tribunal." He explained the legal process of declaring incompetency to Catherine and criticized her for having "made no effort to have him adjudicated incompetent for more than eight years."

Implicit in Hursh's investigation was the assumption that drunkenness was a behavioral trait in the expression of manhood. Consumption of liquor in moderation was a manly virtue. In Dunphy's case, Hursh viewed excessive drinking as a bad habit that could be governed with determination, a conclusion supported by Dunphy's presentation as competent and intelligent. Also, Hursh viewed claims of mental illness as requiring judicial scrutiny to verify. Even if the Dunphy home environment was worse than he found it, he would not interfere with Dunphy's pension, as doing so would humiliate and emasculate the veteran even more than his amputated arms had done. Hursh required no physical examination of Dunphy by a doctor that might have revealed the degradation of his body or other insights into Dunphy's health. Any pain he endured was not recorded. No one asked if the phantom sensations became more tolerable under liquor. Perhaps a physician's examination would have negated the dignity of manhood and humiliated Dunphy no matter the findings.

LEADING CITIZEN AND ARMLESS VETERAN

The 1900 census listed Dunphy, now fifty-eight, as head of a household that included his wife; sons Henry D. and George, both in their twenties; and daughters Mary, Teresa, Annie, and

Elizabeth, their ages between thirteen and twenty-three. Henry worked as a machinist, and George was employed as a blacksmith. Importantly, the census stated that Dunphy owned his home with no outstanding mortgage. Family peace remained elusive as the new century started with a bang: in 1901, son James W. shot and killed one Edward D. Stanton. The news coverage of the killing described James W. as the son of "a well-known armless pensioner living at Vallejo."[54]

James stalked Stanton because he had been "intimate with his [sixteen-year-old] sister and that he refused to marry her." Stanton had married another woman a month earlier. The newspaper stated, "The murder was an unusually ferocious one and was admittedly premeditated by the assassin." The trial took place barely two months later and concluded in a not-guilty verdict. The jury felt that the act was justifiable given the threats to James made by Stanton and his supporters. "When the jury was discharged, Catherine, who was seated beside him, threw her arms round his neck and wept while friends crowded round to congratulate him." Why the necessity to identify the armless veteran in the context of this homicide? Perhaps the reader was to infer that violence among Irish men should be expected or even that it was hereditary. The public mind connected a man whose body had been violently torn and disfigured in wartime with a son who avenges family honor by shooting a man down and then discharging five more shots into his prostrate body.[55]

Richard Dunphy's veteran body made another appearance in the press, this time as the True Cross in an article titled "Armless Veteran." At a meeting of navy veterans, Dunphy was cheered and celebrated as "the only armless man now receiving a pension from the Government." Comrades on either side of him held up his sleeves to reveal his stumps to the accolades of comrades. The same piece told a short story of love, dedication, and pride. While serving on Farragut's flagship, Dunphy was wounded by a shell fired from *Tennessee*, but "upon recovering he returned home and the girl who had promised to be his wife before he enlisted kept her promise and they were married." Ten children resulted from the marriage, and two of his sons were wounded in naval service during the Spanish-American War. "He receives a pension of $100 a month and is one of the leading citizens of Vallejo."[56]

In 1903, the leading citizen and armless veteran was in the news again, this time for suffering a violent attack under peculiar circumstances. Multiple newspapers reported that Dunphy and fellow veterans Michael Dorsey and Dan O'Sullivan gathered at the latter's house to drink. Once all three had become inebriated, an argument developed about the war. O'Sullivan, angered by the talk, produced a pistol and fired four shots that missed his companions, whereupon he drew a knife and began slashing. Newspapers reported that O'Sullivan "stabbed" Dunphy seventeen times, and another stated, perhaps more accurately, that he "was badly slashed on the face, neck and body and is weak from loss of blood." Another reported that Dunphy, "an armless veteran, a well known character in Grand Army [of the Republic] circles, was so severely stabbed that he may die."[57]

It is not known to what extent these knife wounds impaired Dunphy's health over the next year, but they might have contributed to his death at age sixty-two in San Francisco on November 23, 1904.[58] His health had deteriorated rapidly over the previous two months, and his cause of death was registered as "Hypostatic Pneumonia" with "Asthenia, Senility" given as contributory causes. "Hypostatic" referred to fluids pooling in the lungs, a condition suffered by some people who have been bedridden for long periods. "Asthenia" referred to lack of strength or energy, weakness. And senility? The description of senility in this context may have meant little more than diminished general health with age.[59] Thus died Dunphy's civic body. Dressed in a Prince Albert suit, Dunphy's body, per custom, remained at his home for the funeral service and was then moved to St. Vincent's Church in Vallejo where "a high requiem mass [was] celebrated for the repose of his soul."[60]

The date of death for Dunphy's pensioned body is ambiguous. Dunphy had received his last hundred-dollar monthly payment on September 4, 1904. A form in Dunphy's pension file certifies that he was duly "dropped because of death." Within two weeks of Dunphy's death, Catherine or her lawyer began another conversation with the pension authorities. As a widow, Catherine had to prove her bona fides as a veteran's wife. She duly filed a sworn statement by the assistant pastor at the Milwaukee church where she married her husband. She also filed an affidavit attesting that she had not been married before Dunphy and had been married to him for about forty years. Other relations contributed affidavits in which they swore that they had observed the wedding and asserted that Catherine had not been married previously. The Special Examinations Division of the pension office issued a report that recapitulated the 1899 investigation and its rejection of her plea to gain control over the pension. Catherine repeated her previous claims to highlight her family's situation as dependents of a deceased veteran. Her standing had eroded because of her husband's death.[61]

Reopening the Dunphy file, the pension office took depositions once again. Catherine deponed that her husband conveyed the deed to all real property to her in 1903, that aside from the house and its furnishings, she had no other assets and no money in the bank. She recounted the troubles of 1899 and said that she could have done more to protect the family but had been bedridden with a broken ankle. Unmarried and living at home, son Henry, thirty-three, a machinist when he could get work, deponed that when the two wage-earning sons were living at home, they contributed to the monthly income, but at present, they contributed nothing. The Vallejo wharf manager and neighbor attested to the family's looming penury and believed that the Dunphy home might realize some rental income from boarders, but the property was unattractive and needed repair. Catherine's deposition framed the family's financial difficulties as related to Dunphy's alcoholism and apparent selfishness.[62]

The pension examiner who deponed the family members wrote a "credibility report" to the commissioner of pensions. Importantly, the examiner was not involved in the 1899 inquiry and stated:

> I do know personally that Dunphy ought to have had a guardian. I myself saw him on the streets of Vallejo drunk a number of times and remarked . . . that I thought Dunphy ought to have some one to protect him from the leeches that were hanging about him, the men with Dunphy would actually put the whiskey glass to his mouth and take the money out of his pocket and pay for the drinks. He always wore a cape and though he had no arms he was considered quite a scrapper when drunk and about two years ago was cut up so badly in a drunken brawl that he lost about a gallon of blood and was too weak to talk for some time.

Citing Dunphy's earlier assessment of the value of his real estate as being about $5,000, the examiner wrote that Dunphy must have come up with that amount "while either drunk or otherwise irresponsible." He estimated the value at just above $1,000. Further, the house was not conveniently located for boarders who worked in the city. "Claimant's house is old and sadly lacks paint and repairs. It does not look attractive and is not what might be termed an easy renter." Finally, the examiner summed up the pension office's view throughout Dunphy's entire pension history: "Much was overlooked in the conduct of Dunphy because he had lost both arms and generally he was considered truthful, but there is no denying that he was a drunkard and when drunk was a tough character and irresponsible."[63]

Catherine Dunphy, a widow who earned a small amount of money cooking and housekeeping for others, was granted a pension of eight dollars[64] per month in May 1905, thus ending her claims on the federal government. Later that year, the Dunphy family received more press, which, to some readers, probably reinforced opinions about the family. The local paper reported, under the title "Government Drops Unpopular Employee," that George Dunphy, a workman at the navy yard, "a son of the late Richard Dunphy, who lost both arms in the battle of Mobile Bay," and a deserter from the navy, had been blacklisted by the Department of Labor for perjuring himself on government documents. He had also informed on rules violations of a popular foreman at the yard, yet another example of poor behavior from a son of the notorious armless veteran of Vallejo.[65]

A few years later, in November 1909, Catherine died at age sixty-four, and her husband's pension body died as well, file closed. The pension agency had increased her pension payment to twelve dollars.[66] She claimed her final payment on September 4, 1909.[67]

CONCLUSION: A DISCORDANT BODY

In the early twentieth century, many people believed that maimed veterans ought to receive the best medical attention and be integrated into the workplace as soon as practicable. Those matters settled; veterans should just get on with their lives. Veterans' visible wounds still elicited wariness, pity, and avoidance among people. Invisible wounds were not ignored; they were just not acknowledged. In Dunphy's case, Catherine's persistent claims of mental illness and insanity went unheeded. Pension authorities left the armless veteran alone and relegated his antisocial behaviors to Dunphy and his family to sort out. It is tempting to apply modern standards of psychology, its classification of disorders and therapies, to Dunphy's era. Because of the apparent lack of psychological judgments by pension doctors, some historians perceive that Civil War veterans just found their own ways to deal with things. This is not necessarily a correct assumption.[68]

Those soldiers who were not survivors of grievous wounds but who nevertheless got through the war found ways to come to terms with the deaths they witnessed or caused. There was no mention of posttraumatic stress disorder in the medical literature of the time because no one in authority—whether medical or political—asked veterans for their views. Those veterans who faltered in later years were boosted by fellow veterans, usually through their fraternal association, the Grand Army of the Republic. There are several references to Dunphy in the contemporary press that attest to some participation in the GAR or similar organization. We can infer that in this environment, Dunphy's sanity was never doubted, his alcoholism was tolerated, and his manhood was respected.

In Dunphy's time, the pension office was the closest institution to today's federal Department of Veterans Affairs. Its medical intervention into the lives of former soldiers was limited to that which supported a pension increase or sustained a current pension. The term *disability* is mentioned frequently in nineteenth-century pension documents, but the evolving meaning of this term "was a contributory process" that began with the initial debility claimed by the soldier, verified by a physician, and endorsed by the pension office. Later, examining doctors appointed by the pension office modified or restated the description of the disability. Finally, the pension office made a decision that constituted the governing benchmark of disability in the veteran's health history.[69]

"Disability does not equal ruin and despair." Richard Dunphy lacked the supportive environment of his home in Kilkenny, Ireland, but he chose to serve the Union cause despite clear risks, and for the rest of his life, he viewed his stumps as a bodily Medal of Honor. We have no evidence of his living under a pall of self-pity or using his disability to gain sympathy. He viewed his pension without shame: the government, in his view, was fulfilling a contractual obligation. He owned a house and bought adjacent lots to develop them to make money, and he had a menial but honorable job at the navy yard as a courier. He maintained visibility in a community of fellow veterans. And he married and raised a family. This, then, was his civic body.[70]

There is no question that Dunphy's drinking increasingly put his self-image as a patriarch at odds with the views of his wife. He failed to admit that his drinking created a perception within his community that he was mentally unstable and allowed himself to be taken advantage of. His staggering gait was embarrassing to witness. Dunphy exaggerated the worth of his estate, and his property lost value. His home fell into disrepair. The sources of additional income that he cited to pension authorities either dried up or were nonexistent. But through all of his adverse circumstances, it was impossible for him to pass as an average workingman. His stumps told anyone all that they needed to know about his life. He was the "armless veteran." That is all that he could ever be: his disability defined him despite anything he might have done to change that image. His body would forever be a static, mutilated thing; manhood nearly evaporated when that shell exploded near him in 1864.

We have seen how Dunphy's bodily narrative partially comported with the facts. His body, however—and the bodies of the other men examined in this book—presented a complex narrative for anyone who cared to look closely, as Mitchell did. Even Dunphy's civic and pension bodies, though, cannot be trusted absolutely. To doctors, the amputee's body was a static relic. To fellow citizens, it was a threat to social order. Social unease could be mitigated by a pension for the discordant body. Over time, all actors—veterans, doctors, families, and communities—engaged with damaged civic, pension, and veterans' bodies through a haze of nostalgia resulting in a loss of focus on the meaning of the war, even at places of Civil War destruction and memorialization. These places include those locations where civic and veterans' bodies were on display at commemorative events, GAR celebrations, and images of benign, bearded old men on patriotic postcards. Dunphy may have continuously reinterpreted the meaning of his bodily Medal of Honor with the times.

Thanks to Mitchell, we know that Dunphy's body was not static: his stumps altered shape and size over time. Phantom sensations were always present. An outsider may have seen Dunphy on the sidewalk wearing a cape to protect (or conceal?) his stumps, but no one would realize that he still sensed the phantom presence of his arms. No one would know that Dunphy still felt his hands, his fingers curled around his thumbs. He claimed to have experienced no pain with these sensations: perhaps his excessive drinking was due less to having stumps for arms than to the incessant, exasperating sensation that his arms were still there.

In November 2019, the week of Veterans Day, the local Vallejo paper ran a feature on Richard Dunphy showing one of his carte de visite poses with pinned-up sleeves on his naval uniform. The article presented an overview of his life both before and after his wounding aboard *Hartford*.

The article was titled "Tough Times for Armless Civil War Vet in Vallejo." Dunphy's armlessness even preceded his name in the article's title. What his body lacked had become his perennial identity to a posterity with its nostalgic view of the war.[71]

SIX

PRESTLEY DORSEY/DAWSON

(1842?–1907)

VERY DANGEROUS PLACES

In early August 1864, Private Prestley Dawson marched to an encampment near the miles-long entrenchments surrounding Petersburg, Virginia, an engineering spectacle that must have astounded him. He was becoming accustomed to Virginia's intense, sizzling summer heat though he perspired heavily under his blue woolen sack coat and the knapsack and bedroll he carried on his back. Four months earlier, in Lancaster, Pennsylvania, Dawson swore his oath of allegiance to the Union as a recruit before Captain Thaddeus Stevens, the namesake of his famous abolitionist uncle in the Congressional House of Representatives. Dawson had come from an obscure background, likely one of slavery, to serve the cause of the Union and achieve his freedom.

Throughout the spring and summer of 1864, General Ulysses S. Grant's Overland Campaign had been grinding south through Virginia, forcing relentless battles and skirmishes that diminished and pushed Confederate forces into a defensive corridor from Richmond, the Confederate capital, to Petersburg, thirty miles away. By the time Dawson arrived, a protracted siege had been in progress around Petersburg—Richmond still in Confederate hands—to eliminate the town's transportation nexus for trains supporting troop movements and supplies. Dawson's regiment, the Forty-Third United States Colored Infantry,[1] had departed understrength from Camp William Penn near Philadelphia, the first and largest federal training camp for black soldiers. Once Dawson's Company H had achieved full strength, it was sent south to join the regiment. Near Petersburg, black soldiers, including the Forty-Third, were present in great numbers to constitute the Fourth Division, Ninth Corps. One division surgeon, Francis Minot Weld, who entered military service to advocate for the emancipation of enslaved people, wrote, "Negro troops are in high repute here, and are almost universally welcome. Even the copperhead element, which is very small indeed, is willing that the poor blacks should shield them from bullets."[2]

Sergeant John C. Brock of the Forty-Third described this welcome in more personal terms: "The very people, who three years ago, crouched at their master's feet, on the accursed soil of Virginia, now march in a victorious column of freemen, over the same land. The change seems almost miraculous." Many soldiers of the United States Colored Troops (USCT) expressed amazement at the constant stream of refugees from enslavement and the omnipresent, oppressive landscape of war. To be seen as rescuers, as kin to Virginia's refugees and as empowered men in the same uniforms as white soldiers gave black soldiers a particular surge of pride, power, and agency that their white comrades did not experience. Dawson would have agreed with Sergeant Brock: "We have been instrumental in liberating some five hundred of our sisters and brethren from the accursed yoke of human bondage. The slaves come flocking to us from every part of the country. You see them coming in every direction, some in carts, some on their masters' horses, and great numbers on foot, carrying their bundles on their heads. They manifest their love for liberty by every possible emotion."[3]

Once bivouacked with the rest of his regiment, Dawson greeted old comrades, learned of their adventures, and hurried, head down, along the trenches to see the crater that his fellow soldiers excitedly told him about. Enemy sharpshooters waited for enemy heads to bob up into view, and Confederate cannons and sporadic gunfire threatened incessantly. Dawson was amazed at the large gathering of black soldiers in this forbidding and foreign landscape. Massive earthworks lined trenches, and the outward slopes were studded with sharpened tree poles to disorient and stall attacking troops. The inner side of the trenchworks rose high to support gun platforms, which were relatively secure behind breastworks supported by horizontal stacks of logs that were held in place by shorter uprights. Sandbags stacked on the earthworks permitted artillery crews to work their weapons without exposing themselves to sharpshooters. At dawn on July 30, Union soldiers detonated a mine planted under rebel trench works mere yards away. The explosion immediately killed hundreds, opened a breach in the defenses, and created the crater. When Dawson saw the crater, it was strewn with battle debris and human body parts. The hole was about 30 feet deep and 170 feet wide by 80 feet broad, roughly the size of half of a football field. Dawson was proud of his regiment and the role it played that day.

Major Matthew R. Mitchell, who served with another regiment in Dawson's division, the Twenty-Seventh United States Colored Infantry Regiment, and had fought at the Battle of the Crater, recalled "marching in double quick up that approach to the crater and through it, stepping over dead and wounded, and taking a position on the right of the crater." He remembered the parallel advance by Dawson's regiment. "With great bravery the officers and men of the Forty-Third charged the enemy's fully manned entrenchments, which they took and there captured two hundred prisoners, who exceeded in number the men remaining in their regiment. They also captured a stand of rebel colors and re-took colors which had that morning been taken from a regiment of Union troops." Shortly, however, the attack faltered: troops were led into the crater with no place to go and could not climb out. Despite black troops training for this assault for weeks, at the last minute, fearing criticism should the troops bear high casualties, generals sent in white soldiers untrained for the assault who made sporadic attempts to prevent the rebels from regrouping. But regroup they did, and the counterattack drove the Union back with many losses, the rebels shooting or bayonetting wounded black soldiers on the battlefield. As in other battles where black troops fought, Confederate soldiers were enraged and insulted at having to confront them and exercised no quarter on the battlefield. Afterward, captured black soldiers were either sold into slavery or executed.[4]

Exhausted from this futile battle, soldiers of the Forty-Third were put to fatigue labor, digging trenches, building breastworks, creating casemates and bombproofs (shelters built into or against berms lining the trenches), occasionally returning taunts yelled from enemy lines. The weather was ghastly: unrelenting heat, high humidity, and endless dust. Dr. Weld wrote home, "We have not had a drop of rain for three weeks. I think not for four, and the whole country is like an oven. Sunstrokes among the soldiers are common, and they suffer very much from the heat." Even for soldiers accustomed to grueling labor, Petersburg was a nightmare of fatigue, broken bodies, malnutrition, dehydration, and sunstroke. Sergeant Brock wrote, "Our division has built two immense forts, connected by a long chain of breastworks. Sometimes [our soldiers] were in the trenches; in very dangerous places, the bullets whistling over and among our troops all day and all night long, while the men were engaged in digging."[5]

On or about August 28, under the sporadic shelling of Union trenches and while possibly building a bombproof, Private Dawson was working under a disintegrating section of breastwork when the retaining posts gave way and released a load of heavy tree trunks, one of which crashed into his right leg, dislocating his patella and crushing parts of his tibia and fibula.

Civil War physicians defined a dislocation or luxation of a bone as "the escape of its articulating extremity nearest the trunk from the corresponding surface [that] may be caused by a direct force knocking the head of the bone into its false position, or by violence acting upon the distal end, the whole bone forming a lever by means of which its head is displaced." The recommended procedure in such a case was to anesthetize the patient and then carefully straighten the limb. The surgeon would gently push the bones back into place. "Failing in this, he should divide subcutaneously the fibrous structures which hinder the reduction, cutting if necessary even the ligamentum patellae."[6]

When Dawson enlisted on April 21, 1864, the army recorded a physical description and a brief personal history. The latter consisted of three statistics: age, birthplace, and occupation. If Dawson had been enslaved before the war, his sole recorded identity in any governmental record would have been in a slave schedule to the federal census. With rare exceptions, names of enslaved persons were not given, only age, sex, and race. The latter category overwhelmingly listed these people as black, with fewer as mulatto, or light skinned. Doubtless, no white person had ever asked Dawson for his personal history before enlisting. The army began its administrative categorization of Dawson's body by listing his age as twenty-four, his birthplace as Howard County, Maryland, and his occupation as laborer. Signing with an X, Dawson agreed to serve for three years and swore allegiance to the United States of America, also something no one had ever asked of him.

On the day of his enlistment, Dawson underwent a medical examination. Enlistment examinations could be brief and cursory or, if army regulations were to be observed, take up to a half hour. The physician who signed the "Volunteer Enlistment" form attested that Dawson was "free from all bodily defects and mental infirmity, which would in any way disqualify him from performing the duties of a soldier." The army now possessed his body for military service and described him as being five foot, eight inches tall and having dark hair, a yellow complexion, and hazel eyes. He also had a scar on the outside of his left thigh.[7]

When Dawson began his training at Camp William Penn, he evidently displayed leadership ability because he was promoted to corporal on April 29. In July, as his company marched out of camp to Virginia, the army reduced his rank to private. This reduction may have been the result of misbehavior, or the army might have intended the higher rank as a temporary expedient. That Dawson was nonliterate may have made him ineligible for promotion. The military record shows no reason for the demotion.

When Dawson collapsed in the trench under the falling breastworks, comrades came to his aid to move the logs and assess his injuries. Dawson apparently showed that the damage was minimal by standing up and walking, now with a limp that became a permanent lameness. His comrades likely took him to the regimental surgeon. If so, the doctor may have advised a short period of bed rest in camp or prescribed a medication to reduce pain or relax muscles. Whatever transpired, the army has no record of any hospital treatment for Dawson's leg and knee injury during the war or at any time after.

Sometime in August, however, while Dawson labored in the trenches, a female *Anopheles* mosquito, recently bred in nearby stagnant water near the shore of the James River, landed on Dawson's neck or arms and drank his blood. Earlier, the mosquito had feasted on a soldier whose blood infected the insect with a malarial parasite that evolved into sporozoites, which entered Dawson through the mosquito's bite. These sporozoites infected his liver cells and became schizonts, which burst and released a mutation called merozoites into his red blood cells. There they matured and destroyed those cells. Some of the merozoites became gametocytes that entered feeding mosquitoes, where male and female gametocytes mated and began the cycle again. Once Dawson's blood became infected, the clinical symptoms of *Plasmodium falciparum*,[8] the most severe and common form of malaria in the South, expressed themselves. "Illness is the night-side of life. . . . Everyone who is born holds dual citizenship, in the kingdom of the well and in the kingdom of the sick." Dawson would live with this dual citizenship for the rest of his days.[9]

From the time of the mosquito bite, within only a week, he developed feverish sweating alternating with chills and suffered episodes of vomiting, weakness, body aches, and general lassitude. Without treatment (which, apart from quinine, was palliative), malarial fever could degenerate into blindness, epilepsy, or a worse mental deterioration. The symptoms might abate for long periods, then recur with disabling attacks that lasted for hours at a time.[10]

Civil War physicians did not realize that mosquitoes were not only a vector of the disease but also a cohost with humans in a complex cycle. Dawson's regimental surgeons understood malaria through the behavior of its associated fevers. Fevers, in fact, constituted a category of disease at the time and were classified by their duration and recurrence. *P. falciparum*'s fever was classified as tertian because it appeared in cycles about two days apart. Nevertheless, physicians understood that quinine, a derivative of cinchona bark, reduced malaria's symptoms and apparent impact. To understand malaria (as identified by the tertian appearance of the symptoms), the surgeon would have been frustrated to find no discussion of diseases experienced by black bodies in a medical textbook.[11]

One of the most inventive and brilliant minds in the army medical service, assistant surgeon Joseph Janvier Woodward published a guide on diagnosing and treating diseases in military camps. He found that three "influences" framed the most prevalent and troublesome diseases there: "malaria, crowd poisoning, and the scorbutic taint [scurvy]." Worse, these diseases cooccurred and were rarely distinct from one another. Seasonally recurring malaria, observed Woodward, "or *marsh miasm*, is a cause of disease . . . with which very few facts are actually susceptible of demonstration." He noted its "intermittent and remittent" nature with recurring symptoms and explained that "the essential condition of its existence is usually affirmed to be vegetable decomposition . . . [that] acting upon the economy through the respiratory tract chiefly, produces the disease."[12]

Despite this assertion, Woodward conceded that the precise cause remained unknown. Most opinions on the matter were "all as yet equally undemonstrated, and without any actual foundation in fact." If vegetable decomposition was not the cause of malaria (etymology: "bad air"), it must at least "be *one of the most important of the determining conditions.*" In Dawson's case, a diagnosis of malaria was probably strengthened by the belief that "dry and prolonged hot weather of great intensity is most generally the condition which accompanies [malarial symptoms'] unusual frequency." The patient might experience diarrhea and dysentery via malarial poisoning, "a sallow or yellowish complexion, generally accompanied by more or less emaciation, with disturbed bowels, disordered appetite, yellowness of the conjunctiva, torpor of the intellectual functions, debility, and a disinclination to exertion of every kind; oedema [swelling] or dropsical effusion."[13]

The military leadership in Washington preferred to deploy black soldiers to the South because of the widespread belief that black bodies were inherently immune or resistant to tropical diseases such as malaria and yellow fever. For example, in 1863, the military governor of New Orleans requested black soldiers to garrison forts because of white soldiers' susceptibility to these diseases, to which the army surgeon general agreed. Some authorities believed that soldiers from northern states might be susceptible because of the rarity of malaria in their districts, including Maryland, Dawson's home state. The mix of white and black soldiers compounded misunderstandings about the origin and spread of malaria and associated fevers. Plantations, for example, with a nucleus of white people and a community of enslaved people, constituted public health nightmares. The living environment of impoverished enslaved people harbored an endless cycle of diseases often characterized by fevers and respiratory and digestive maladies. As we know now, mosquitoes spread malaria, flies proliferate typhoid and cholera, an army of parasitic microorganisms infect water sources, and parasitic worms afflict animals and people.[14]

As a general prophylactic measure—apart from daily doses of quinine—Woodward recommended that soldiers "shall have coffee and biscuit immediately after reveille in the morning and before proceeding to any exercise or exposure." Otherwise, a restorative diet and rest were prescribed until the patient returned to health. Dawson would have followed the command to "fall out for quinine" and lined up for a cup of the mixture (naturally bitter). Despite this ration, he nevertheless experienced sporadic returns of symptoms for the rest of his life.[15]

With Dawson's onset of alternating chills and fevers, the surgeon of the Forty-Third recognized malarial fever on September 18 and sent him to the Hospital for Colored Troops at nearby City Point (Hopewell, Virginia), an enormous, temporary military depot and staging area where General Grant maintained a lodging. The hospital complex with its streets of tents was an organizational marvel. Edward B. Dalton, a surgeon with the US Volunteers and chief medical officer of the City Point Hospital, submitted to his superior a report noting that by the end of 1864, the hospital could manage 10,000 patients in 110 hospital buildings and 1,200 tents spread over 200 acres. Based on a compilation of daily reports, Dalton determined that between mid-May and the end of October 1864, 68,540 soldiers were hospitalized for at least two days. Of this number, 51,313 were transferred to general hospitals in several northern cities. Dalton described the predominant sicknesses treated to include "dysentery, diarrhea, and malarial fevers." Many of these cases, he continued, were comparatively mild ones that "do not properly come under the head of either of the recognized classes of malarious fever, but were rather cases of a depressed condition not inaptly expressed by the term malarial malaise. A large proportion of these recovered rapidly and entirely under the influence of rest, cleanliness, and good nourishment, together with moderate administration of quinine and iron." We see by Dawson's longer-than-usual hospital convalescence that his was a severe case.[16]

A wartime nurse, observing the Union wounded in the hospital, wrote, "Illness is itself an occupation . . . how did [hospitalized soldiers] ever get through the long and weary hours?" Dawson endured a long hospital stay for "Malarial debility." He probably found his hospital a wonder. If he had any association with hospitals, he would have thought that poor people died in them. Here, however, an African American doctor and several nurses may have been in attendance. At this time, around a dozen black doctors had been appointed to the US Bureau for Colored Troops, although most black regiments were medically understaffed. Also, wards in white hospitals for black soldiers or the few hospitals devoted to black soldiers received second-class status, being inadequately supplied and not as clean as white wards. Dawson sufficiently recovered to return to his regiment on November 30, marking a hospital stay of nine to ten weeks. Six weeks constituted an average length of stay for serious illnesses.[17]

Dawson returned to the trenches having recovered from a malarial attack but without any treatment for his leg or acknowledgment of his limp (no mention of it occurs in the muster rolls). His leg healed to some extent over time, but a later examination revealed unhealed bone fractures pushing against the skin. His knee and lower leg remained painful to the touch to the end of his life. A later deposition by Dawson's second wife described him as walking with a limp as his right foot turned out to the side with each step.

In November, the regiment was posted along the James River and remained there until black troops were organized into a single large unit, the Twenty-Fifth Corps. In January 1865, in the last action in which Dawson participated, his regiment opposed Confederate gunboats trying to sail south on the James River to attack Union ships and shore fortifications and capture City Point. Just before General Robert E. Lee surrendered at Appomattox, Virginia, in early April, the men of the Forty-Third were among the first troops to enter Richmond. For the newly liberated black citizens of the city, the sight of black soldiers was emotionally overwhelming. Shortly thereafter, the regiment was ordered to City Point to await transfer to Texas. Dawson and his comrades embarked on steamboats headed for a posting along the southern Rio Grande to protect the border against any attempts of Confederates who might mass in Mexico for an attack.

However Dawson managed his recurring malarial symptoms, he evidently saw himself as fit for duty—as did his supervising officers—while embarking to Texas for an indefinite period. Three weeks after departing City Point, the Twenty-Fifth Corps arrived at the barrier island of Brazos Santiago at the mouth of the Rio Grande, a waste about five miles long and half a mile wide. Soldiers fortified a small fort on the island erected during the Mexican War almost two decades earlier, set up camps on sand dunes, and organized patrols along the border in the vicinity of Brownsville, a small town upriver opposite Matamoros, Mexico. The Forty-Third was ordered to march to camp in Brownsville. The town had switched sides a few times during the war. For the Confederacy, it served as a conduit for sending cotton south into Mexico to export to Europe, thus avoiding the Union blockade. The twenty-five thousand men of the war-worn Twenty-Fifth Corps were in no condition to meet their new duty. Chief of Staff and Major General Henry Halleck had stated before their departure to Mexico that the entire corps was "poorly officered and in bad discipline, and altogether unfitted for the military occupation of Virginia."[18]

The army effectively abandoned the troops. Sent to a distant outpost of the reunited country, the soldiers were not resupplied and were left to fend for themselves. Just two weeks after landing at Brazos Santiago, Private Noah Davis, Eighth United States Colored Infantry Regiment, entered the military hospital in Brownsville with scurvy. He and his fellows had eaten little beyond salt pork and hardtack and contended with reduced rations of water, as no fresh water source could be found on the island. Assistant Surgeon Ida Perry recorded that Davis's "gums were red and bled occasionally; his legs became swollen and shortly after ulcerated. . . . He was somewhat emaciated and so weak as to be confined to bed. He had a diarrhoea of eight to twelve evacuations daily." Dr. Perry used a local remedy, pulque, a thick white drink made from fermented maguey (*Agave americana*) sap, popular throughout central and northern Mexico. Despite taking pulque, Davis died a month after entering the hospital.[19]

A comrade from the Forty-Third, Timothy Shaw, who enlisted at the end of June, was patrolling the border opposite Matamoros. In a letter home, he complained of the vanishing rations and mentioned the heat, insects, lack of vegetables, and scurvy cases. He noticed the declining number of soldiers fit for duty, and, although feeling scorbutic symptoms himself, he avoided reporting to sick call because "I thought him [the regimental surgeon] no good and took the best care I could of myself." Nevertheless, by October, the month his regiment was due to leave Texas to muster out, he was ill enough to attend sick call. Over the summer, scurvy was epidemic. Between 60 and 80 percent of all black soldiers had come down with it.[20]

On August 20, 1865, "Prestley Dorsley" was admitted to the Brownsville hospital for "Malarial Fever." A handwritten note in Dawson's pension file, apparently a continuation from another document and undated but presumably written by either a pension officer or examining doctor, gives a clue to Dawson's recurring symptoms: "in Fall of 1865 at Brownsville Texas lasted 3 weeks. Has had 4 attacks upon an average each year lasting a week to 10 days. Lost 1/3 of his time." The description is consistent with the long-term effects of *P. falciparum* and *P. vivax*.

Whatever treatment Dawson received enabled him to convalesce among his bedridden scorbutic comrades. In its first weeks, the hospital logged 842 patients, half of whom had scurvy. For those who died in the hospital, the common cause of death was diarrhea caused by scurvy and compounded by dysentery. The Forty-Third's camp nearby was a hellish place. The black soldiers were forbidden to forage for food. One soldier described Brownsville as "one of the most forsaken looking holes you ever saw."[21]

The army's neglect of its black troops remains unfathomable. Army leadership recognized the salutary effects of fresh vegetables and fruit (which could be provided canned) but failed to supply the Twenty-Fifth Corps. "Hundreds of men died without seeing a single hostile action, and the army's response was to deny and cover up its officers' obvious malfeasance . . . but its taproot was a callous disregard for the 25,000 black men transferred there without adequate food or water." The neglect of black soldiers in Texas is hardly mentioned in histories of the war, mainly because of the army's reluctance to acknowledge it. But former army surgeon and influential physician in the United States Sanitary Commission Sanford Hunt criticized the army for not doing enough "to prevent one of the most remarkable and extensive prevalences of scurvy that the world has known, from occurring in the Rio Grande Expedition after the war had closed. . . . The latter instance is one for which there was no sufficient excuse."[22]

The army, however, had an excuse: it blamed the black body. Provost Marshal General James B. Fry wrote a report that confirmed common stereotypes about black male bodies, noting how they were "less able than the white to endure the exposures and annoyances of military service." That black bodies failed to hold up to white ones was due to moral causes, "that the great susceptibility of the colored man to disease rose from lack of heart, hope, and mental activity, and that a higher moral and intellectual culture would diminish the defect."[23]

On October 14, just days before Dawson's regiment was due to muster out of military service, the hospital released him, nearly two months after he had entered it. He found the Forty-Third packing up to leave, accounting for equipment and absent soldiers, and submitting final paperwork to the corps commander. Dawson may still have had scurvy symptoms and was not free of malarial ones. Nonetheless, he was hustled out of service.

If Dawson continued to suffer malarial symptoms upon leaving Brownsville and was possibly still recovering from scurvy, the trip home for mustering out proved a threat to his entire regiment. Soon after, he boarded a ship from Brownsville to Philadelphia. The ship leaked and eventually flooded and stalled the steam engine. For days, Dawson and his regimental comrades bailed water and threw overboard both horses and supplies to lighten the ship. Finally, the pilot ran the steamer aground at the mouth of the Mississippi. Troubled by the near sinking, the noncommissioned officers requested to travel by train and offered to buy their own tickets. Dawson and the other lesser ranks remained with the ship. By late November, he found himself in Philadelphia where the regiment received its final pay and mustered out.[24]

A SPECTRAL MAN

Dawson's narrative reveals inconsistencies and questions about his identity. Consequently, within the historical record, he fades in and out of focus. As he was nonliterate, there is no written personal account, except when he marked an X to confirm his identity. His enlistment document gave his surname as Dawson, and subsequent military records maintained the identification,

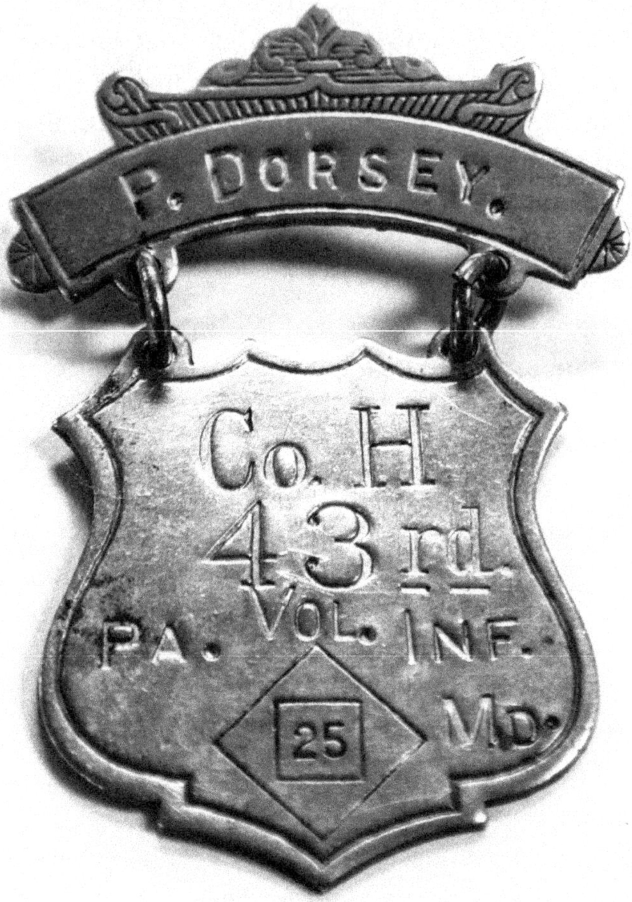

Veterans' badge inscribed for Prestley Dorsey/Dawson, Company H, Forty-Third Pennsylvania Volunteer Infantry, Maryland (home state), Twenty-Fifth Corps. *Credit: Dawson family, courtesy Gail A. Dawson.*

but pension and other public records list his surname as Dorsey. His first name was spelled Prestley or Presley, but in pension depositions by friends and relatives, he was called Press. Dawson was the name chosen for his military service. In civilian postwar life, he went by Dorsey and placed his X on sworn statements as

Dorsey. When his family members gave depositions to support pensions for his second wife, they used the surname Dawson. The name Dorsey was used in most census counts.[25]

Although Dawson enlisted in Lancaster, Pennsylvania, it is not known how he came to be there. We know nothing of his prewar relatives or friends; pension and other public records link no one to his prewar past. The only friends and relatives listed in the record date to after the war: neighbors, business acquaintances, and Dawson's immediate family. He gave his birth year as early as 1840 and as late as 1842. While in a later deposition his son recalled Dawson's mention of a Maryland boyhood, there is no evidence of his birth there. Military and pension records show his birthplace to be either Harford or Howard County in Maryland. His grandson, Thomas Dawson, said that as he grew up, his grandfather's background was never discussed, and he knew that it was not to be discussed. Thomas Dawson admitted the possibility that his grandfather may have been enslaved before the war.[26]

It is reasonable to infer from the scant available evidence that Dawson had been enslaved on a farm in what became Howard County, Maryland (created as a district in 1839, then a county in 1851). Although Dawson gave his birthplace as Howard or Harford County, a map of the latter from the 1870s shows no residences with the name Dorsey. In Howard County, however, the name abounds: Dorseyville, Dorseys Switch Station, Dorseys Run Station, Dorseys Mill Station, and at least twenty farms named for a Dorsey. Dawson might have appropriated the name Dorsey from a previous owner. He may have used other surnames aside from Dorsey.[27]

Most of the slave owners in the northern counties maintained small farms that produced cereals, unlike the labor-intensive tobacco farms elsewhere. Many of the slave-owning Dorseys in Howard County possessed only one or two enslaved persons. If this was Dawson's enslaved background, he must have performed generalized work as a "laborer," meaning that he performed various types of manual labor. Veterans who described themselves as laborers changed jobs more often than skilled men, but Dawson does not seem to have moved frequently or far from his place of birth. He may have developed farming skills with cereal crops that enabled his postwar success. Soon after the war, he identified himself as a farmer.[28]

If enslaved, Dawson might have been known to a white master by only one name. Many enslaved African Americans during this time had different surnames than their owners. Many used surnames hidden from white people. "Neither their owners nor their Yankee liberators usually realized that many slaves carried surnames into freedom." Research on black Civil War veterans shows that many who had entered service from enslavement abandoned their slave owners' surnames and adopted new ones, taking "names that reflected family connections through the male line. . . . Former slaves adopted their fathers' last names even if they had never known their fathers, and even if they were white." Perhaps Dawson's father was a white Dorsey.[29]

The different dates and places of birth in Dawson's records do not mean that he equivocated when this information was demanded of him. He had little contact with white people who required this information. If Dawson had been enslaved, his identity would not have been of interest to anyone. Judging from slave schedules in the federal census, many Maryland Dorseys were slave owners, but the schedules recorded only age, sex, and race. If Dawson was free and had been interviewed by a census taker, he may have provided information that a white notetaker would have considered to be inaccurate.[30] All historical records featuring Dawson's name were documented by white individuals who transcribed it phonetically.

Dawson may have faced another challenge in communicating with white people in authority, particularly military ones: his speech may have been difficult for white people to understand.

Although white officers commanded black troops, little camaraderie existed between them. To many white officers, black soldiers were boys, despite their bravery and battlefield honors. White doctors, possibly the only white military men with whom Dawson communicated directly, would likely have assumed that a nonliterate black man lacked intelligence and believed superstitions about his body and health. Even in the USCT regiments, white doctors were of uneven temperament and ability. Some openly abused their patients. Some would not touch black bodies. In private correspondence, Dr. Weld expressed his reservations about one of the doctors administering to black soldiers. This doctor, an assistant surgeon to the Twenty-Seventh United States Colored Infantry Regiment, was "not a very brilliant man. He does not allow men to have anything but rheumatism or pneumonia. His treatment for them is one and the same, viz. Dover's Powder[31] frequently repeated till death or recovery ensues."[32]

Those doctors who cared about the health of their black patients might still confront cultural barriers. Aside from a negative response to the patient's blackness and racist associations with physically and morally dirty living, white doctors distrusted their black patients, whose emotional expressions through prayer meetings (known as "shouts") and when in the company of comrades seemed excessive. Masculinity among white men connoted emotional control, not extremes of expression. This perceived excess of emotion was seen as contributing to poor health, a "mental suggestibility as inherent in the black body [that] flourished in the proslavery scientific racism of the 1850s and appeared regularly in medical journals."[33]

In comparison with the white soldiers whose lives are examined in this book, Dawson's body seems difficult to bring into focus. The ambiguous nature of the malaria that twice put him in the hospital reflects how malaria was broadly defined at the time, particularly its consequences for black soldiers. A medical axiom dictated that black bodies were resilient to southern diseases arising from miasmas, particularly malaria. Physicians associated malaria with the southern states that, they believed, constituted an environment distinct from northern states. Worse for black soldiers, prevailing medical belief viewed quinine as unnecessary for them. Yet black soldiers experienced on average 2.4 cases per soldier with a 3 percent mortality rate, compared with 2.7 cases for white soldiers and a 1.73 percent mortality rate. Typho-malarial cases increased the mortality rate to 2.6 percent for white soldiers and 5.0 percent for black soldiers.[34] These data are grounded in the medical parlance of the 1860s that classed malaria as a periodic fever. The specific disease by that name was not defined until the 1880s.[35]

The ambiguous nature of Presley Dawson's body also derived from his skin color. Given the military description of his hazel eyes, light skin color, and wavy hair, he may have been a mulatto, the epithet of the day that described people of mixed white and black blood. The federal census by 1860 offered mulatto as a racial category. Based on military statistics, mulattoes constituted a higher percentage of USCT soldiers than in proportion to the civilian population. White society viewed a mulatto man as occupying "a sort of junior manhood." Dawson was aware that his body undoubtedly discomforted white people.[36]

If Dawson had difficulty communicating with a white physician and vice versa, there was no way for him to understand his body, the white doctor's methods and ways of perceiving illness, and the precise meaning of malaria. Success in a medical interaction depends on shared assumptions and values about health and illness between patient and doctor. As a social construction, "disease is at once a biological event," a cultural history of medical ideology and practice, and a component of personal and professional identity. In all of Dawson's interactions with physicians, "disease concepts mediate[d] and structure[ed] relationships."[37]

Based on Woodward's book on camp diseases, the regimental doctor relegated most diseases to the zymotic class, which has "ill-understood causes" but nevertheless "modify profoundly the normal condition of the whole system." Woodward divided this class into three orders, one of which was miasmatic diseases or those arising from the decomposition of vegetable or human bodily matter. This order included malaria and the range of fevers associated with dysentery or yellow fever. Within Civil War practice, however, debate about the nature of and limits to contagion challenged the zymotic theory. The debate weighed the sources of miasmas against individual susceptibility to disease. The anticontagionists believed that decomposing matter generated miasmas that contaminated the air and posed risks to people with susceptible constitutions. Contagionists located communicable diseases within the exhalations of sick people and therefore focused on appraising the human body holistically, considering personal habits, the constitution of the body, diet, and environmental factors.[38]

Northern and southern doctors and plantation owners agreed on the resistance of black bodies to fevers, a heightened tolerance to extremes of heat and cold, and an increased susceptibility over white bodies to intestinal and respiratory diseases. These views still prevailed after the war in the practice of physicians who aided newly emancipated people through the Freedmen's Bureau, a new institution devoted to acculturating formerly enslaved people via grants and other aid. Bureau doctors viewed black bodies as inferior to white bodies and served freed black people "through the highly charged ideological prism of the South as a distinct region with its own peculiar etiology." Additionally, veterans who claimed disabilities owing to disease were treated by authorities with suspicion. Disease held a lower moral connotation than the bullet-wounded body with scars and amputated limbs. If Dawson had been enslaved before the war, his diseases or injuries would not have been treated by a white doctor. Slave owners were the medical arbiters when their enslaved workers claimed illness or injury.[39]

If Dawson grew up enslaved on a Maryland plantation, his understanding of his health and bodily functions would not have been the same as that of white people. Emancipated African Americans rejected the authority of white medicine as a component of freedom. "Pharmocosm" describes a worldview of enslaved people that "emphasizes the healing and harming capacities of spiritual power." This power embraced people, animals, and objects. The material manifestation of this perspective in healing therapies must have confused and annoyed white doctors who perceived them as superstitious humbug. A practitioner in a slave community may have promoted cures such as pine tar for frostbite and white sassafras root tea for blindness or remedies expressed through amulets, incantations, dreams, and fortune telling.[40]

Enslaved black Americans embraced "a relational vision of health" whereby the health of an individual was contingent on community spiritual health. *Conjuring* referred to healing practices that drew on the pharmocosm to restore health to a community through the reincorporation of a sick person made well again. "Sickness was not a condition to be endured alone; neither was individual healing possible without the consideration of extended social relationships." Conjurers understood this well: anything in the pharmocosm that induced sickness in one person exerted that influence on the larger community unless it was halted by sympathetic magic. The conjurer was particularly useful in detecting if spells or curses were at work. In the early twentieth century, African American doctor John Donalson found that many southern rural black people attributed disease to an affliction conveyed by spells. His practice reckoned with the pharmocosm and its attendant relational universe of health "in a world where spiritual matters, personality, and local flora all informed a healer's knowledge and combined to give a healer medical power. His understanding connected the body with a larger environment and cosmos."[41]

A SPLENDID SPECIMEN OF PHYSICAL MANHOOD

Many of Dawson's comrades in the Forty-Third came from enslavement; others were free black men from the North. The training he received at Camp William Penn introduced a disciplined mode of life that forged a military community with a hierarchy of rank. His training took place under a spotlight. The camp, just north of Philadelphia, received many visitors and spectators to the soldiers' drill. Nestled within an abolitionist community on land owned by the son of Lucretia Mott, a pioneer abolitionist and advocate for women's rights, the barracks and ancillary buildings were praised by the press for their cleanliness, order, and neat appearance. A water fountain even graced the commanding officer's house. Drilling in formation, Dawson must have been conscious of a new sense of self: as an object of pride and admiration, even envy, from onlookers and visitors.[42]

In common with other black regiments, the Forty-Third employed civilian teachers and chaplains to teach literacy. At enlistment, only seventy soldiers could read and write to varying degrees, but after several months, over half had achieved the ability.[43] That Dawson was not one of those could be due to many factors. His two hospital sojourns might have put him behind his comrades, or perhaps he was reluctant to meet the challenge of reading in addition to coping with the new military environment.[44]

Around the time Dawson mustered out in Philadelphia, he befriended a younger man, Armstead (later, Armistead) Williams, who was enslaved in Virginia. The two men moved to rural Maryland, not far from the Delaware line. They chose to live in different communities in Caroline County, Dawson to pursue farming near Goldsborough (Goldsboro), and Williams to reside and work in the county seat, Denton. The only details about their postwar relationship come from a tribute to the still-living Williams in a 1924 newspaper that acknowledged his leadership in the black community and profiled him as a "highly respected colored citizen . . . whose cheery salute of his white friends always had with it a tip of the hat." The article recalled the arrival of Williams and "Pressly Dorsey" in Denton in the 1860s, "two splendid specimens of physical manhood, [who] made diversion for and created vast admiration among both the white and colored youth of the town for their feats of prodigious strength." Dawson performed a crowd-pleasing stunt by hoisting a barrel of flour over his shoulder and strutting about. The limp of his imperfectly healed right leg did not seem to have inhibited his upper-body strength. The newspaper article also signaled Dawson's name change to Dorsey.[45]

The postwar picture of health for veterans was not an encouraging one. Relevant to Dawson and supported by his latter experience, "soldiers who had contracted at least one illness while in the service tended to become disabled as they grew older with more frequency than those soldiers who had never become ill in the service." Over half of all black veterans in the several northern Maryland counties had been enslaved prewar. By 1890, 42 percent of those veterans still alive had claimed debilities to pension authorities. "Clearly, service in the Union Army did not elevate or ennoble these men; they were actually worse off than African-Americans who had never served."[46]

The decision to live and work in Caroline County was a wise one. Williams's leadership role helped build a reputation for independence and self-reliance in the black community around Denton. This reputation may have bolstered Dawson's standing among his white farmer neighbors. Before the war, about 79 percent of all African Americans residing in the county were free, and its operation of the Underground Railroad was the best organized and operated of any in the country. Today, although Dorsey is an uncommon name in Caroline County, Dawson is common. The choice of Dawson for his wartime identity might have been an effort to dissociate himself from slave-owning Dorseys and embrace a name associated with a free black community.[47]

Among the social world of African American Caroline County, Dawson found a mate: in 1868, he married Sophia Grace. By 1870, "Press" Dorsey, thirty, and Sophia, twenty-one, lived in the town of Goldsborough. They lodged with a laborer, William T. Sparks, his wife, two daughters, and another woman. The marriage proved troublesome. The couple divorced or separated for good after several years, and the lack of documentation of the marriage (later remedied) and the subsequent divorce created impossible obstacles for the widow—Dawson's second wife—after his death. For many black veterans, especially those who had married by "common law" while enslaved, no record of their marriages exists. Where pensions were at issue, pension authorities resorted to depositions from knowledgeable people to compensate for the lack of official records.[48]

Before the decade passed, Dawson married again. The circumstances of his separation from Sophia did not become clear to white authorities until decades later. On February 9, 1875, minister A. Grinage married "Press Dorsey," thirty-five, to Mary J. Benton, thirty-three, at a place called Ford's Hall. Mary, who went by Janey, was also nonliterate and came from an enslaved background. At the same time, Dawson's friend Williams, a "farm laborer" according to the census, resided on a farm in Denton owned by a white couple. He lived in Denton for the remainder of his long life, dying at about age one hundred in 1942, "a credit to his race."[49]

NOT RATABLY DISABLED

By 1880, "Preston Dorsey," thirty-eight, was listed in the census as head of house and "farm laborer" with a family of four children—George W., William H., Mary E., and Samuel P.—all born after 1870. They lived in Henderson, a few miles west of the Delaware line. After leaving the Sparks family, Dawson and Janey became tenants to a physician and war veteran, William Henry Winslow, and his wife, Annie Traquair Winslow. In 1881, "Preston Dorsey" purchased a farm of sixty-two acres for $200 from the Winslows who had acquired the property for $7,000 in the 1870s. On the same day as the deed was executed, Dawson sold the lot for $200 to one M. J. L. Purvis. This may have been a single three-way transaction. Perhaps Purvis was also a war veteran and the cut-rate sale was Winslow's effort to boost fellow veterans. A few years before his death, Dawson purchased more property in Queen Anne County.[50]

Despite Dawson's farming success, his body suffered to the extent that he began petitioning pension authorities for help. He engaged a pension attorney, W. H. Wills & Co. of Washington, DC, to represent him. Nonliteracy discouraged many worthy applicants from applying, and obtaining a pension would have been impossible without a lawyer or pension agent. The usual form of remuneration to pension attorneys was a fee recouped upon issuance of the first pension check. Dawson may have traveled to Washington to consult with his attorney. He must have been prepared to pay travel expenses, notaries, and court fees and meet with a medical board to have his disability assessed and rated.

The central barrier to nonliterate applicants, particularly black ones, was establishing identity. Doing so involved obtaining birth certificates and testimonials from neighbors, and of course the cost of sending lawyers' staff to take depositions or appear with deponents in court. If military records were insufficient, former soldiers' comrades or commanding officers were sought for statements attesting to applicants' identity and eligibility. African American applicants also faced a barrier in their own communities, which valued images and narratives about the "fully masculine black figure"—healthy, vigorous, and patriotic men—and avoided images of their disabled own. Black lives were shown as oriented to the future and constructing citizenship. Black veterans who claimed pensions effectively vied for citizenship, their status affirmed by returning from war with visible wounds. The black veteran, in effect, achieved citizen status "by submitting to violence." With these contradictions, it is no wonder that far fewer black than white veterans applied for pensions.[51]

The pension system challenged black manhood in important ways. Both white and black communities honored veterans with visible disabilities, at least within certain boundaries. Pinned-up sleeves or pants legs were acceptable; scarred or disfigured faces, diseases, and invisible injuries were not. Claims of disability without apparent physical causes were viewed suspiciously. Such injuries might be due to moral lapses or, as pension officials said, "vicious habits." Pension documents cautioned that pensions were not intended to compensate immoral behavior or moral degeneration through alcoholism. For black veterans, these challenges were exacerbated by changing times: with enslavement, white men were all equal on a substrate of inferior black bodies. During Reconstruction and the Jim Crow era, for white men to continue with a prerogative of superiority, they devised new efforts to subvert black manhood. Pension authorities subjected black applicants to heightened scrutiny. The system's gatekeepers placed additional obstacles before them. Yet the achievement of a pension constituted recognition of citizenship, a powerful motivator.[52]

In 1885, Dawson appeared before the Caroline County Circuit Court to swear to the facts itemized in his pension application. At forty-three, Dawson listed his service particulars and described himself as five foot, nine and a half inches, light-complected with black hair and gray eyes. He stated that on August 29, 1864, near Petersburg, Virginia, he "contracted rheumatism and incurred injury to right leg caused by a log slipping from breast works and dislocating his knee. He has been lame from said injury ever since. He claims pension for disability resulting from rheumatism and lameness." He listed his two episodes of hospitalization from which any reader would infer that they resulted from this injury. No mention was made of malaria. Two witnesses attested to Dawson's identity, one of whom was Armstead Williams.[53]

Within weeks, pension officials had placed a record of the application—a card—in the new pension file for "Presley Dawson" of Ingleside, Maryland, with a description under "Alleges" of the rheumatism and leg injury. The army rejected his claim, and the reverse side of the card noted that Wills filed a new claim in 1896, "Rejection adhered to," and again in 1898 with new documentation. The documentation was "carefully considered. Claim for rheumatism referred. Rejection of injury to right leg adhered to."[54]

By the turn of the twentieth century, veterans' pensions consumed about a third of the federal budget. Almost one-third of all white men over fifty-five were receiving pensions for Union army service. An immense bureaucracy was required to administer the system that included profiles of thousands of men's bodies. The massive compilation of all that had been learned about medicine and surgery during the war, *The Medical and Surgical History of the War of the Rebellion*, published by the federal government, required detailed bodily histories that also informed pension claims.[55]

Pension authorities responded according to the malady presented by the claimant. Once the panel of examining physicians saw the applicant, they modified or revised the description of the malady according to their professional judgment. That judgment, submitted to the pension office, was either approved or disapproved. For Dawson, this process meant multiple requests for reviews of his pension status as Congress continued to amend and expand pension benefits into the early twentieth century. Through Wills, Dawson submitted a "state of the body" report periodically to permit others to scrutinize him under evolving rules. In all his claims, Dawson was undoubtedly coached by

Wills to shape a narrative likely to elicit a pension. On average, a veteran submitted twelve applications before 1900 because of periodic changes in applicable laws. Each time he did this, Dawson presented himself with a diminished civic persona. For instance, although he apparently succeeded in farming, he represented himself in the original 1885 pension application as an unskilled laborer.[56]

Based on the latest legal requirements, Wills encouraged Dawson to reapply following a rejection. The original pension law of 1862, known as the "general law," awarded pensions with a set amount to veterans unable to perform manual labor owing to war-related disability and to their dependents. Congressional acts of 1866, 1872, and 1873 elaborated on the original act by creating a rating system based on the measurable extent of disability (e.g., the loss of a hand, leg, or eye was rated for a given amount per month). The Act of June 27, 1890, constituted the next significant milestone in the liberalization of pensions. Any soldier who served at least ninety days and received an honorable discharge could be compensated for disability, no matter how the cause. No longer did debilities have to be war- or service-related, although a higher rating was likely if the veteran had been injured or wounded in service. This liberalization resulted from the powerful congressional lobby of the veteran's association for former Union soldiers, the Grand Army of the Republic. Most senior statesmen had served in the army during the war and were GAR members.

A comprehensive study of the compensation of Union veterans found that between 1862 and 1890, 43.9 percent of white veterans applied for a new pension, whereas only 19.7 percent of African American veterans did so. Owing to the liberalization of the 1890 law, between 1890 and 1907, the year Dawson died, 91.6 percent white and 93.6 percent African Americans applied for new pensions. Dawson's light complexion may have been an advantage because "examiners were considerably less likely to recommend a dark-skinned African American for a pension." Nevertheless, compared with white applicants, light-complected African Americans saw their chances of obtaining a favorable rating drop 40 percent, and for dark-skinned men, 50 percent.[57]

Just as black veterans presented themselves as diminished in their civic identities when asking for pension hikes, white applicants retreated from their ideals of manhood by appealing to pity: unless they received an increased pension, they could not truly be men. Because of cited grievances or misfortunes, they verged on desperation and helplessness. African American applicants, however—and Dawson was an example—did no such thing, despite struggling against prejudices that assumed their lack of responsibility, their failures as role models for young people, and their inherent "Sambo" personality.[58]

Dawson dutifully submitted the requisite paperwork via his attorney, but the journey to an adequate pension was challenging, particularly when his widow presented herself to pension authorities. Claiming disability for a leg and knee and related rheumatism required Dawson to overcome official skepticism about invisible injuries. Pension authorities invested no small resources to determine Dawson's eligibility and need, thus requiring an ongoing, intimate assessment of his habits, background, associates, and particularly his two marriages.[59]

In response to Dawson's application for a pension, the pension office requested his medical record from the surgeon general's office. The office verified Dawson's two rounds of hospitalization, at City Point for "Malarial Debility" and Brownsville for "Malarial Fever." The request for this information supplied the veteran's name as "Presley Dawson," but the response used the surname "Dorsey" and stated, "This soldier's name [Dorsey] is not borne upon such records as are on file bearing on the case." Company records of the Forty-Third verified the hospital stays but noted both surnames and instructed the War Department that "records on file do not show disability or injuries alleged nor do they show any specific disability during service."[60]

Over the next few years, nothing was issued from the pension office. In 1890, attorney Wills applied again because the pension law had changed. The form to be submitted, "Application for Invalid Pension under New Law," advised claimants that, to succeed in their pension application, they must have problems "of a permanent character" and "not the result of vicious habits." Again, Wills stated Dawson's disability as "Weakness of the Breast—lame in Knee and hip from Rhumatism [*sic*] caused [in military service and a] knee dislocated from the hurt of a log fell off Breast Work." As of July 10, 1890, Dawson had received six dollars monthly[61] for the specific disability of rheumatism and leg injury. The documentation in Dawson's pension file included a stamped text: "Partial inability to earn or support by manual labor." The "partial" qualification meant that the pension amount would remain fixed until the pension authorities determined that Dawson had become completely disabled.[62]

Dawson's first disability pension might have set a benchmark for his future, but in 1894, the government rescinded the pension. According to the pension authorities, Congress's Act of June 27, 1890, intended to liberalize pensions, worked against Dawson. The pension office's Board of Revision visited extant pensions to determine whether the monthly amounts should be revised upward. In a letter to Dawson, authorities cited various administrative orders to deny the pension. In a second notification, they stated that Dawson's name was dropped because he was "not ratably disabled for earning a support by manual labor, under the act of June 27, 1890."[63]

SIX DOLLARS A MONTH

By this time, Dawson may have distrusted the workings of a government whose faceless administrators seemed to exist in another world. The cancellation of his pension spurred Dawson to push his claim, but various government offices affirmed its rejection. A medical referee stipulated that a physical examination of

Dawson would be "immaterial," and the initial pension rejection remained: "No pensionable disability from alleged rheumatism and injury to right leg."[64]

Dawson and his contested body took a new path in 1897. His attorney reopened the claim, and the pension office sent "Presley Dawson" of Ingleside, Maryland, a questionnaire about his marriage and family. Dawson responded that no record existed of his marriage to Janey and admitted to a previous marriage to Sophia Dawson who by that time had died, although he could not recall the date. His children and their ages came next—William H., Mary E., Samuel P., John H., and "Arbessie" (Arline). In the 1900 census, "Preston Dorsey" listed his occupation as farmer and head of household, age sixty, his wife "Jane," age forty-five, and their small family (a son and a servant) at Church Hill in Queen Anne County. At this time, four of his six children were still alive.[65]

In 1902, Dawson appeared before a medical board in Easton, Maryland, which recommended that the pension be continued. That year, Dawson had undergone a comprehensive physical examination for the first time since the war. In Easton, Dawson was examined by three physicians. If he mentioned his hospitalization for malaria, the doctors did not record it as material to determining disability. Following the examination, Dawson's monthly pension of six dollars was resumed. The next year, the government increased it to eight dollars.[66] As was the prevailing practice, newspapers reported the names of pensioners and the amounts of their pensions.[67]

The record suggests that Dawson and his family enjoyed self-sufficiency as tenant farmers. The disposition of the property Dawson owned in Queen Anne County remains unknown. Following the war, he waited two decades before requesting a pension, enduring repeated rejections as his health worsened. His farm sustained his family, and Dawson earned enough capital to purchase more land. For $1,000, he and his wife mortgaged twenty-seven acres in Caroline County. All parties to the sale signed legal documents with an X. Dawson was planning for self-sufficiency.[68]

In 1904, thirty-nine years after the war's end, the pension office summoned Dawson to Dover, Delaware, for an examination by another panel of physicians. The surgeon's certificate generated for Dawson provided the most detailed information about the state of his body on the occasion of his sixty-fifth or perhaps sixty-fourth, sixty-third, or sixty-second year (Dawson was never consistent). Through his attorney, he requested a new assessment of his pension due to worsening rheumatism, although his leg and knee injuries remained unchanged. The increase of his pension to eight dollars monthly was determined by the 1902 examiners' consensus that Dawson was "disqualified for manual labor two thirds of his time."[69]

This examination furnished new data on Dawson's body: five feet, nine inches, 172 pounds, black complexion (a change from mulatto), bald, brown eyes, temperature 98 and 2/5, and respiration and pulse rates taken when sitting, standing, or after exercise. On inspiration, his chest measured forty-one inches and on expiration, thirty-eight inches. His occupation was listed as farmer and his birthplace as Harford County. Under "Names of disabilities," a physician wrote, "[injury] to right leg Injury to right hand Dis[ease] of heart Partial [loss] of right hand. Injury to Rt Knee Gen Debility and affection of breast."

The medical observations and conclusions were listed under several categories. Under "Rheumatism," the report described "Crepitation" (cracking) stiffness in the shoulders, hips, and knees and noted no attendant swelling or inflammation. Other joints appeared normal.[70] "Lumbar muscles are stiff rigid with painful and impaired motion. Unable to reach the floor with palms of his hands. Pain in stooping and upon pressure." Muscles, however, had not atrophied. Under "Injury to Right Leg," the examiners noted a linear half-inch cicatrix (raised scar) over the right patella, but "at the inner condyle of right knee,"[71] the bones appeared to have been crushed at one time, and a "boney prominence" could be felt under the skin above the condyle. The periosteum,[72] the bones' "outer skin," appeared to have been "denuded," and the skin was painful to the touch. "It is a condition of exotosis[73] but is not inflamed." The examiners found that "rheumatism was very stiff and has some pain on motion . . . in right knee cannot flex knee upon thigh and to that extent impaired motion." Presumably, the examination required Dawson to walk a short distance, turn, and walk back. The doctors surely noted his limp and turned-out right foot each time he took a step. As the crushed bone healed without medical intervention in 1864, new bone growth created spurs that inhibited motion and caused pain.

A subsection, "Injury to Right Hand Partial Loss of Right Hand," introduced a new injury, presumably a by-product of postwar farm life. Dawson displayed a stump of a thumb: a half-inch of the "distal phalanx" of the right thumb was gone and a half-inch linear cicatrix cinched the stump. He was unable to grip with his right hand, and the muscles around his wrist and extending to his hand and forearm had atrophied. The disuse of his right hand must have afflicted him for some time because it no longer showed the evidence of manual labor that the left hand did. He also showed some loss of sensation on the outside of his right hand, apparently related to irritation of the ulnar nerve.

A separate discussion of "Disease of the Heart" highlighted "irregular and intermittent action of heart" palpitations and an "area of percussive dullness" over the apex of the heart. Dawson exhibited dyspnea (labored breathing): "He does have . . . smothered breathing upon exertion."

Dawson's lungs appeared normal, as did his stomach, spleen, liver, and bowels. While the report cited no specific disease, it noted that Dawson's "age alone [is] accountable for feebleness." A urinalysis revealed healthy kidneys. Under "General Debility," the examination concluded, "The aggregate permanent disability for earning a support by the performance of manual labor is due to rheumatism Injury to hand and partial loss of hand. Injury to knee Disease of heart and not due to vicious habits and warrants a rating of ten dollars per month." If Dawson's malarial symptoms had recurred, the medical report does not mention it. The weakened heart might have been the result of the long-term effects of *P. falciparum*. About malaria, the doctors did not inquire.

Dawson may have received the raise in pension. Three years later, on March 12, 1907, he died.

SURVIVING BLACKNESS

Because of pension authorities' skepticism about claims with no visible evidence, veterans like Dawson without such obvious afflictions as amputee stumps were less likely to pursue pensions. Dawson may have waited for two decades because of his suspicion about the process. Mindful of the manual labor benchmark for determining who was pension-worthy, authorities viewed veterans who received pensions for disabilities but still earned wages as anomalies or misfits. All the veterans profiled in this book, however, received pensions for disability but continued to work for pay. Veterans' relationships with pension authorities followed prescribed rules that were inapplicable in all other spheres of life. This fact was even more confusing because Dawson and other pensioned veterans inhabited three bodies, each with distinct social expectations: a civic body, a pensionable body, and a veteran body.[74]

Dawson and his pension body's experiences with the pension office were similar to those of white veterans in that the manual labor standard was rigidly observed yet examiners distrusted bodily phenomena that were not visible, such as recurrent malarial fevers and pain. Prevailing attitudes regarding the black male body, however, may have affected some pension decisions for black veterans. The legitimization of slavery depended on a view of black bodies as inherently disabled by inferior intelligence and capacity. The introduction of "insane and idiot" categories in the 1840 census enabled slave owners to list black bodies as such. Predictably, the highest percentage of people listed in this category were black. "Slavery advocates pounced on this data as proof of the incapacity of African Americans, the deleterious effects of freedom, and the nation's moral obligations to maintain the practice." For African Americans after the war, these prejudices were still endemic and difficult to overcome.[75]

Over time, black veterans who persisted in disability claims were examined by a board of three physicians (and later, one). For men like Dawson who perhaps had never received help from a white doctor apart from his hospitalizations, the medical examination might have been both disturbing and revelatory. The white doctor may have assumed that trust was implicit in all conversations with veterans. Black veterans, however, may have seen white doctors as a potential enemy and dreaded the encounter. Some soldiers feared the "night doctor" in the folklore of the Deep South, the thief of bodies. Additionally, language obstacles were part of larger cultural barriers that proved particularly rigid when black men with enslaved backgrounds underwent examinations but had debilities that were not apparent, thus placing a linguistic burden on the veteran to explain and justify the problem. Doing so, however, led to suspicions "of fraud and malingering." The veteran's disclosure also risked the intensification of prejudice because "it was a short step from evaluation of an applicant's character to ascription of assumed group characteristics to the individual."[76]

Since attributes of manhood included economic and political power, many black men enlisted in the war to develop these powers by soldiering for the Union. One avenue open to soldiers before the war was participation in voluntary societies including Freemasonry, and after the war, the GAR. Even if some societies promoted segregation, black men could still organize and advance their collective interests, including perennially memorializing their contribution to saving the Union. This memorialization became more strident as the public forgot black veterans' contribution to the war. The postwar Lost Cause myth provided a new narrative that promoted the reconciliation of honorable white foes who endured a brotherly spat, the promotion of the Confederacy as a noble, romantic experiment, not as a deep-rooted disagreement about the maintenance and expansion of slavery. Organizers of blue-gray reunions did not invite black veterans, thereby ensuring their public invisibility. "The struggle of black Union veterans for manhood appears to have encompassed six discernible areas: politics, veteran-government relations, economics, family and marital life, interracial and intraracial veteran relations, and historical memory." Dawson's veteran body, unlike the civic and pension bodies, relied on the nonjudgmental camaraderie of fellow black veterans to recognize and affirm his injuries and sacrifice for his country.[77]

For Dawson, the exercise of manhood through veteran status may have taken the form of GAR participation. In Maryland, there were twenty-three black GAR posts and no integrated ones, so there were many opportunities for fellowship among black veterans. The two Dawson artifacts that have survived in family custody are a faded carte de visite photograph and a badge. The photograph was poorly fixed when it was created, so the image disappeared during Dawson's lifetime, but the family kept it nevertheless. The badge was a common type, made up by the vendor on demand for sale at veterans' events. Stamped on the badge are Dawson's regimental and corps affiliations; his name appeared as Dorsey. Dawson certainly wore this badge on many occasions, particularly those that commemorated the wartime sacrifices of black soldiers. His widow, Janey, cited both artifacts in a pension deposition and mentioned that her husband had been active in GAR activities. Presenting these artifacts to pension authorities meant owning material pieces of Dawson's identity to establish her own. If Dawson possessed GAR-issued decorations, none have survived.[78]

During its first years, the GAR did not attract many veterans, but membership grew substantially by the 1880s and 1890s, and the organization became a major political lobby. Initially, the GAR observed no color line and welcomed all honorably discharged veterans, but soon problems developed: GAR affiliates, called posts, did not always accept black applicants for membership, particularly in the southern states. At the national level, however, there was no policy of discrimination. Inclusion "made the Grand Army special among fraternal societies in the post–Civil War period, in which racial segregation or total exclusion was the norm." Toward the end of the nineteenth century, the reconciliation ethos stressed the GAR's policy of inclusion. Many white Union veterans accepted Jim Crow as the prevailing reality, even at the expense of their black fellow veterans. Dawson would have experienced this tension if, as Janey deponed, he had remained active in the GAR. White veterans "could remember . . . emancipation, without believing in . . . equality."[79]

The GAR was able to sustain an interracial community precisely because most Union veterans had not forgotten the role played by black soldiers in a war that had eliminated slavery. "Black veterans were the political and social equals of white Americans in one of the most prestigious organizations in the United States. In an era in which race trumped virtually all other social identities, black and white veterans created an interracial organization at both the national and local levels." In this environment, black veterans were quick to access federal benefits as they became available. Black and immigrant veterans "outpaced native whites" in their pension claims and persistence in applying despite administrative obstacles or rejections.[80]

The single reference in the pension documents to Dawson's GAR participation may indicate a wider social sphere of mutual support and political activism. For example, both white and black GAR posts were affiliated with women's support or auxiliary groups. In collaboration with the activities of veterans, posts created a larger network of social relationships and mutual assistance in the form of charitable relief. For black posts, the Women's Relief Corps of the Ladies of the GAR was particularly productive and popular. Other comparable organizations that operated tangentially to faith communities were the Sons and Daughters of Lincoln, United Sons of Love, and Colored Odd Fellows.[81]

An analogous sphere of life that conferred fellowship, equality, mutual aid, and charity was faith, a dimension of Dawson's civic body. There is no direct reference to church affiliation or involvement in any of Dawson's military or pension documents or in depositions by family members, yet its absence from records does not mean it was absent from Dawson's world. By contrast, Dawson's comrade in the Forty-Third, Sergeant Brock, who, like Dawson, had been a farmer and later a gardener, described in his correspondence his family's participation in the African Methodist Episcopal Church; in particular, his secretarial duties for the church Sabbath school. Toward the end of his enlistment, Brock noted that most of his comrades attended school in camp during winter months under the "superintendence of our able and efficient chaplain, who manifests a great interest in our soldiers." This might have been the same chaplain who doubled as the quartermaster sergeant of Company C, of whom Brock wrote, "We find that he has lost none of his enthusiasm but is still as eloquent as ever. He held the audience spellbound, for almost one hour, listing to his stirring remarks." Dawson might have been in that audience.[82]

There are no explicit references to spiritual life in the documents pertaining to any of the Union veterans examined in this book. The experience of war might have led these veterans to adopt "providential pragmatism." In other words, the war did not dissolve soldier's prewar spirituality or eliminate a Christian deity from their universe, but perhaps each soldier's journey of loneliness for home, exhaustion from the march, and terror of battle united them "by a spontaneous philosophy best described as providential pragmatism, which enabled a soldier to think in the moment without giving up on God."[83]

JANEY'S AND DAWSON'S PENSION BODY

Prestley Dawson's civic (and physical) life ended, but Janey strove to acquire a dependent's pension by keeping her husband's pensionable body viable. By enlisting in the army, Dawson's body entered an administrative zone that recorded data essential for his identification, including his marriage(s) and family and his location while in army service. As Janey would discover to her disappointment, the apparently unrecorded first marriage and its termination stalled pension authorities from acting on her behalf. Achieving a pension, as other African American wives could attest to, constituted governmental recognition of the wives' identities as citizens.[84]

Despite the avowed intention of the pension office to treat white and black veterans equally, the equitable application of administrative rules precluded some African Americans from participating in the system even though they deserved compensation. Just as white Americans struggled to recognize black soldiers as civic equals by virtue of their service, black Americans had difficulty recognizing that the fact of enslavement did not diminish their character or moral personae. Some black veterans may have passed the invisible tests of proving moral worth to receive a pension. Some white pension authorities—in common with many other white people—linked poverty with personal failure. Wives of soldiers, particularly if they came from backgrounds of poverty or enslavement and lacked literacy—like Janey—struggled to convince pension authorities to grant awards. They proved their status as spouses and hence their standing to receive pensions.[85]

The culture of African Americans and the discretion of slave owners shaped marriages and divorces within enslaved communities. Marriages and divorces, then, did not necessarily carry identical meanings or boundaries with those understood by white people. Most marriages within enslavement, however, still required the community recognition that they had occurred. Dawson married twice postwar at a time when the clerk of the circuit court should have recorded the first marriage, the divorce, the subsequent marriage to Janey, and their children. Pensions could not be granted to claimant dependents who could not prove a legal relationship to the deceased veteran.[86]

Just weeks after Dawson's death, Janey (through attorney M. Garrett) applied for a widow's pension. In anticipation of having to prove her identity and standing, she swore an affidavit that declared her wedding date, the location of the marriage ("Fred Halls House"), and the presiding minister, the Reverend A. Grinage. Her two witnesses were neighbors who attested to having known the couple for thirty years. At this time, Janey was sixty-five and lived with five children. A year later, the pension office denied the claim.[87]

Congress introduced a new law in 1908 that required evidence of cohabitation and affidavits of two credible witnesses. Credibility was determined by a pension officer's judgment. As discussed in Richard Dunphy's case, pension examiners were assigned to investigate a claim by taking depositions of friends, neighbors, and local officials. On a cover sheet listing all depositions, the examiner rated deponents for credibility. The pension office notified both Janey and her attorney of the new law and, in October 1908, wrote attorney Garrett with a detailed list of instructions. In addition to submitting Dawson's death certificate, the authority required

> a verified copy of the public or church record of the claimant's marriage to the soldier, or if no public record exists, a certificate to that effect, under seal, from the clerk of the court, and, if no church record exists, the affidavit of the person who performed the ceremony, if obtainable, or, if not, claimant's statement to that effect, under oath, together with the testimony of [two credible witnesses] present at the marriage, showing the date thereof; the best obtainable evidence, record if possible, showing the date of death of Sophia Dawson, with whom the soldier lived but to whom it is alleged he was never lawfully married; the testimony of two competent witnesses showing whether claimant and the soldier lived together from the date of their marriage to his death, and, if not, whether they were divorced; also the testimony of credible persons having the requisite knowledge, showing whether claimant has remarried since soldier's death, and, if so, to whom and when and where such remarriage occurred.[88]

The letter implicitly criticized Janey for not having obtained the requisite legal documentation of Dawson's previous marriage. The lack of documentation of a previous marriage (and divorce) reinforced notions of black moral inferiority. By this time, however, pension authorities recognized that public records of marriages or divorces might not be obtainable, so affidavits of witnesses and people who presided over ceremonies sufficed. While these rules applied to all veterans, by 1908, authorities had had enough experience with the differences in marriage and divorce practices among African Americans to request other legal evidence. Janey wasted no time in gathering it. The same week her attorney received the letter, the pension authority sent her a questionnaire to verify vital statistics regarding her late husband (age at enlistment, place of birth, occupation, physical characteristics). If Dawson had been enslaved, the questionnaire noted, she needed to name his owners, particularly those present at the time of marriage. Dawson's postmortem, civic body still required justification, verification, and reification.[89]

Into the early months of 1909, Garrett corresponded with pension authorities, initially by submitting an affidavit by one Charles Lewis that he had known Sophia Dawson for about thirty years and could attest to her death, as he had dug her grave. By this time, because there was no marriage certificate, pension authorities did not expect to receive a marriage or divorce record and stressed the need for eyewitness affidavits of a marriage service, cohabitation, or Sophia's death. Garrett obtained an affidavit from a neighbor who had attended her funeral and burial. Meanwhile, the pension authorities thought that contacting Dawson's still-living fellow soldiers might yield more affidavits and settle the matter of the first marriage and divorce.[90] If the divorce could not be verified, then, as far as the pension office was concerned, Janey had no standing as a claimant. Accordingly, by spring 1909, Janey's pension was denied with the terse explanation "that claimant never was his lawful wife."[91]

The same week that Janey's pension claim was denied, a pension officer referred the case to the board of review and suggested that the claim be examined further. The officer noted the confusing file of names for the deceased soldier—Dawson or Dorsey—and explained, "The date of [Sophia's] death should be ascertained. All the witnesses except one who testifies to cohabitation, are unable to write and appear to be illiterate and this testimony should be [examined and if] they have no personal knowledge of the facts to which they have testified the testimony of other witnesses should be procured . . . [and other considerations] appear to be established and case prima facie established."[92]

Pension examiner R. P. Fletcher came to the Maryland community to investigate and gather depositions. All the deponents were nonliterate, none had known Dawson before the war, and none knew of his home or work before the war. Few could attest to having met the first wife. Those who knew that the couple had separated nevertheless believed that there had been no formal divorce. The records included the inconsistent spelling of names, for example, and because many of the deponents were nonliterate, they could not correct these misspellings. The scribes recording deponents' words, therefore, wrote down what they heard.[93]

Janey and her children's depositions clarified some aspects of the Dawson story. They were unacquainted with Dawson's prewar life and knew little of his military service. They knew that

Dawson's true name was Dorsey and that he had changed his surname while in the army but could not explain why. Janey claimed that Garrett was not her attorney of record on this matter and that she had engaged one R. E. Graham to prosecute the claim, but despite paying him, he "has done [nothing] for me." Janey stated that she had been enslaved before the war and had been owned by Samuel and Charles Walls, now deceased, but she had obtained a statement from Charles's son that gave her a birthdate: October 1, 1841. Janey recalled the circumstances of her marriage at the house of her uncle, Fred Hall. She listed wedding guests (and, therefore, witnesses), most of whom were deceased by this time.

Outside of the army records, Janey was the only other person to acknowledge Dawson's malaria. She told Fletcher that "he had an attack of fever while in the army" and confirmed that he had an injured hip and lameness. She could not recall any mention of a single army friend, why Dawson enlisted, or why he enlisted in Pennsylvania. The only Dawson artifact she presented to Fletcher was "the only photograph I have of him . . . a tin type [not a tintype but a carte de visite]—which is so faded—you can not discover whether the man was black or what he looked like." She also presented Dawson's veteran's badge and noted that he "use to wear [it] when he attended GAR post meetings which shows his service." Janey also recalled that Dawson had met Armstead Williams in Washington, DC, after the war when both men moved to Maryland. Dawson, she continued, "had been sent out to the Eastern Shore near Denton MD by the Freedmen's Bureau shortly after his discharge." This is the only mention of the Freedmen's Bureau's involvement with Dawson in any document. At Dawson's death, the couple owned no property except for acreage that he mortgaged, and yet she had no widow's income. Dawson died without a will. The only personal property upon his death was a horse, a cow, and some farm tools worth $200.[94]

Fletcher discovered from neighbor Peter Goose that Dawson's son, Tennessee, by his first wife lived nearby. Goose also said that Sophia had subsequently married William Thomas, who attended her funeral. Goose signed his affidavit with an X. William Thomas also witnessed Goose's affidavit with an X. Tennessee Dawson, a laborer in Caroline County, recalled little about Dawson since the latter had been married to his mother for less than two years. He attended his mother's funeral with no help from an undertaker. He maintained that his parents never divorced.[95]

Fletcher's diligence in pursuing the case led to success in one respect: the Caroline County Circuit Court clerk found the "certificate of license of marriage" for Sophia and Prestley Dawson and provided a copy. The clerk also affirmed that the couple had separated and that Sophia later remarried, but the clerk did not find a divorce record. Just before he received the marriage record, Fletcher wrote a status report to his supervisor. He was aware of the difficulties of proving marriages and divorces among African American communities consisting of formerly enslaved people. He wrote:

> I have found this . . . often [to] be the case with colored ministers in years past; that is they secured the license, but made no return of the marriage performed by them. I found one old negro preacher who kept all licenses and he has a whole trunk full never having made a return of any marriage ceremony performed by him, but retained the licenses as his record. Years ago, and at intervals since, I made search for a private record or church record of marriages performed by the Rev Asbury Grinage, but no such record exists, and until the last few years of his life he made no return of marriage ceremonies performed by him . . . I do not see the necessity of securing further testimony . . . I recommend that the papers be referred to the Chief of the Board of Rev. for his consideration.[96]

Since 1907, Janey, through her attorney, filed multiple documents with pension authorities, mostly affidavits by witnesses to Dawson's first marriage and separation, his subsequent marriage to Janey, and their cohabitation until his death. Some had known Janey since childhood and reinforced the certification of her identity and standing to make a claim.[97]

Janey's persistent claims recalled her husband's status as a war veteran and offered redundant evidence that, by community if not legal standards, Dawson had been married once, divorced, and remarried, and he had remained so until death, producing several children. The pension office, however, remained unmoved. The obstacle was the previous marriage with no demonstrable divorce per Maryland law: "The widow's claim was rejected, on the ground that at the date of the soldier's attempted marriage to claimant he had a wife who was never divorced from him, and therefore claimant was never his lawful wife and has no status as his widow."[98]

With a new attorney, Herman W. Grant of Washington, DC, Janey applied again in 1911. The pension office remained adamant. More letters of rejection followed, the wording of which no doubt cut deep: "Your above cited claim for pension filed June 15, 1911, is rejected on the ground that you were never the legal wife of the soldier, and are not entitled to pension under any law of which fact you were advised May 26, 1909 upon the rejection of your claim under the act of June 27, 1890 and the act of April 19, 1908." Janey continued to look for new attorneys to press her claims: John Wainwright & Co., a Baltimore firm, later renewed the fight, only to be told in the final pension document in Dawson's file that "the claimant never was his lawful wife and has no status as his widow."[99]

Janey then gave up her pension claims. Her husband's pension body faded into memory, no longer providing a way for her to seek financial help from the government. In 1910, she lived in Henderson with her son, John H., and his wife, Mary, but by 1920, she had moved to West Chester, Pennsylvania, to live with her daughter Bessie and her husband. No longer responsible for a farm, she worked as a day laborer doing housework. She died in 1922 of apoplexy, likely cerebral hemorrhage.[100]

CONCLUSION: THE BADGED BLACK BODY

Following his war service, Dawson chose a stable and advantageous rural environment within which to create a postwar existence, marry (twice), rear children, and remain self-sufficient. Permanent land ownership—the universal signifier of independent manhood—eluded him. His interest in his health and body was shared by significant others from family members to physicians who could facilitate or block access to government assistance. As we have seen, black veterans and their spouses found it more difficult than white ones to receive federal pensions. Even before Dawson's birth into (presumed) slavery, the United States defined him as representing a "degraded" race not intended for citizenship that, according to a 1790 naturalization law, was reserved for white people. To white doctors, black men could never be fully autonomous beings because of the inherent deficiencies of their bodies, thus the necessity to command them.[101]

Dawson not only grew to adulthood recognizing his separateness; through army experience, he may have realized that white medical authorities viewed his body as inherently unhealthy, inferior, and prone to failure. It is telling that his physical reminder of the war—lameness—was due to a brutal accident not recorded in his wartime medical record. Perhaps the regimental surgeon regarded it as a superficial injury not worthy of hospital treatment. The surgeon might have assumed that a black body was inherently inured to the leg's pain. It is also possible that no surgeon examined the leg at the time of injury.

However Dawson arrived at the recruiting office in 1864, he evidently presented a healthy body and was almost immediately promoted to a temporary supervisory position. If he had been enslaved, then most of his ideas about how the body functions and how illness occurs would have been shaped by fellow enslaved people. The lack of literacy interfered with the government's documentation of his body: Dawson's name changed to fit the circumstances, and his other vital data remained vague. As Dawson could not write, the documentation of his body both within service and later was necessarily subject to the vagaries of white men whose medical parlance sounded like a foreign language.

While in the war, Dawson would have practiced self-care to a degree equal to that of most white soldiers. Primary medical care was self-care: "Self-care could include eradicating pests; constructing protective shelters; intervening in camp terrain; supplementing rations, especially with fruits and vegetables; locating suitable water for drinking and bathing; attending to sanitation and dress; obtaining regular exercise; and straggling for relief. It was often a group effort: soldiers taught each other techniques or learned from officers, formed communal messes to share food, cared for one another when illness did strike, and reached out to civilians at home and at the front for advice, supplies, and comfort."[102]

Mainly surrounded by black soldiers, Dawson shared and absorbed ideas of health and specific therapies outside the boundary of military medicine. Dawson and a white physician both determined that his knee was dislocated, but their healing therapies derived from different perceptions of how the black body worked. His two long-term hospitalizations for malarial fever were never mentioned in postwar conversations with doctors. His lameness was the sole focus of pension examinations, although he was not hospitalized for it during the war. The lack of wartime documentation of his leg injury doubtless influenced the pension rejections later. Dawson likely communicated his symptoms to doctors who interpreted them through a filter of stereotypes about black bodies.

When Dawson first received a pension, S. Weir Mitchell and John Mitchell circulated their questionnaire to three of the white soldiers profiled in this book. The fourth white soldier was in the same social circle as the elder Mitchell and volunteered relevant information about his body. No black soldiers participated in that study and therefore contributed no record to posterity about the state of their aging bodies beyond pension examinations. The poorly healed leg would have contributed to the Mitchells' study of nerves, although the other enduring malady afflicting Dawson, malaria, would have fallen outside of their purview. Research into the causes and modes of transmission of malaria continued over the final decades of Dawson's life. A decade before Dawson's death, a Nobel Prize was awarded for the discovery of the role of mosquitoes in the transmission of the disease.

To Dawson, malaria meant a recurring fever. In the year following the war's end, he suffered multiple returns of symptoms, a pattern that may have persisted throughout his life. In his later years, he might have moved the fever into the category of illness he presented to doctors as "rheumatism." It is also possible that his recurrences had all but disappeared as he aged. Dawson never presented his fever specifically as a disease category nor did he seek help for its symptoms. The single newspaper article that recalled Armstead Williams and Dawson performing public feats of strength tells us that Dawson, despite his limp and war injury, was a robust man. He pursued hard manual labor postwar, which gradually diminished over the years as his body deteriorated. His knowledge of his body shaped his perception of his postwar health. He entered the world of white medicine only for pension purposes.

Dawson's account of his illnesses and injuries might have been unintelligible to doctors and pension authorities. White people in authority asked Dawson questions about his health but may not have understood his responses, particularly since Dawson did not share the same vocabulary and philosophy of healing. Dawson's second wife, Janey, experienced a similar communication obstacle. Names, dates, and places appear inconsistently in the record as if the government agent made a guess based on a poorly understood conversation.

The existence of Dawson's veteran's badge, a common souvenir of veterans' meetings and events and not a medal awarded by the government, attested to a commitment he made to his country, achievement of a new kind of manhood, and tangible proof that he had fought to preserve the Union. The badge attested to Dawson's veteran body and embellished it, indicating that his body served to protect the country. It conferred an honor readily understood by white and black people; it placed his public body in a higher social stratum. This badged body offered a record, "the surest validation of fading and uncertain memories." While the badge embodied memory, it also allowed people to forget the struggle for emancipation, for example, or the challenge of proving one's worth in a Union uniform on the battlefield. For black Americans, "their efforts to carve out a social and political space in the United States demanded a different set of forgettings and rememberings." The badged black body carried a heavy weight of multiple meanings.[103]

One of Janey's depositions stated that Dawson participated in GAR activities. Black veterans were welcome to GAR membership by policy, but Dawson would have traveled far to join a post. Dawson's lack of literacy would have kept him from participating as an officer of the fraternal order, but he may have enjoyed and benefited from the camaraderie. If he had joined an integrated post, he might have socialized with white people for the first time in his life. "Nowhere else during this era did African Americans stand as political equals to white Americans." The discourse of patriotism and service to country and other veterans and public remembrance of wartime sacrifice must have resonated with Dawson's sense of self as veterans continually redefined their identities in a changing world. "Soldiering destabilized treasured assumptions of a world steeped in the culture of sentimentalism and Christianity."[104]

Despite Dawson's medical examination a few years before his death, he probably saw himself as a success. Although doctors identified many of Dawson's maladies, his civic body achieved a central ideal of manhood and self-sufficiency to raise a family. His body beat the odds. Most single black soldiers left the service and gravitated to cities, especially after the end of Reconstruction. Those who returned to rural areas typically experienced lives of poverty. Not surprisingly, many black veterans whose prewar work was listed in military records as "laborer" were bound by that role for the rest of their lives. By 1890, about 23 percent of white veterans were unskilled laborers, and about half of black ones were.[105]

Dawson's pension body succeeded only briefly. As proud as he must have been about his military service, the full benefits of citizenship did not come easily. He waited years to apply for a pension. Suffering many rejections, he received a pension for only a few years before his death. As we have seen, Janey and her attorneys gathered all the existing evidence to support her claim to legal marriage, but the pension office remained adamant in its rejection. Enslaved backgrounds and the recollections of non-literate people forced Janey to meet a higher standard of proof than white claimants. Policies appeared nondiscriminatory, but the presumption that claimants' histories were documented by common records (births, baptisms, marriages) presented overwhelming obstacles to many black claimants. Consequently, pension office "agents placed a greater burden of proof on blacks that required more special examinations and evaluations, rejected a higher number of African American applicants, and suggested lower payments for the approved claimants." Pension officers may have held the moral view that black people living in poverty deserved it because of their nature. Changing surnames, for instance, from Dorsey to Dawson and back again may have been perceived as moral laxity.[106]

Dawson's body, however, indirectly influenced military policy about recruiting, training, and deploying black soldiers during World War II. Any information the army collected about

Dawson's body entered the vast compilation and analysis of medical data generated by the army during the war, *The Medical and Surgical History of the War of the Rebellion*. Its multiple volumes featured graphic displays of data that constituted the second government compilation of statistics regarding the health of African Americans. The first published data on the health of black soldiers, however, was prepared under the auspices of the US Sanitary Commission.

Before the end of the Civil War, government and business leaders wanted guidelines for occupational insurance to be formulated on the presumption that many discharged soldiers would seek employment in manufacturing plants. The commission therefore sponsored a study in 1864 that required the distribution of kits to army doctors containing instruments for anthropometric measurements. Vital data were collected by measuring black and white bodies. The commission competed with the federal government to produce the most reliable picture of the health of black and white soldiers.

A key tool of the Sanitary Commission's kit was the spirometer, which measured lung capacity, a simple measurement fraught with cultural assumptions and embedded bias. For example, the spirometer data seemed to show that black bodies appeared to have smaller lung capacity when compared with white bodies, thus substantiating a view that black bodies were inherently deficient. Two studies resulted from an analysis of the data submitted to the Sanitary Commission, one in 1869 and the other in 1875. The earlier report normalized whiteness as the baseline standard of health. The latter examined the measurements in all their complexity and concluded that no statistically significant difference existed between the performance of black and white bodies during the war. The 1869 study considered black people to be a subordinate race with measurable shortfalls in physical abilities such as lung capacity. Both studies, however, combined clinical measurements with value judgments and opinions about black bodies based on "'well-known facts' or 'beliefs' or universal opinion." The tools and methods of these studies established anthropometry as a credible tool for analyzing race, thus giving "legitimacy to racial science and the validity of its conclusions about race and racial inequality."[107]

When bodily phenomena translate into numbers, they acquire an authority and truthfulness at the expense of qualitative data. As ambiguous a figure as Dawson presents as a historical actor, as a statistic in medical studies, his case supports arguments both for and against the integrity of the black male military body well into the twentieth century.

SEVEN

JOHN SHIELDS
(1839–1923)

A RED BALL OF FIRE

Amid the fighting in and around Gettysburg, Pennsylvania, on July 2, 1863, Captain John Shields ushered his men forward to join other Union soldiers massing along high ground known as Cemetery Ridge. A large force of Confederates had marched toward Gettysburg the day before, and Union troops began a running battle that rapidly surrounded the town. By July 2, Union troops had established a strong defensive line facing west along the ridge, stretching from the outskirts of Gettysburg south to the hills of Big and Little Round Top.

Shields and his regiment arrived at around eight in the morning and had little time to familiarize themselves with their surroundings as they awaited orders for battle. Regiments on either side gathered and pushed west from their hardened lines of defense, deploying within a peach orchard, farm fields, and forests enclosing half-buried boulders the size of wagons.

Shields's regiment, the Fifty-Third Pennsylvania, had come north through Virginia following a punishing campaign in locations that became milestones of the war's gains and losses: Fredericksburg, Malvern Hill, and Fair Oaks in Virginia, Antietam in Maryland, and Chancellorsville in Virginia. Shields knew firsthand the terror experienced by disorganized troops who were surprised by an enemy force in unfamiliar territory. One humid late-spring night in 1862, having waded through shoulder-high water across the Chickahominy River east of Richmond, Virginia, Shields and his company pushed through the swampy growth to the site of a day's battle, hearing "moans of the wounded and dying, and men running to and fro with lanterns, gathering the wounded together." After a night's rest, the Fifty-Third and other regiments advanced toward the supposed location of the enemy. Soon, the line stopped to clear obstructions, and the Fifty-Third rested for a few minutes. "At that instant," Shields wrote, "a tremendous volley was fired into us. My Captain fell through the ranks, severely wounded in the head." Shields assumed command of his company.[1]

The previous December in Fredericksburg, Shields had participated in an ill-considered uphill charge on frozen terrain, fired on by well-fortified rebels. During his advance ahead of his company, a rifle bullet struck Shields's right inner thigh inches from his testicles, passing through and out his leg. He was hospitalized for about ten days, after which he arranged a leave of absence to return home to Mauch Chunk, Pennsylvania, to recuperate. Shields had experienced surprises on the battlefield: the sudden appearance of rebels shooting at him, hoarse voices shouting orders or curses, the air polluted by the sulfurous steam of gunpowder, the thud of distant artillery rounds, and the incessant rattling of rifle fire.

Today, July 2, Shields was alert, ready, confident, and wary. During the hot afternoon, he and his regiment hid behind a low stone wall within sight of a farmhouse to the north across a dirt road. The line of soldiers was backed by a gentle creek, and the sound of flowing water disappeared in the murderous thunder of artillery and rifle fire to the left, ahead, and to the right. He looked along the wall to survey the quiet soldiers awaiting orders. Shields's regiment, only 124 men strong, nestled alongside several other eviscerated regiments as a brigade in reserve. His own Company E numbered only thirteen soldiers, including himself. Peering over the wall, through trees and beyond another road, he saw an open field of dried and trampled wheat under a "sulphurous canopy." He could not easily discern uniforms or battle flags. Soldiers appeared to be shooting at muzzle flashes in the miasma of dust and gunpowder. His brigade faced the setting sun, its glare reduced to a descending "red ball of fire." Three Union brigades had already advanced across the field and held positions on high ground facing Confederates arrayed alongside another creek. The word was passed that the three brigades had suffered severe losses and were running out of ammunition.[2]

A rebel artillery battery had located the reserve brigade and "had become very annoying." Determined to take or eliminate it and having just received orders to advance, John R. Brooke, the twenty-five-year-old colonel of the Fifty-Third and also the commander of the patched-together brigade, dismounted from his horse and yelled at his soldiers, "Boys, remember the enemy has invaded our soil, and the eyes of the world [are] upon us and we are expected to stand up bravely and do our duty." With a subdued response, the reserve brigade rose and marched into the field. As a soldier later said, if one has "had the nightmare and attempted to scream and could not," then one understands why soldiers emitted shrieks instead of manly cheers.[3]

Into a tornado of lead, shouts, blood, and dirt, Shields led his dozen into a battle most "desperate and sanguinary." Each side attacked the other, firing rifles with "unyielding tenacity." Soldiers advanced shoulder to shoulder, aware of each other's bodies, their smells, and their sounds. "Soldiers generated other kinds of noises themselves. As pulse rates spiked, the mechanisms of personal self-control crumbled, producing loss of bladder and bowel control, along with other ordinary cultural inhibitions." Men in the brigade shouted, cursed, displayed a red-hot killing frenzy, and shrieked with laughter. Soldiers experienced the dull

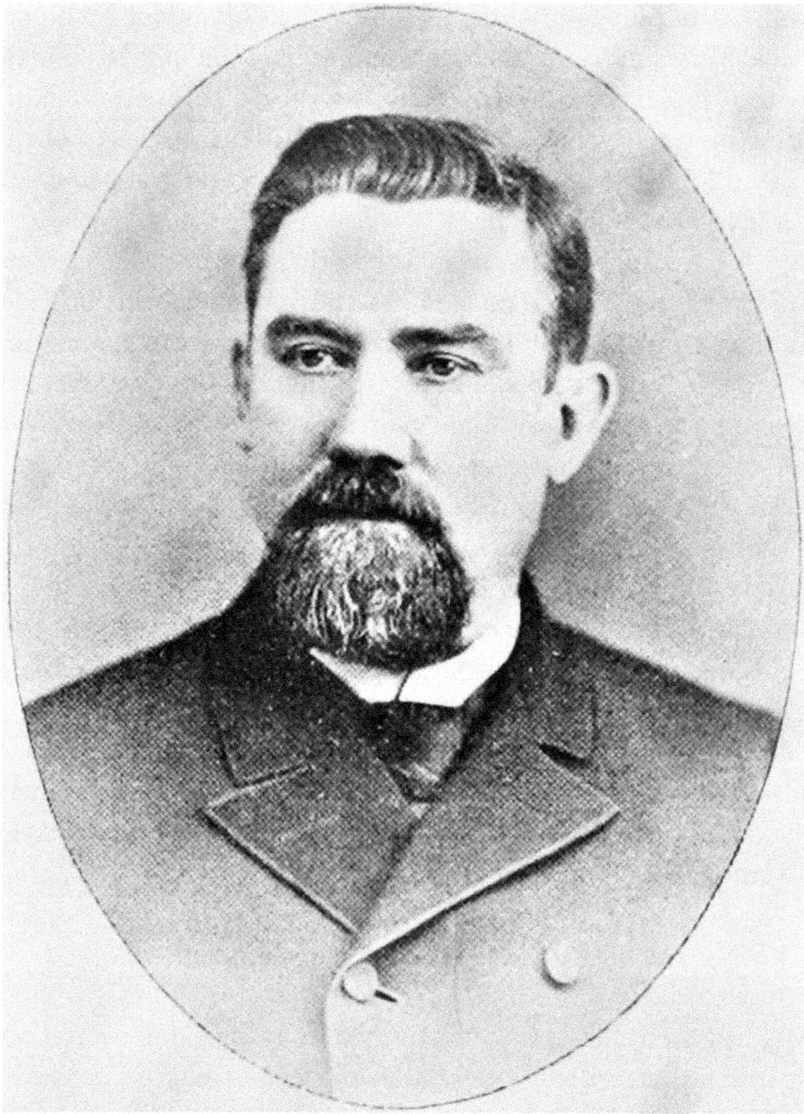

Captain John Shields, 1860s–1870s. *Credit: William Henry Powell, ed.,* Officers of the Army and Navy (Volunteer) Who Served in the Civil War. *Philadelphia: L. R. Hammersby, 1893.*

impact of bullets or shrapnel felling their comrades accompanied by peculiar but distinctive sounds like "the weird harmonic ring of bullets striking fixed bayonets, the clicking of the locking ring on the bayonet when fixed on the rifle's muzzle . . . or the metallic clink when [bullets] struck bone or the dropped china crack when they hit teeth."[4]

In the lead, Brooke reached the other end of the wheatfield only to discover that in the haze and excitement, his brigade, almost out of ammunition, had outdistanced the supporting Union brigades on his left and right flanks. The Confederates were moving to encircle his men, so Brooke ordered a retreat. About the time Brooke came to this realization, Shields, still advancing but holding his head down, took a bullet in the neck. The bullet smashed through the thyroid cartilage[5] just below the Adam's apple and passed through the larynx, the voice box, a complex intersection of cartilage, ligaments, and membranes that governs air flow to the lungs and speech. The bullet compromised the larynx and disappeared into the right shoulder, possibly underneath the scapula, where it remained. As Shields fell, his comrades noticed his profuse bleeding. They helped him to the rear, and he was soon taken to a field hospital "where simple dressings were applied."[6]

PERMANENT DISABILITY MAY RESULT

By July 4, the battle was effectively over as the Confederates began their retreat to Virginia. Shields's hemorrhaging stopped a few hours after he was shot, and doctors observed that he was breathing normally. At this time, orderlies placed him on a train to Baltimore for further treatment. By July 5, he was admitted to Jarvis Hospital under the supervision of Dr. Dewitt C. Peters. The initial assessment verified the trajectory of the bullet downward through the larynx into the shoulder. Early in Shields's recovery, doctors noticed evidence of damaged nerves, such as a weak right arm, sensitivity to heat, and absence of perspiration on the right side of the face, neck, and upper right arm.

At 9:00 a.m. on July 5, the duty physician "found him bright, breathing easy . . . and able to converse without difficulty." Swelling appeared minimal; "the wound had closed and no emphysema existed." Later that afternoon and evening, Shields's condition rapidly worsened. He had fallen asleep while sitting, and his breathing was labored and stertorous. His pulse rose dramatically, and his "chest and face were covered with a cold perspiration, and his expression was exceedingly anxious. The symptoms indicated that the officer was in a critical condition, and active steps were demanded to save his life." Emphysema became pronounced, and swelling had set in.[7]

The duty physicians reviewed Shields's condition and decided to perform a tracheotomy. Anesthesia was administered, and Dr. Peters cut the skin over the cricoid cartilage located opposite the bullet wound, at the back of the windpipe. "The thyroid gland was exposed and found greatly distended and infiltrated by air and bloody scrum, as indeed were all the tissues." Dr. Chris Johnson inserted a tenaculum—a long-handled instrument with a hooked end—to pry apart tissue so that he could introduce a knife to pierce the trachea. The first cut yielded no result, so the surgeon made a deeper cut, which was "followed by the escape of a bubble of air. The fresh wound was cleansed. . . . Very little blood escaped into the trachea, and one or two explosive efforts cleared it of these small clots and a quantity of tough mucus. The patient breathed easily through the opening."

To support the lacerated throat, one of the surgeons inserted a metal stent, "Dessault's tube," that kept its position without sutures. Shields felt better immediately, his pulse returned to normal, "and he was soon enjoying a pleasant sleep." By the next day, Shields took liquid nourishment, including flaxseed tea. By July 9, the swelling had disappeared, and the stent was removed. He could now breathe normally without surgical aid. By the eighteenth, the wounds appeared to be healed. "The patient walks about, and his voice is as strong as ever. Being anxious to return home, he was discharged cured." On the eighteenth, Shields returned home to Mauch Chunk (renamed Jim Thorpe in 1954) to convalesce.

At eleven, Shields had immigrated to the United States from County Donegal, Ireland, and joined his family: father Patrick, mother Anna, and sister Anna. The town was only a generation old when John Shields arrived. The small community occupied a narrow portion of the Lehigh Valley and became a major canal—and later railroad—nexus for shipping anthracite.[8]

The year before the war began, at age nineteen, Shields performed work as a laborer (his occupation as listed in the 1860 census) while living with the Isabella Bowlen (widow) family, her two adult sons, and three other young men, all boarders, in Chester County, Pennsylvania, about seventy-five miles south of Mauch Chunk. When the war began, Shields enlisted in the Fifty-Third and trained in Harrisburg at Camp Curtin. On October 16, 1861, he was appointed to the rank of first lieutenant. Nothing is known of Shields's education or what qualities impressed the recruiters, but events proved that the recruiters' appreciation of his abilities was justified.[9]

Shields's wounding at Fredericksburg marked the beginning of a lifetime of periodic examinations by physicians and sporadic hospital stays. For the remainder of his life, whether in or out of military service, he remained in constant negotiation with the government to recognize maladies he viewed as interconnected products of his war experience. The beginning of this negotiation was his thigh wound, then the bullet in his neck. Shields perceived his degradation of health during the following decades as deriving from both wounds. He also claimed bodily suffering due to possible nerve injuries of the type studied by the Mitchells. Of all the soldiers profiled in this book, only Shields was examined by both John K. and S. Weir Mitchell in Philadelphia.

On December 13, 1862, once Shields quit the Fredericksburg battle and limped—or was later removed and carried by a stretcher party—to a field hospital, the physician he saw described the thigh wound as "serious" in a casualty report, and Shields was removed to a hospital in Washington, DC. The next day, he formally requested a leave of twenty days because he was "unfit for duty." He wrote, "I think a visit to my home in Penna would tend to secure my speedy recovery." His leave was granted, and Shields departed around December 22 for home, where his healing was supervised by a local physician, A. Leonard. Various entries in the military record at around this time do not adhere to any army standard of precision. By the time Shields reached home, his wound had been described as located in the thigh or hip, qualitatively as "serious," "severe," or categorized as simply a "flesh wound." Curiously, although the surgeon's certificate for sick leave required a notarized statement of confidence in Dr. Leonard, the same document stated that the authorizing surgeon removed the "ball" from Shields's thigh, leaving him "in a fair way for recovery." Later reports by examining doctors for pension purposes identified both entry and exit wounds on Shields's inner thigh, so any mention of the ball removal was in error.

Shields returned to his regiment in late January or early February 1863—when he was promoted to captain—but he was back in the hospital on March 9 and 10 for a new malady: gonorrhea. His discharge from the hospital was premature, as he returned for another stay between March 23 and April 3 for the same reason. Gonorrhea and military camps were synonymous. Dr. Samuel D. Gross, one of the renowned physicians of his time and the author of *A Manual of Military Surgery*, stated that preventing gonorrhea among soldiers was impossible. Despite their knowledge of the consequences, soldiers risked getting the disease and "often pay a heavy penalty for their indulgence." At first, treatment consisted of "rest, low diet, active purgation, and a mix of antimony and salt plus copaiba."[10] Next, the penis and scrotum were periodically bathed in warm salt water, and once the gonorrhea discharge lessened, the doctor injected into the urethra "lead, sulphate of zinc, or nitrate of silver, at first very mild and gradually increased in strength, repeated every six, eight or twelve hours" for about five days, at which time symptoms were expected to disappear. Shields evidently never mentioned either case of gonorrhea to government doctors. If he had symptoms of this disease following army service, Shields could have seen private physicians whose confidentiality was unquestioned.[11]

From July 18, 1863, the day Shields arrived home after Gettysburg, his disability leave was good for twenty days. He was required either to return to duty or obtain a doctor's sworn statement that he would need another twenty days. In early August, Dr. Leonard supplied the statement with its pro forma wording, "I hereby certify that I have carefully examined said officer + find him unfit for duty in consequence of said wound I further certify that in my opinion he will not be fit to return to duty for a less period than twenty days by reason of the above mentioned wound." Leonard repeated this statement in documents dated September, October, and November. On December 12, he did so again. On the same date, Shields married Anna M. Curran (b. 1845) at the Immaculate Conception Church in Mauch Chunk. Another Irish immigrant, Anna went by "Annie."[12]

In January 1864, Dr. Leonard submitted his final "not fit for at least 20 days" sworn statement. Shields returned to his regiment in February, but it soon became apparent to him and his fellow officers that his neck wound precluded the full exercise of his military functions. On March 2, Shields submitted a memorandum of resignation from the army "on account of [his] health" accompanied by a surgeon's certificate. The next day, Surgeon George W. Jackson of the Fifty-Third endorsed Shields's letter, stating, "I do hereby certify that I have carefully examined this officer and find him suffering from effects of Gunshot wound of the Larynx received at Gettysburg July 2nd, 1863, which impairs the voice to a considerable extent." Jackson added that Shields might not be able to resume duties for "a considerable length of time." He concluded with his "belief that if he be retained in the field permanent Disability may result." Shields's final appearance in the regimental records is found in the Company Muster Roll for March and April 1864: "Discharged at near Stevensburg Va March 13, 1864, on surgeons certificate of disability for wounds received at the Battle of Gettysburg July 2nd, 1863." Shields received a pension of twenty dollars[13] a month in 1864.

Shields returned to his family in Mauch Chunk and considered his future.

FUGITIVE PAINS

As Shields was en route to Baltimore, contract assistant surgeon S. Weir Mitchell arrived in Gettysburg and was stunned to encounter death and suffering on an unimaginable scale. Here and at Turner's Lane Hospital, Mitchell saw cases like Shields's with either enduring, fleeting, or evolving symptoms of pain from apparent nerve damage. His case notes reveal views apparently not shared by the doctors Shields had consulted. Mitchell would have applied a holistic appraisal, but military and later pension doctors could not rate Shields's pain (for a pension) because they found no associated lesion or trauma. Outside of Mitchell's methods, medical practice did not have a way to locate or rationalize pain if a lesion could not be identified.[14]

In a comparable case illustrating worse outcomes for a neck wound, Mitchell evaluated Sergeant J. C., who, at Gettysburg, was shot in the left side of the neck, the bullet angling downward into the right shoulder, "splintering" the clavicle before coming to rest in the trapezius, a triangular-shaped muscle anchored to the back of the skull, the clavicle, and over the spinal column. Shortly after being wounded, J. C. experienced chills followed by fever, with "darting and aching pain" throughout his swollen left arm.

To Mitchell, "he showed very plainly that the mind as well as the body had suffered—his memory being impaired, and his temper excessively irritable."[15]

In another comparable case, nineteen-year-old Private John C. Drye, Seventy-First Pennsylvania Volunteers, was struck by a bullet while fighting at Gettysburg on July 3. It pierced the skin at the upper neck behind the left ear and traveled downward; it was never located. As a result of the wound, Drye appeared to be paralyzed on the left side of his body. Mitchell was particularly interested in Drye's speech difficulties attendant on the paralysis. The doctor's detailed notes far exceeded the attention given to the paralysis by military doctors, who, in fairness, lacked the time and perhaps expertise with nerve injuries to proceed further. Mitchell electrized the soldier before evaluating the wound's effect on speech. Drye "pronounces letters with difficulty or imperfectly. . . . The labials are of course affected, but the guttural sounds are also imperfectly executed." Mitchell continued the electrization, but there was no improvement in Drye's speech. Over time, Drye learned to compensate for some speech difficulties but still "talked 'thick' and lisped." These two cases illustrate Mitchell's interest in mapping anomalies of the nervous system by accepting soldiers' descriptions of pain when specific physical causes remained unidentified.[16]

Mitchell examined Sergeant L. P., who, like Shields, was shot through the thigh. L. P. reached Mitchell's ward a week after being wounded. Mitchell surmised the damage to the sciatic nerve. Within a day or so under Mitchell's care, the sergeant developed chills followed by sharp pains and a burning sensation in his foot. The onset, duration, and intensity of pain astounded Mitchell, who wrote, "He begged at times to be killed, at others, to go home; while sometimes he would lie open-eyed, regarding ferociously the passers-by who shook his bed as they walked, every movement seeming to add to his torment." The pain lessened over months, the burning sensation ebbing more slowly.

Mitchell watched L. P.'s personality change: "From being a man of gay and kindly temper, known in his company as a good-natured jester, he became morose and melancholy, and complained that reading gave him vertigo, and that his memory of recent events was bad." Mitchell warned fellow physicians of the danger in not recognizing nerve damage consequent to wounds because of the potential for long-term difficulties. How the damage resolves "must depend, to some extent, upon how soon it is recognized, how boldly and skillfully treated."[17]

NEW MANHOOD

As he convalesced in Mauch Chunk, Shields considered pursuing a position in business. With the war over and industrial expansion offering opportunities, business shaped the new masculinity. The postwar–model businessman lived by his own rules, created his own opportunities, and enjoyed the reward of wealth. Veterans, still young men in the late 1860s and 1870s, adopted the ethics of ambition and competition. A flood of self-help books inspired business schemes and adventures. Self-made men of business became the ideal, and "with assertiveness, greed, and rivalry set free in the marketplace," those who succeeded in wealth and influence were celebrated. Those who did not realize their ambitions faded into irrelevance and obscurity.[18]

Veterans who bore the visible marks of their wartime sacrifices found it difficult to view their wartime experiences as a form of masculine competition. That is, the world of business employed war metaphors to articulate ambition and business strategies. This world depressed those veterans who had lost limbs and, unless educated, skilled in nonmanual labor, and socially connected, found themselves placed on a shelf to age gracefully as symbols of the preservation of the Union. Their sacrifices were applauded on Decoration Day and the Fourth of July but were otherwise absent from public discourse and the business world.

Shields wasted no time in securing his veteran status with a pension. A government pension provided the equivalent of 30 percent of the earnings of an unskilled laborer. Pension authorities did not rate disabilities as permanent unless a soldier was obviously incapable of performing *any* type of manual labor. Dr. Horace P. Moody of Scranton examined Shields in April 1864 and certified that his wounds constituted a "probably permanent" disability. Of the Gettysburg wound, Moody wrote, "It has seriously affected the air passages and may lead to confirmed tuberculosis." The lack of a reliable voice to exercise command was probably a major reason why the army discharged Shields. Subsequent physical examinations over the following decades confirmed that Shields's neck wound had never completely healed. He could speak clearly for several minutes but would inevitably cough, become hoarse, and feel irritation in his larynx. The surgeon's statement supplemented Shields's "Declaration for an Invalid Pension" (April 20, 1864) and an affidavit by John Patton, formerly first lieutenant, Company G, Eighty-First Pennsylvania Volunteers, who witnessed Shields's wounding at Gettysburg.[19]

Of all pensions issued to veterans by the late 1880s, about a quarter, like Shields's, were given because of gunshot or shell wounds. A much smaller percentage, between just over 8 to 12 percent, were issued because of rheumatism and chronic diarrhea. Shields's Irish origins likely were part of the discussion with pension authorities. Generally, in the Union army, Irish immigrants enjoyed better health throughout their service than other soldiers, native-born or not, and Irish (along with German) soldiers required fewer hospitalizations than others; therefore, the muster rolls showed greater attendance among their regiments.[20]

Until the end of the war, the army retained Shields on the payroll in a largely nominal capacity as deputy provost marshal for Carbon County. Concurrently, he found a new career as a railroad contractor, possibly prompted by the growing importance of railroads in his home community. By 1870, Shields headed his household in Mauch Chunk at age thirty-one, with his wife, Annie, daughter Anna, and son John, five and two years old, respectively.[21]

Shields moved his family to Flemington, New Jersey, where he farmed and maintained a peach orchard. The same character and abilities that merited an officer's commission transferred to his new community. His captain's rank and honorable wounds constituted a résumé that enabled him to join the local elected governing elite as president of the Board of Street Commissioners, the body that supervised all local government functions.

By the early 1870s, as pension laws and his body were changing, Shields sought a new surgeon's certificate to prompt a pension review followed by, hopefully, a payment increase. The form gave Shields's description as five feet, ten inches, 175 pounds, and with a ruddy complexion. The examining doctor noted that a skin discoloration was evident over the spot where the bullet presumably came to rest. He also observed that Shields "complains of weak voice subject to frequent Hoarseness" plus shoulder pain. Shields continued to receive his monthly pension of twenty dollars.[22]

Shields traveled to Leighton in Carbon County in 1873, 1876, and 1877 for medical examinations, taking advantage of every significant change in pension law to reapply, despite risking his current pension being reduced or taken away. By 1876, Shields had gained five pounds, and an examining surgeon added new information to buttress a claim for an increase. Shields "states that the right-side of his neck does not perspire and always feels numb + disagreeable noticed particularly in Summer—much troubled with burning pain from dryness + much discharge from throat especially in the morning deep down in throat near sternum." Aside from the bullet wounds, the examining doctor could only repeat Shields's assertions of difficulties connected, as he claimed, to wartime wounds and privation while in the army. The surgeon concluded that Shields was entitled to his pension but did not suggest an increase. The next year, in another surgeon's certificate, Dr. N. B. Reder repeated the description of the two wounds and through inspection verified the "inflammation of the mucous membrane of the throat." He quoted Shields in confirming rheumatism in the right shoulder, "numbness of the right side of the face," and lack of perspiration in hot weather. The embedded bullet had begun to irritate Shields. When he exercised his right arm, he felt the bullet. Shields also invoked his Fredericksburg wound and cited stiffness and rheumatism of his right leg. For the first time, the surgeon's form included a front-back diagram of the body on which was noted the location and appearance of thigh and neck wounds.[23]

By the 1880 census, the Shields family was living in Raritan, Hunterdon County, New Jersey, adjacent to Flemington. The family had increased by two more sons, Robert E. and Henry G. The next year, Shields was appointed to the board of directors for the new Flemington National Bank. By 1885, another family was boarding with them, Clarence J. and Elizabeth W. Hamilton and their three children. Shields's migration was not unusual: rebuilding the United States after the war in a burst of industrial expansion created opportunities in growing communities. Whether Shields was sympathetic with the ideals of Gilded Age self-made businessmen, he found leadership roles in business and fraternal organizations.[24]

Within this decade, Shields became active in the Grand Army of the Republic (GAR). Veterans had begun to place monuments at the sites of their battles and congregated in encampments for days of lectures, tours, and socializing. A photograph dated 1887 shows veterans of the Fifty-Third posing in the wheatfield on a summer's day. Shields may be seated next to a man holding a national flag. In September 1889, a small group of veterans attended the dedication of the Fifty-Third monument, a vigilant and determined-looking bronze soldier atop a stone plinth facing the enemy, placed adjacent to the wheatfield at Gettysburg. By this time, over half the veterans in Shields's regiment had died.

Doubtless, Shields had helped to raise funds for the statue and plan its dedication on "Pennsylvania Day." Continuing problems with Shields's throat no doubt interfered with public speaking, including making monument dedications.[25]

Periodic medical examinations attest to Shields's trouble with speech. He continuously exhibited symptoms of catarrh, an inflamed, irritated, and painful throat. He could converse for very short intervals before he became too hoarse, with resurgent pain in his neck that required a period of silence before he spoke again. In a suit with a high collar, Shields's wounds were not visible. When he spoke, however, listeners perceived his difficulty. While his speech would not have interfered with his prestigious role as a bank board trustee, his ability to make public speeches probably worsened. No local newspaper article reported any speeches Shields made after the war. He turned down invitations to speak on commemorative or civic occasions. In some business transactions, his limited speech probably disadvantaged him. Further, his developing rheumatism in his right leg forced him to limp. When walking, he might have favored the right side of his body where the nerves of the neck and arm caused pain and perhaps impaired motion.

The GAR promoted an ideology of soldierly manhood around activities that ensured the visibility of veterans and an ever-present reminder of their sacrifice and dedication. In public, members wore GAR badges and distinctive military hats. The national network of local posts was organized around military lines with commandants, adjutants, and the issuance of general orders. Gathering members and political momentum during the 1880s, the GAR promoted a "millennial, republican" worldview. Conservative socially as well, the GAR was not sympathetic to evolving rights for immigrants, African Americans, and women. African American veterans were admitted and sometimes enjoyed equal social status, but where they were unwelcome (as in the South) or for other reasons, they set up and ran their own

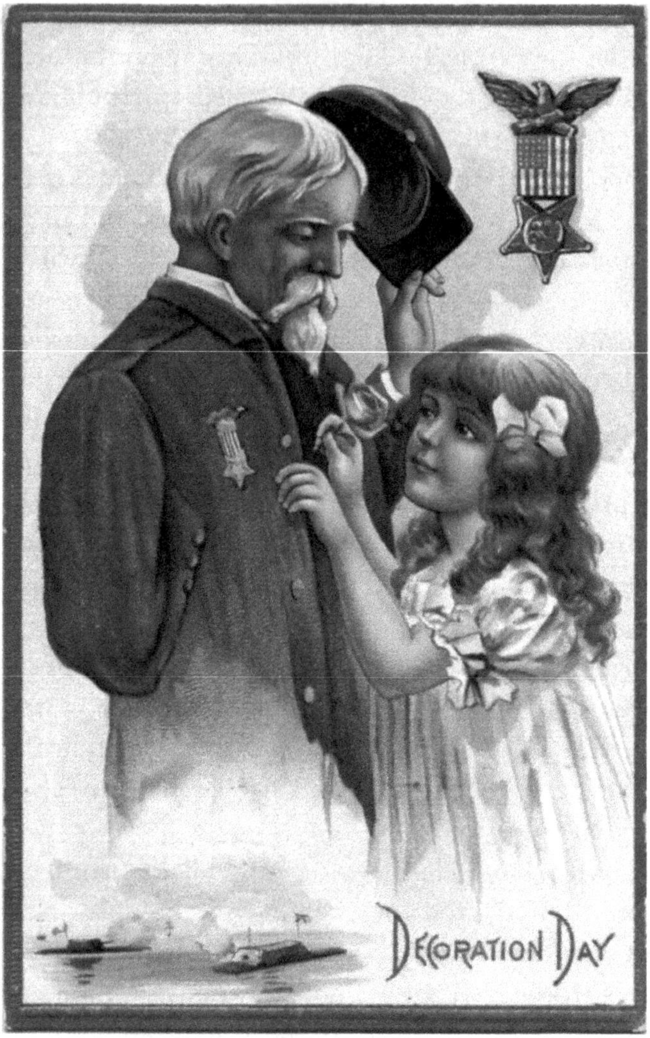

Decoration Day commemorative postcard depicting an armless veteran, c. 1910. *Credit: Author's collection.*

local posts; segregation paralleled the larger segregation of civil society, as Prestley Dawson possibly experienced. When immigration caused national concern that newcomers would supplant white people, the GAR put forth strident views against open immigration, even to the extent of race-baiting and taunting newspapers that opposed expanded pension benefits as being owned by "Jews and Gentile aliens."[26]

The stance on immigrants and the self-consciousness about bringing military discipline into all facets of working life were probably related to a concern shared by the wider public that the luxuries of middle-class life and the lack of war to galvanize young men threatened national manhood. A sure remedy for "the soft, pampered life of the business and professional classes after the [Civil] war" was another war. The Spanish-American War answered the call to rid manhood of "flabbiness." Public imagery in the form of popular postcards celebrated the aging Union army veterans but now conflated these images with those of young volunteers to fight in Cuba.[27]

Whether Shields also approved of segregated posts and opposed immigration of nonwhite people, the record does not say. Shields did promote the image of veterans, even destitute ones, as dignified members of the community and opposed the characterizations of pensioners as lazy, alcoholic, or vagrant. He was well informed about changes in pension laws over time and not only sought to benefit from them himself; he also advised impoverished or suffering veterans. Generally, indigent people, if they received any aid at all, obtained it at the local level. Localities supported their own asylums and almshouses. The GAR was one of the few national organizations that offered temporary assistance to needy veterans, administered locally via GAR posts.[28]

In late 1889, Shields filed another request with the pension office. He acknowledged his current monthly rate of twenty dollars but stated a growing need for more because of "increased disability resulting from the [neck wound] for which pension was granted as it has resulted in rheumatism which interferes with my right arm which has been slowly increasing since I left the army also in large veins on each leg which troubles me very much." Shields articulated possible and unhealed nerve damage consequent to the neck wound and persisted in treating these phenomena as related miseries. Pension authorities remained skeptical or rationalized the rejection of his claims as being outside the purview of legislation. By this time, Shields had engaged Soule & Company, pension attorneys, to act on his behalf.[29]

MEETING THE MITCHELLS

In 1890, Shields underwent an exhaustive physical evaluation of his body. His importuning of medical authorities brought him to Philadelphia, where John K. and S. Weir Mitchell examined him. Shields was not a later recipient of their health questionnaire; rather, he and his private physician responded to the elder Mitchell's published plea to veterans to write to him about their wartime injuries or wounds and answer specific questions.

In February 1890, on letterhead reading "John Shields Railroad Contractor, Flemington, N.J.," Shields related his wounding at Gettysburg to Mitchell, named both Drs. Peters and Johnson, and noted that his "voice has never been what it was before the wound." Shields asked his physician, A. Parish, MD, of Henington, New Jersey, to write to Mitchell in more detail about himself. Parish repeated the now-standard narrative of the wounding and noted that the bullet remained lodged somewhere near the brachial plexus. Of the neck injury, Parish wrote that the "wound of larynx and surrounding structure has caused a decided stricture of trachea and this gives much trouble in breathing on active exercise—a cold gives much trouble by persistent hoarseness . . . pharyngitis and post nasal catarrh" remained chronic. He outlined the nerve-injury phenomena of lack of perspiration on the right side of the head; deafness in the right ear; atrophied right shoulder, arm, and forearm; "and more [or] less constant pain." Mindful that the threshold for any pension was the inability to perform manual labor, Parish described Shields's failure to "carry weights" in the right hand or use it in any way to perform manual labor. He also added new ailments, such as varicose veins in the legs and varicocele[30] of the left testicle.[31]

Possibly in early February, Mitchell examined Shields in Philadelphia. Undated, rough notes in Mitchell's idiosyncratic phrases and abbreviations document Shields's description of his symptoms, his history, and Mitchell's points of interest. Given the traumatic injury to Shields's neck and shoulder, Mitchell suspected an additional injury to the eyes. He arranged an interview with Dr. George E. de Schweinitz, an ophthalmology professor at Jefferson Medical College. Dr. de Schweinitz examined Shields and reported the results to Mitchell in a letter. Mitchell directed de Schweinitz's attention to the behavior of the pupils and the associated muscles controlled by the sympathetic nerve. While the ophthalmologist found the pupils to exhibit normal responses, he described Shields's optic nerves as "rather 'sick,' and that the blurring of their edges, especially on the nasal side, was more marked than should be the case." De Schweinitz said that Shields would visit again for more tests, but there is no record that he did so.[32]

Later, Shields appeared in Somerville, New Jersey, before a three-physician medical board for a physical examination to support a new surgeon's certificate. All certificates began with the claimant's explanation of his debility, which, in Shields's case, included worsening rheumatism of his right shoulder and arm, numbness, pricking sensations, varicose veins, and varicocele. Next, the panel recorded body measurements. At fifty-one, Shields weighed 206 pounds, and his neck scar was described as straddling the median line of the neck one inch below the Adam's apple. "Fully 1/3 of trachea has been removed materially [and the damaged area is] tender + greatly interferes with respiration on forced exertion." The examiners' physical inspection of Shields included asking him to move his limbs or his head in specific ways and describe any pain, discomfort, or impaired function.

Examiners proceeded category by category. To investigate the numbness of the right arm, they measured limbs; the right arm and forearm had shrunk in comparison with the left. Turning the head from side to side induced rheumatism in the right arm from the shoulder down. Next, a hearing test was administered using a ticking watch. Slight deafness was discovered and "thickened + inflamed tissue [in the] eustacian canals," particularly in the right ear. Then the legs were examined and found to have enlarged, distended veins with a higher temperature than the surrounding body. The varicose veins "bid fair to ulcerate." Major organs appeared to be normal.

The doctors' summary of Shields required precise language because pension adjustments would be based on it. Shields, they stated, was "entitled to a total rating for disability," based on a point system that assigned weights to the neck wound, rheumatism, slight deafness, "varices" (enlarged veins) of the legs, and varicocele. The examiners added a handwritten note that expressed difficulty in reconciling Shields's apparently interconnected maladies with the pension rating system. "We have not made our opinion as clear as we wish owing to the number of disabilities for which we were obliged to rate, + losing sight of the fact that these ratings could not be added for . . . a total we would herefore state that in our opinion the claimants condition is equivalent to loss of arm at shoulder."[33]

The panel offered the pension office an uncomplicated way forward: just aggregate Shields's maladies and rate them as if his arm had been amputated at the shoulder. A few months later, a pension office authority stamped the examiner's notes, "Rejected." The pension remained at twenty dollars per month.

After Mitchell examined Shields and referred him to the ophthalmologist, John K. Mitchell examined him in Philadelphia. His findings did not serve pension purposes but would have given Shields some insight into his cluster of ailments. He measured both arms and forearms and noted the differences. Like the later pension examiners, he tested Shields's responses to body movements but had difficulty articulating minute cause-effect phenomena. Shields himself had a similar difficulty. John K. Mitchell wrote, "Certain positions, which he could not describe, and which I was not able to find by experiment, give a sudden shock down the right arm like that from a battery. Usually these are postures in which he is leaning back, neck stretched, and head somewhat back, as, for instance, in a barber's chair. Sometimes sharp rotary movements of the head cause a similar pain."

The younger Mitchell had seen the medical report of Shields's injuries and subsequent hospitalization and tracheotomy. He had also seen Parish's letter. John K. Mitchell recounted Shields's history of the various difficulties that he described as emanating from nerve damage related to war wounds. The doctor therefore investigated and tested claims about lack of perspiration on the right side of the face, movements of limbs, and deafness ("decidedly less acute in the right ear than in the left"). While he noticed that Shields's speech seemed to be unaffected by the neck wound, the trachea had suffered "a partial stricture which causes some trouble in breathing on active exercise." He concluded that Shields had "chronic pharyngitis and post-nasal catarrh."[34]

John K. Mitchell's overall reaction to Shields's condition was puzzlement. He suspected a lesion had caused the strange perspiration pattern. Although Shields maintained that the weakening of the right arm had begun at the time of the neck wound, if the nerves had been injured, the doctor reasoned, there should have been immediate pain and loss of power in the right arm. If the sympathetic nerve had been damaged, how could the trajectory of a single bullet have affected it? "The case leaves much to the imagination." Despite his confusion, John K. Mitchell did not question Shields's account: "The witness is a good one, and his statements entitled to absolute belief." He did not examine varicose veins or the thigh wound, as he was interested in the phenomena of the nerves, not pension rates.[35]

A MODEL REPUBLICAN

Early in 1891, Shields submitted another "Declaration for the Increase of an Invalid Pension." He acknowledged his current pension as twenty-four dollars a month[36] (apparently, his twenty-dollar pension had increased marginally since the previous year) but requested more because of "increased disability resulting from the one for which pension was granted." Sporadic "severe pains" afflicted his right arm from his shoulder to his fingertips. Breathing difficulties had worsened; even walking or casual exercise brought them on. Deafness had increased. "By reason of above disability and its results he is entirely unable to perform any manual labor." The pension file does not contain a response.[37]

In the civic sphere, Shields remained active as a leader, manager, and administrator. The trustees of the Hunterdon County National Bank elected him president. Over the decade, his GAR activities intensified. Working with the local Major Boeman Post Number 48, Shields and other leaders raised the funds to create a memorial to Civil War soldiers from the area. Installed at a crossroads in Flemington, the monument (which still stands) emulated the design of many memorials installed on or near battlefields during the last quarter of the nineteenth century. A sculpted stone soldier, hands resting on his rifle, stands alert and resolute atop a stone plinth. A photograph still exists of Shields and fellow GAR leaders reverently observing their silent sentinel.[38]

By the mid-1890s, the GAR had grown into a powerful lobby. The fraternal bonds enjoyed by its members extended to all reaches of politics, government, and business. The photograph showing Shields and colleagues at the new memorial in Flemington includes the commander of Post Number 48, Andrew A. Connett.[39] In the early 1880s, Connett, the original commander and charter member of the GAR post, was also the president of the Flemington Fire Company, chaplain for the Darcy Lodge,

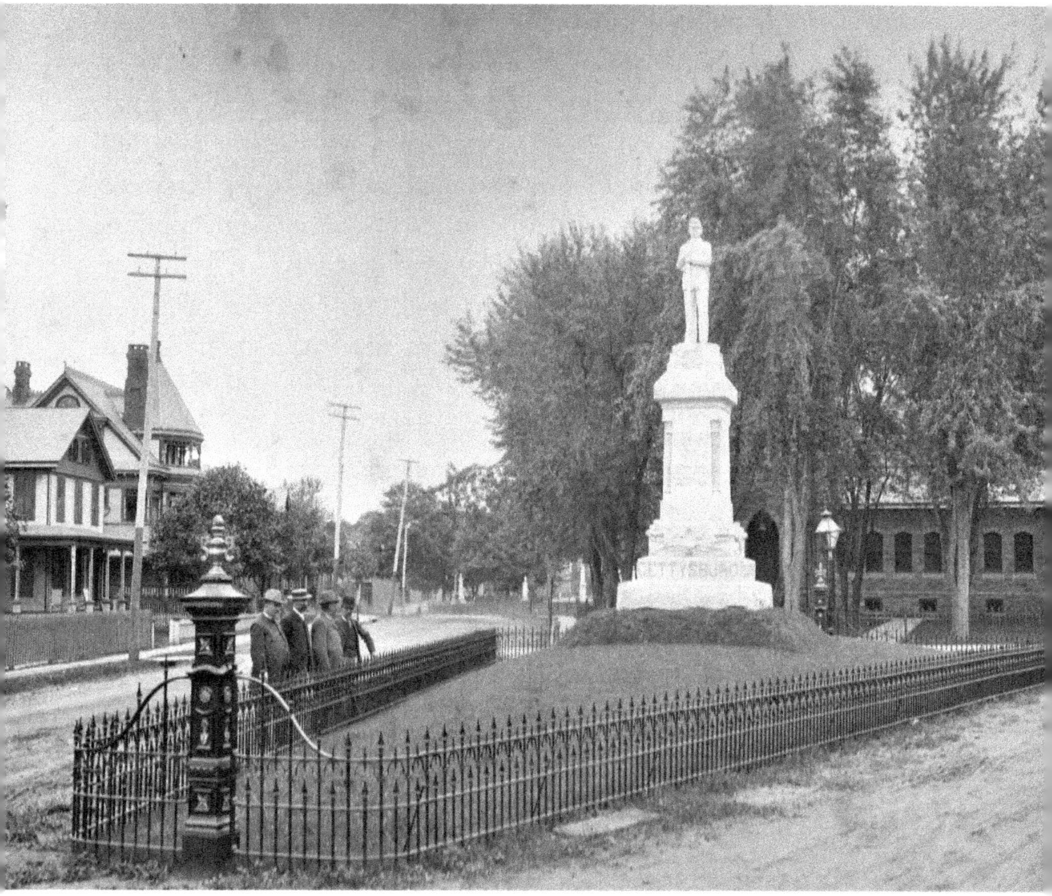

Soldiers' monument, Flemington, NJ, erected in 1892 and sponsored by the Lambert Boeman Post No. 48, Grand Army of the Republic. Of the four men shown, John Shields stands at the far left, and next to him (wearing the boater) is Andrew Connett. *Credit: From the collections of the Hunterdon County Historical Society, New Jersey.*

Number 37, Free and Accepted Masons, and director of the Flemington Building and Loan Association.[40]

Living and working within a GAR network, Shields and other veterans with disabilities did not need to be shy about their wounds. In obtaining pensions, however, all set aside their dignity and claimed an inability to earn a living by manual labor. Without this assertion, no disability pension was possible. Yet under these circumstances, by the 1890s, "claiming a pension implied an affirmation of manliness." Receiving a pension constituted the federal recognition of one's body and manly sacrifice. By this time, too, an increasing number of foreign-born veterans were applying for pensions. Under the original general pension law, in proportion to their numbers when in active military service, relatively few immigrants applied in the 1860s. Shields appears to have been an exception in pursuing a disability pension immediately upon resigning his commission.

In 1894, Shields's GAR comrades elected him as department commander. After he was sworn into office, he selected Andrew T. Connett as his assistant adjutant general. Shields's visibility in this role led to his nomination as the Republican candidate for state senator. The newspapers, however, highlighted the Republican state platform resolution "in repealing legislation which had created unnecessary offices and expensive sinecures." As a result, Shields lost the election.[41]

The physical evidence of Shields's standard of living in the late 1890s was on display to the world. A local publication, *Flemington, New Jersey, Illustrated,* was a privately printed, hardbound booster to highlight community attractions to newcomers and stimulate commercial growth. Among the buildings of note was the "Shields Building . . . a handsome structure near by [*sic*], and also has stores, offices and residence rooms." Shields owned this multipurpose building. In a gazetteer of the finest homes in town, two pages feature Shields's home, a large three-story house on a hill with a wrap-around porch, belvedere, various outbuildings, and a tall flagpole flying the national colors. Interior views show a well-appointed Victorian home with stylish furnishings, gasoliers, potted plants, bookcases, and elegant wallpaper. Mr. and Mrs. Shields doubtless entertained business colleagues and friends here. In fact, the Shields home was the only one the publication featured.[42]

Despite his successes, Shields continued to have difficulty speaking, including hoarseness, irritation, and coughing. He also experienced the progressive atrophy of part of the right side of his body. Although he presented his body holistically to pension officials, authorities persisted in dividing his physical phenomena into categories sorted by decreasing relevance to Shields's wartime wounds. In 1898, he submitted himself to another medical examination. Dr. E. D. Leidy of Flemington had practiced medicine for thirteen years and had known Shields for six. For two months before Leidy swore his affidavit for the pension office, Shields had been under his care because of "entire loss of power to deltoid muscle of right arm." Leidy stated his belief that the atrophy was due to the wartime neck wound. "The bullet—which is still in the region of the back either pressing on the nerves or the nerves being involved in the cicatricial [scar] tissue in track of the bullet. In his present condition [Shields] is totally disabled from performing manual labor."[43]

The next year, New Jersey created one of its first state-funded homes for indigent veterans and those unable to care for themselves, the Home for Disabled Soldiers, Sailors or Marines and their Wives, in Vineland. The first inmate (the term used at the home) entered the institution on January 2, 1900. Initially, married applicants must have been wedded for at least twenty-five years, but by 1903, this limitation dropped to fifteen years. Shields evidently had a role in creating the home, as he was mindful that for years, GAR members led the effort nationwide to create such institutions and serve as board members. Shields was selected to serve on the first board of managers for the home.[44]

Dr. Leidy's affidavit for the pension office accompanied other documentation submitted by Shields to obtain an increase. In early 1899, Shields submitted an "X ray photograph which may aid your Medical Board in arriving at a proper decision." During the same year, Shields underwent another round of applications, certifications, and a medical examination. A new surgeon's certificate acknowledged possession by the pension office of an X-ray and confirmed the current pension of twenty-four dollars a month. The certificate repeated much of the information that had appeared on earlier ones but highlighted increasing pain in the right thigh and attested to the total uselessness of the right arm. Shields, now fifty-nine (mistakenly listed as forty-nine), weighed 224 pounds. The certificate also stated incorrectly that the fugitive bullet "has been removed . . . at the end of the scapula." The examining surgeon concluded with the observation that Shields ought to receive a pension increase of thirty dollars monthly, but given the need for a full-time personal assistant to help perform vital functions, fifty dollars was justified. And Shields showed no vicious habits.[45]

The 1899 surgeon's certificate led to a full-scale review of Shields's circumstances. He received a questionnaire from the pension office in July (essentially identical to the one sent to him in January 1898) to confirm family circumstances: marriage, to whom, by whom, where, and when, affirmation of no previous marriage, and a list of children living (Annie, John H., Robert E., and Henry S.). At the same time, the pension office requested Shields's "full military and medical history" from the War Department. The data provided by the latter identified the two hospital stays for gonorrhea, the only mention of the disease in Shields's pension file. One or more pension officers, having reviewed Shields's previous medical examinations and their recommendations, ordered another to ascertain the status of the neck wound, rheumatism, catarrh, and deafness. The internal pension office order stressed the need for a "thorough test examination. . . . Ascertain the facts and report them fully. You are not at liberty to accept claimant's statements of pain, loss of motion +c unless fully confirmed by your own repeated + varied test, made when his attention is diverted." Clearly, the pension office treated pain complaints with skepticism.[46]

Over time, pension authorities were able to elicit from examining doctors more numerical data to accompany qualitative remarks, the latter judged insufficient by administrators in rating debilities. Authorities wanted descriptions of pain and assertions about restrictions in bodily movement quantified. In November 1899, at sixty, Shields appeared in Easton, Pennsylvania, for another examination before three physicians to support a new surgeon's certificate. Shields recited the familiar story of his wounding at Fredericksburg and Gettysburg and stated that although rheumatism had occurred at intervals only over the past ten to fifteen years, he had suffered catarrh and deafness since his wounding. Doctors recorded his pulse and respiration while sitting, standing, and exercising and recorded his weight at 215 pounds. The new report recorded a detailed examination, including precise measurements and locations of the scars on Shields's neck and thigh. The examiners noted that the bullet in the neck remained "encysted somewhere in the tissues of the neck," thus creating "a traumatic paralysis of the shoulder and upper arm to the extent of all those tissues supplied by the branches of the posterior cord of the right brachial plexus; the resulting atrophy is well evidenced in the contrast of the two shoulders as shown by comparative measurements."

The examiners provided the most precise statement yet of the debility of the right arm: "The paralysis does not seem to extend beyond the elbow joint, beyond the fact that the grip is materially weakened; the outward, upward and backward movements of the shoulder joint are all greatly impaired, the shoulder droops and the claimant cannot elevate the right arm above the horizontal. There is partial anesthesia evident particularly over the anterior and lateral surfaces of the shoulder and upper arm. The atrophy of the deltoid, biceps, and pectoral muscles has been progressive to the extent that to-day the right arm is wholly and permanently disabled for the performance of any manual labor."[47]

With similar detail, the examiners evaluated Shields's claim of rheumatism (by inspecting the joints, muscles, and tendons), his heart (no evidence of "murmur, oedema, dyspnoea, cyanosis, dilatation, or hypertrophy"), catarrh, deafness, and the thigh wound. For the last three categories, the examiners provided pension ratings. The report concluded that the partial paralysis of Shields's right shoulder and arm was disabling and recommended a thirty-dollar monthly pension based on Shields's inability to perform manual labor but suggested that fifty dollars ought to be considered because of Shields's "frequent (daily) and periodical aid of another person to assist in putting on his collar, cravat and coat."

During the same month as the Easton examination, Shields's pension attorney at Soule & Co., Washington, DC, received notification that Shields's previous "Increase Invalid Pension" application had been rejected, apparently based on the preceding medical examination. In fact, the reviewing pension officer wrote on the form, "Alleged resulting rheumatic pains, deafness and catarrh of throat referred to Medical Referee," presumably the examining panel that had just thoroughly inspected Shields's body. The rejection confirmed the neck wound, difficulty in breathing, and severe pain in the arm but could not overcome the "alleged" nature of Shields's difficulties and recommend a pension increase.[48]

NEW CENTURY, SAME BODY, AND THE GAR

In 1900, Shields, sixty-one and working as a railroad contractor, was still living in Raritan on a farm with a mortgaged house with his wife, Annie, adult sons Robert and Henry, and servant Maggie Crowley. His daughter Anna had married and moved away.[49]

In January, the state legislature confirmed Shields's appointment to the board of managers for the new Vineland home for disabled soldiers. The new century would see Shields's participation in and reliance on the GAR to provide him with his last professional identity, one that collected his life's experiences into one final act of service to the Union.[50]

For the first fifteen years after the war, GAR membership remained low. A fraternal order among many others, it offered three founding principles: charity, fraternity, and loyalty. These did not distinguish the GAR sufficiently from the many other fraternal societies available to American white men, including the Freemasons, Odd Fellows, Knights of Pythias, and the Independent Order of Good Templars. Estimates vary, but during the last half of the nineteenth century, about 40 percent of white men belonged to at least one order.[51]

By the 1880s, membership in the GAR increased and new posts were established. For some veterans, the new generation comprised younger people and those who would follow them had no direct experience with the war and might not share veterans' values of patriotism and duty. Veterans sought like company in a setting that ensured that the republican virtues espoused during the war years would be maintained. GAR members who entered public office attached veterans' interests and commitment to the Union to political platforms. During the 1880s and 1890s, as the myth of the Lost Cause of the Confederacy came to define the war among both major political parties and blue-gray reunions, the GAR became a crusade. "The war's place in popular culture as a successful crusade allowed Union veterans to assume the role of savior, and they did not hesitate to do so." Within the storm of emerging civil rights for African Americans and other changes in American society, GAR veterans held the skirmish line firmly at distinguishing between what was appropriate, proper, and lawful in American society and the terrifying consequences of disunion.[52]

The GAR projected itself as the nation's savior and embraced Christianity as part of its ethos, unlike most other fraternal societies. The notion of what the United States meant to the world as a nation was fixed to an 1860s vision. Whatever paths veterans took ideologically and spiritually in the coming years, in the work and rituals of its posts and encampments, the GAR held to a national ideal of the Union in peril. This dedication to veterans' sacrifices to avoid the collapse of the Union intensified as public indifference to the relevance of the veteran increased. Shields would have been annoyed to see veterans caricatured in popular print as useless old men whose only audiences were children eager for a heroic story.

As a senior official in the GAR, Shields must have shared a "deadly addiction to truth," an obsession with compiling official records and regimental histories to demarcate the dimensions of the war and enshrine its meaning. Veterans also created narratives in the song sheets they sold to make money for their indigent comrades. This compulsion was strengthened by the rituals the GAR adopted for the conduct of its meetings and encampments. The rituals and the compilation of data strengthened but also made static the core narrative of the war. Shields participated in these activities to fix his invention of self as an American, one with unimpeachable credentials of moral vision, ethical conduct, discipline, and loyalty, all subsumed within a burgeoning business career in building a twentieth-century nation. Part of Shields's narrative was inscribed on his body, as was the case among other veterans. In comparing narratives with comrades, he may have tilted his head up and held his collar down to show his neck scars that supported his version of the wheatfield and the lifesaving surgery that placed a metal stent in his trachea.[53]

Meeting comrades at Major Boeman Post Number 48, Shields entered an exclusive space with performance rituals unseen by the public, "one in which veterans even developed their own lexicon and sense of time." Closed to outside distractions, the environment of the post evoked military activities, sentries were posted, bugle calls announced the day's milestones, and members observed inspections and drills. Entering the post, Shields would have been enveloped in military imagery. Flags adorned the walls, as did framed photographs of military leaders and President Lincoln. Upon entering, Shields comported himself with a military bearing and a willingness to submit to the orders and protocols of veterans appointed above him. In the room's center was an altar, the dynamic center of the post universe, the place where matters were addressed and policy was decided. Post officers, mimicking regimental roles, sat near the commander, who presided from an ornamental chair on a dais. The officers—chaplain, quartermasters, surgeon, and adjutant—looked on while seated in distinctive chairs in specific locations within the room. Shields would have been challenged by a sentinel for a password, and this challenge was issued several times in succession as he was permitted to enter deeper into the sanctuary. "The confounding of military and quasi-religious imagery suggested an army life that was somehow sacrosanct, orderly, and hierarchical, not an actual army camp but an idealized model of it—the camp as sanctuary."[54]

GAR members wished to halt or mediate some forms of social change, but the onslaught of postwar industrialization roughly treated veterans who lacked the will or skills to compete. Many veterans who could not return to agricultural life or general labor were forced to work for wages in the cities. Families were increasingly unable to care for their own. In industrial manufactories, family connections seemed to disappear as wage earners found themselves to be interchangeable with many others in search of work. Other social changes confused veterans: changing gender relationships, the national government asserting power in distant oceans and countries, and the worship of wealth. Veterans were indeed "trapped in a developing notion of manhood." The physical evidence of war on veterans' bodies was insignificant in industrial settings except when veterans were eliminated from the workforce because of that evidence, the same evidence that was highlighted at GAR encampments.[55]

By the new century, Shields had given himself fully to the new industrial economy. In New York City, construction of the subway had begun. The Rapid Transit Construction Company had subcontracted all facets of the project: Shields's allotted section extended from 124th Street to 125th Street along Broadway. His workers had excavated deep enough to locate and remove fire alarms and gas pipes and shift a twenty-inch water main to the other side of the street before additional excavation could take place. Although fully immersed in a dynamic economy as an employer and manager, Shields continued his membership on the board of managers for the Vineland home. Increasingly, he became a public advocate for the veterans whose intellectual and physical identities could not cope with a rampaging new economy. In an annual report for the home, he wrote the following on behalf of the board of managers to the New Jersey governor:

> As time rolls on the survivors of war for the Union are growing more feeble and lose their earning capacity. Bravely have many of them struggled in the battle of life, handicapped as they are by infirmities and disease, incident to their service on land or on sea in the defense of their country, until now, with tottering steps trembling limbs and feeble sight, they find that they cannot sustain life upon the comparative pittance that comes to them in the shape of their pensions. Their life-partners, too, have arrived at an age when work for the support of the household is no longer possible.[56]

Captain Shields could have been describing himself, given his persistent pension claims for increasing debility of motion and hearing consequent to his wounds. Several of the examining doctors reasoned that some of his maladies were due to aging irrespective of war wounds. Contemplating his health challenges likely prompted Shields to consider similar hardships faced by other disadvantaged veterans. His experience and civic leadership

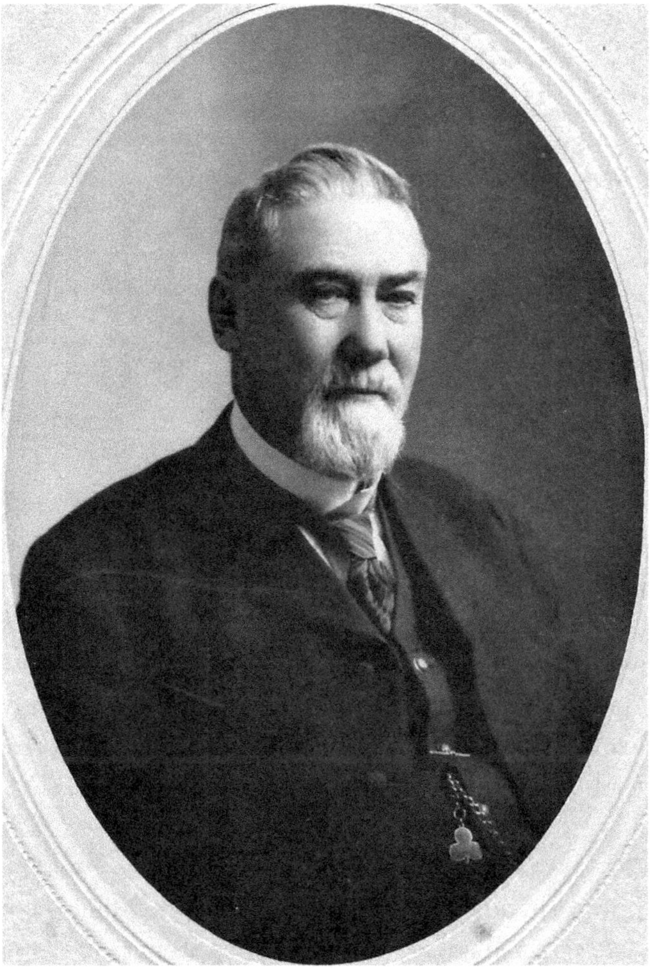

John Shields in the late 1890s or early 1900s.
Credit: Vineland Historical Society, NJ.

combined to give him authority and political influence regarding the growing network of homes for disabled and indigent soldiers. At the Thirty-Fifth GAR National Encampment in Cleveland, Ohio, Shields was assigned to a committee to inspect the other New Jersey home for disabled soldiers in the town of Kearny.[57]

By the early twentieth century, railroad contracting was proving successful for Shields. Further, his GAR leadership had established him as a leading voice for a large home for disabled soldiers. Then, in 1904, at age fifty-nine, Shields's wife Anna died in Flemington of "hepatic carcinoma"—liver cancer.[58]

NEGOTIATING FRAGILITY

Within weeks of his wife's death, Shields applied again for a pension increase. If Anna had been helping to maintain his body, the need for a permanent assistant would have become paramount. Through local Flemington attorney, friend, and business associate John L. Connet, Shields acknowledged a current pension of twenty-four dollars monthly and requested an increase due to "disability" owing to his neck and thigh wounds. A few months later, Connet supplemented the application with a sworn statement by Edwin D. Leidy, MD, the same physician who had examined Shields in 1898. Leidy cited the X-ray that showed the bullet close enough to the spinal column to cause "pressure on the spinal nerves of the right side." Leidy asserted that he had treated Shields's atrophied muscles of the shoulder and back and observed that the right "arm at that time was almost helpless." Leidy noted Shields's chronic hoarseness and inflamed pharynx. Further, "he has dizzy sensations, also weakness of the back. He has been under my care professionally for six or seven years past, and during that time has been unable to perform any manual labor. I consider him totally incapacitated to perform any manual labor because of the injury to his throat and the pressure of the ball on the spinal nerves."[59]

With each pension request, political and cultural circumstances evolved to affect public and medical views of Civil War pensioners. During the first decade of the twentieth century, Union veterans received on average about thirteen dollars per month. By 1915, among the four hundred thousand Union veterans still living, 93 percent received pensions. Disabled veterans had good reason to negotiate raises in payments of only a few dollars. For farm laborers around the beginning of the century, pensions made up about 53 percent of their income. Skilled workers such as Kircher and Shields who prospered as businessmen received 12 percent of their income from pensions.[60]

Increasingly, the pension system—the progenitor of all subsequent government pension systems—worked to reconcile competing interests and challenges. The pattern of industrial expansion and employment in manufacturing necessitated standards as benchmarks for achievement and performance. As war veterans receiving pensions, former Union soldiers embodied patriotism, manly commitment, and sacrifice in the national interest, characteristics that differentiated them from other would-be pensioners. By the twentieth century, the system had developed a preference for veterans in civil service and job training, particularly typewriting, accounting, and telegraphy. Soldiers' patriotism served those who were political candidates, and political candidates wanted the veteran vote and helped older soldiers find jobs. As Henry Kircher had found, visible amputations helped veterans campaigning for office not only for their candidacy but also for Republican politicians.[61]

Pension authorities administered federal funds according to Congress's acts and amendments while trying to remain fair. They balanced congressional oversights, veterans' needs and increasing demands, the lobbying of the GAR and other organizations, and the ever-present pension lawyers. Liberalizing pension laws provided the opportunity to broaden governmental discretion. Since the initial pension law of 1862, nothing changed the system as extensively as the Act of 1890, which permitted pensions for any demonstrable disability, war-related or not, but required that soldiers receive ratings "based entirely on inability to perform manual labor." Despite this legal liberalization, pension claims did not become easier for Shields and other veterans who complained of multiple, related debilities. To receive anything, pensioners had to not only demonstrate an inability to perform manual labor but were also expected to show good moral character and lack of dissolute habits.[62]

During the war, pension rules defined disabilities as "inferior" or "total," but by the twentieth century, the system had evolved other methods of gauging degrees and longevity of disability, thus adhering to a medical model that equated specific bodily losses to dollar values, a "hierarchy of abnormalities." Initially, doctors' certificates linked the disability to specific wounds. A decade later, they inquired into personal habits that by 1890 were established as "vicious habits." In the new century, examining doctors rated the severity of the identified disability according to eighteen types. On average, a Civil War pensioner received about five medical examinations in his lifetime. Shields obtained at least nine surgeon's certificates (each one requiring at least one extensive examination), five letters or sworn statements from physicians supporting his claims of disability, and two examinations conducted by the Mitchells.[63]

Adding numbers in a surgeon's report of examination to arrive at ratings did not equate to the award of a pension for a given amount. Rather, "the emerging meaning of disability after the Civil War was contested terrain—an evolving social construct articulated in the press and in local communities through a myriad of encounters among pension claimants, examining surgeons, pension lawyers, and G.A.R. period politicians." Shields's requests for pension increases required new medical examinations in which he negotiated with the doctor who investigated his claims. Examiners rarely introduced other issues during these sessions. Doctors recorded findings for each claim and suggested a corresponding pension rating. Pension authorities, however, were not bound to honor physicians' recommendations.[64]

Implicit in these negotiations was social class. To examiners, Shields was educated and articulate, and he led a responsible civic life. John K. Mitchell's examination explicitly referred to him as an unassailable gentleman who was undoubtedly truthful in his claims despite confusion about their medical interpretation. No one who examined Shields could dismiss his claims based on so-called vicious habits (they would not have known of the wartime gonorrhea) or any moral failing. No public disapproval was attached to his claims, only doubt about fugitive pains and the compounded nature of the wounds and subsequent behavior of the nervous system.

Physicians responded best to veterans of their own social class and background. Mitchell's clinical notes, for instance, occasionally condescend to soldiers who were uneducated or socially unsophisticated, or lacked communicative abilities. Mitchell and "the Firm" worried that men of lesser social status might be malingerers who could deceive physicians, thus posing a professional challenge. Not surprisingly, physicians sometimes made observations on the character of these men and their right to a pension. Not only pension authorities but surgeons, too, "categorized soldiers based on their personal beliefs about the validity of the men's claims of disability, and their opinions of the men's reputation and character."[65]

Pensions were a matter of public record and appeared in local newspapers. Shields and other veterans were self-conscious about having their pensions made public, which would force them to expose their wounded or injured bodies to public scrutiny and approval, but they had no choice. Local citizens who knew or knew of Shields might have reflected on his standing before pension authorities and wondered if any pensioner thus provided with a government handout might languish in laziness and descend into poverty. Despite a physical disability, veterans were expected to "man up" and show independence and mastery over their bodies. Shields found this increasingly difficult to do.

SUCCESS, FAILURE, AND SUCCESS

By 1905, Shields was still living at his Raritan home, his mortgage paid off. At sixty-six, Shields lived alone except for Maggie Crowley and another household assistant, Florence Kern. The John Shields Construction Company had just obtained a major contract with the Pennsylvania, New Jersey & New York Railroad to build two tunnels under Bergen Hill, New Jersey, as an extension of the railway. The two-million-dollar contract supported work to create tunnels 1.25 miles long for passenger trains traveling to and from the Manhattan station. The two-years-or-less project "will be particularly arduous, since Bergen hill is mostly 'trap rock.'" Work began in May.[66]

By the following January, the contract had been reassigned to friend and business colleague William Bradley because Shields's company entered receivership. Evidently, several bills came due, and Shields was unable to pay them. The newspaper cited Shields's company's assets as about $200,000, while liabilities totaled $350,000. By year's end, however, together with two partners, Shields had reestablished his business as the Shields-Bogart Construction Company and was awarded a contract to build a fifty-mile track in Roxie for the Mississippi Central Railroad. "Colonel Shields will be the active man of the company," which had raised capital stock worth $100,000.[67]

Perhaps affected by the immense anxiety and work required to close one business and open another, Shields's health continued to deteriorate. He became more aggressive about getting the attention of senior pension officials. His congressional representative, Ira W. Wood, wrote a letter on Shields's behalf to the commissioner of pensions, who politely responded without a commitment that Shields had a pending claim for a pension increase requiring a physician's examination already scheduled, and "when said [examination] certificate shall have bee[n] received, prompt attention will be given the claim." As the examination was being scheduled, Shields was in Mississippi building a railroad when a fire broke out at his hotel, destroying his effects, including his pension certificate and voucher for the current payment. He applied for duplicates, a process that took months. When he received new paperwork and the pension office appointed him to appear before another examiner, Shields was forced to miss the appointment because of his work in the South. His lawyer, John L. Connet, approached the pension office for another appointment. Shields had another reason for returning North: he had a new job.[68]

The board of managers at the Vineland disabled soldiers' home appointed Shields, a charter member of the board and recently its president, as the home's new commandant, subject to the governor's approval, which was obtained despite another political favorite contending for the position. "[Shields] has always stood well with the old soldiers, having filled the office of Department Commander of the G.A.R.," reported the Vineland *Evening Journal*. Shields became the home's second commandant.[69]

RETURN TO COMPANY E

Early in the war, the federal government recognized the need for places to house ill, indigent, and disabled veterans who were without family resources. In 1865, Congress created the National Asylum for Disabled Volunteer Soldiers (later the National Home for Disabled Volunteer Soldiers), initially as three homes sited regionally, with more added subsequently. The government changing the title to replace the term *asylum* with *home* was due to public sensitivity to the idea that the government was funding institutions for the dissolute or insane. *Home* connoted family, loving attention, comfort, and stability. Throughout the nineteenth century, people had come to perceive "the idea of home as not simply a dwelling but a kind of support group from which parents and children drew comfort, strength, and stability."

Despite the popularity of state and federal homes, the staff of these homes quickly learned that both physical and mental health problems did not disappear but became worse or evolved into newer, more challenging ones. The disabled soldiers' home was intended to re-create a family environment, but some of the residents had been placed there by their own families. In assuming leadership, Shields was aware of the spectrum of responsibilities and challenges he faced and doubtless identified with his new troops, spouses, and widows. Residents of the Vineland home in 1909 when Shields began his tenure received pensions with fewer restrictions than experienced by veterans soon after the war. He envied some of the services his institution provided, services that he had been unable to secure from pension authorities. The system had become "an open-ended system of disability, old-age, and survivors' benefits for anyone who could claim minimal service time on the northern side of the Civil War." What the law permitted, however, did not necessarily correspond with what pensions were granted.[70]

If the ideal for national homes was to provide a family environment, Shields stepped into a role that treated the home as a regiment. Quasimilitary administrative infrastructure governed Shields's professional life; he was a company captain again. As a longtime board member, Shields knew what he was taking on. The institution had enjoyed little, but mainly favorable, press. The main challenge was to ensure a state budget that permitted growth. The institution had a waiting list. The most newsworthy recent event in the newspapers was an investigation into the quality of the food. Sixty-five "inmates" petitioned to improve the meals: no meat for the evening meal was the predominant complaint coupled with inadequate nursing care and lack of medicines for invalids. A state investigation (covered by the

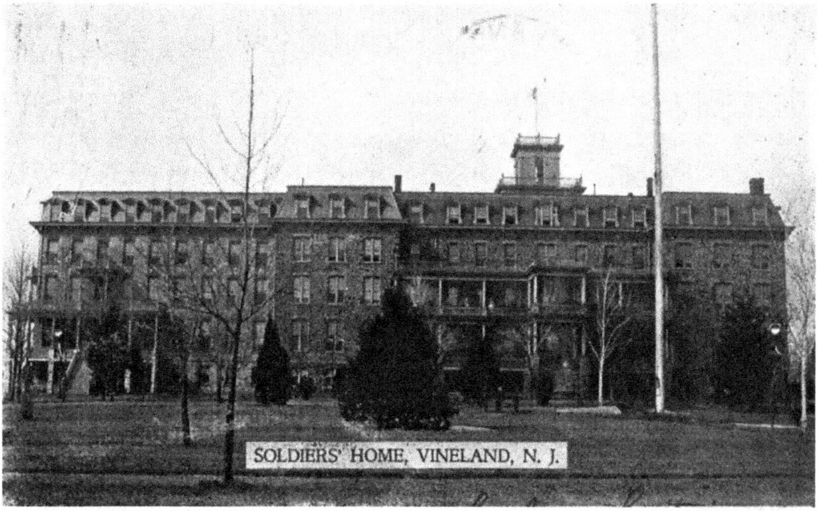

Postcard of the Vineland Soldiers' Home, NJ, 1905. *Credit: Author's collection.*

press) concluded that no systemic changes were necessary, that physicians supervised the diet and had reduced meat because of residents' elderly status and sedentary lives, and that all issues emanated from one "disgruntled former inmate." The use of "inmate" to refer to veterans led to inferences that stereotyped them as alcoholic layabouts undeserving of federal money, a perception that Shields fought.[71]

Shields wasted no time addressing the home's financial needs. He wrote to the governor citing rising expenses for constructing the new wing (in progress during the spring of 1909), noting that before his arrival, the construction costs were borne on credit, and the budget shortfall was close to $11,000. A week later, he wrote to William J. Bradley, who chaired the appropriations committee in the New Jersey legislature. Someone had suggested that deductions be made from residents' pension payments to help with operating costs. Shields found the idea not "very good policy." The likely vocal opposition by the veterans would result in "a very bad effect politically." In the same year, he also authorized the routing of gas and electric lines to the older campus buildings and purchased a new automobile for the home, a five-passenger model with a winter top. Bradley, about a dozen years younger than Shields and therefore not a veteran, was another self-made engineer and politician who promoted the Republican Party. Shields might have made an earlier acquaintance with Bradley, which enabled the Bergen Hill project to transfer to his hands with the means to keep the construction contract viable.[72]

The *Tenth Annual Report of the Home for Disabled Soldiers, Sailors or Marines and Their Wives for the Year Ending October 31st, 1909*, the first publication to acknowledge Shields's leadership of the home, listed his key staff as Edward P. Southwick, adjutant, Emma J. Southwick, matron (Edward's wife), and John S. Halsey, MD, surgeon. Although the home employed about forty full- or part-time workers, Shields relied on his key staff who, in turn, appear to have supported him. The Southwicks became friends. Halsey examined Shields for pension purposes and served as his advocate for an increase. In Shields's first year, the home had reached capacity, with 95 men in residence, 186 women, and a waiting list. Reflecting Shields's priorities, the board stated that it was necessary to install a fire escape, although the 1907 legislative appropriation for this addition fell far below the contractors' bids. More farmland was needed; the home tried to grow as much food as possible.[73]

Shields evidently relinquished his contracting work to perform exclusively as commandant. He sold or sublet his Flemington home. As of 1910, he lived as a tenant on a farm south of Vineland in Cumberland County. The farm was owned by a young Italian immigrant family named Balurio, parents in their twenties with two children. Edward Southwick, who possibly arranged this place for his supervisor, also lived on the farm. It was a busy year for the energetic Shields, who had a fire escape built at Vineland, new plumbing installed, new furniture purchased, and the cemetery enlarged. The board of managers raised his salary from $1,500 annually to $2,000.[74]

At first, state and federal homes included many GAR veterans as board members. In some cases, GAR-affiliated politicians exercised influence in the construction and management of soldiers' homes, including the selection of commandants. The GAR created the military infrastructure for the management of these homes. Shields doubtless saw a seamless link between GAR and his new job. The Vineland home created its own GAR post. Shields appealed to his GAR contacts when he encountered administrative obstacles. For example, given ambiguous wording in the language of the authorizing law, the New Jersey legislature had passed a bill to fund a new wing, but the bill stalled. Shields appealed to New Jersey GAR department commander Jas. P. Connelly: "I cannot understand how this occurs, as the bill passed both Houses and you told me the Governor had signed it. Let me know the reason it has fallen through."[75]

Due to his job as caretaker of dozens of disabled soldiers, Shields's daily conversations with residents must have included constant references to pensions and pension laws. He supported many applications for reviews. He tried again for his own pension increase, this time making his case on institutional letterhead to bolster the claim. No longer did he hide his impatience:

> I request you to take further consideration [of] my claim for increase of pension. Some time ago, I was sent before the Pension Board at Somerville N.J. and they recommended an increase of my pension to $50.00 per month, but Mr. Evans, Pension Commissioner at that time, declined to act on the recommendation of the Pension Board. I was ordered before another Pension Board, at Easton, Pa., and they also recommended that my pension be increased to $50.00 per month, but this recommendation was also turned down. You have the papers in your office and the X ray photograph showing where the bullet is located close to spine. I was 71 years

> of age last May. I would like to know why I should be ordered about from Board to Board and each Board recommend that my pension be increased, and nothing come of it. What is the use of having Pensions Boards if their recommendations are continually ignored?[76]

Shields's impatience—and his stature as head of a veterans' home—prompted a quick response. Evidently, the bureau had kept his file in suspension because of the missed appointment with an examination board years before when he was building a railroad in Mississippi:

> In response to your letter . . . you are informed that after a careful examination of all the papers on file . . . it appears that you failed to appear for medical examination on an order issued (in your claim for increase of pension under the general law filed September 19, 1904), January 9, 1907, and the claim is considered abandoned.
>
> If you believe that you are entitled to an increase of pension, it will be necessary for you to file another application therefor[e], together with competent medical evidence to show that by reason of pensioned cause alone, you are totally incapacitated for the performance of manual labor, when proper action will be taken.[77]

There is no documentation to support an immediate response by Shields. Managing a home for veterans had bolstered his argument with the pension office to heed examiners' endorsement of his claimed maladies and their recommendations for a pension increase. He tied this quest to emphasizing that impoverished, disabled veterans were dignified men who sacrificed for the country and should not be dismissed as society's human waste. He became angry at New Jersey Commissioner of Public Reports Thomas B. Holmes for his dismissive attitude about veterans. Holmes's agency published annual reports on state institutions, including the Vineland home. Shields submitted an annual report that contained a list of residents by name. Holmes objected. Shields's reply says much about his self-image and feeling of solidarity with other veterans. His letter is the only extant Shields correspondence of any depth on a matter other than his own pension increases:

> You say that you see no more reason why the names of the inmates of this Home should be published than the names of the inmates of the Hospitals for the insane and other penal and charitable institutions of the State. Your classification of the veterans of this Home with those persons who are confined in Insane Asylums and in the State Prison is a studied and gratuitous insult to every man who bore arms in defense of the Union. Your classification of this Home as being on a level with the Insane Asylums and Penal Institutions is a most odious and despicable comparison, and is the more so on account of coming from one who holds a commission from the Governor of this State.
>
> You may say that you are open to conviction, but I consider it to be a superfluity on my part to attempt to convince you what is plainly apparent to every loyal and right [ ]thinking man, that the Veterans of this Home, every one of whom holds an honorable discharge from the service of the United States, are not on a level with the insane and the criminal. Nor is this Home a charitable institution, as it was founded, and is maintained, for those who are entitled to its benefits by reason of their voluntary and honorable service to the country.
>
> Every National Home for Soldiers publishes the roster of the inmates. Every State Home for Soldiers of which I have any knowledge publishes the roster of their inmates, and the information made available by this means is often of great importance in locating lost or missing comrades.[78]

There is no record of a response.

ARTERIOSCLEROSIS

In 1911, Shields submitted another request to increase his pension via the firm of Soule & Company. Shields provided the pension office with a new physician's affidavit about his wounds, this time by Dr. Halsey. He offered a familiar description of Shields's injuries and recovery and emphasized his debility based on his impairment of motion and pain. He found that Shields "is unable to put on left stocking and is unable to put on either shoe. Applicant states that he has pain starting from center of spine and encircling body. Applicant upon assuming exact posture . . . is unable to start walking naturally on account of lack of control of limbs, due to incoordination and must travel about 20 or 30 feet before he can strike his natural gait." The report detailed a reduction in

Shields's ability to lift his right arm, twist his right or left arm, or lift any weight, all of which "interferes with dressing and undressing and attending to calls of nature." Halsey also documented how Shields's voice was affected "with increasing weakness and hoarseness" and occasional difficulty swallowing.[79]

The new application for the pension increase and the affidavit prompted the pension office to order a medical examination, and Shields was duly scheduled to appear before three doctors in Millville, a contiguous township to Vineland. Seventy-two-year-old Shields underwent the examination on August 2, 1911. He could not give his occupation as a manual laborer; the form listed his occupation as commandant of the Vineland home. His height had decreased slightly over the years to a bit under five foot ten, and he now weighed 210 pounds. The examiners' report was divided into subsections: neck wound, thigh wound, "sciatica, lumbago," heart, chest, and kidney. The new medical shorthand eliminated qualitative observations (except in summary). Numerical data included pulse and respiration, chest measurements for inhalation and respiration, percussion, palpation, and chemical tests of urine. The health of the heart—or its dysfunction—was recorded in a form of medical Morse code: "Apex [of the heart] beat is not felt or seen, located by ear, 2 1/2 inches below directly, the left nipple, dullness begins mid-sternum opposite upper border of 4th hip . . . cartilage."

Pension rates were recommended (or not) for each category. The veteran's body had become a site for anthropometry. Even Shields's testicles were measured (varicocele of the left one noted, three and a half inches long and one inch in diameter). Shields exhibited an enlarged prostate and light cyanosis of the hands, feet, face, and lips, possibly associated with nerve damage incident to the neck wound. Overall, the doctors concluded that Shields was in a poor state of health: "Debility is marked. Skin is clammy moist, palms soft; general flabby muscular condition. . . . Arterio sclerosis is present and more marked." Importantly, the report adds, "No evidence of vicious habits." This report gave the first indication of arteriosclerosis, a degenerative condition.[80]

Eager to elicit a quick response from Washington, Shields wrote on the Vineland home letterhead to the pension office, included his new surgeon's certificate, reminded the recipients that they had an old X-ray of his bullet lodged in shoulder tissue, and asked, "Do you require anything further in relation to this claim?" Meanwhile, the pension office wrote to the senior physician who had examined Shields, requiring additional information. The letter acknowledged Shields's current pension of twenty-four dollars monthly for the neck wound but demanded an elucidation of other findings:

> Alleges gunshot wound of right thigh as a new disability. Examine carefully. Note in detail condition due to wound of neck. Give points of entrance and exit of missile, size and condition of scars. State what structures were apparently injured, and in what manner this wound now disables. Also describe condition due to alleged wound of thigh. Give points of entrance and exit of missile, size and condition of scars. What structures were injured In what manner does this wound now disable? Has he general rheumatism, lumbago or sciatica?
>
> Report fully condition of the heart, lungs, kidneys, bladder and prostate gland. Is there arterio-sclerosis? Give description of his general physical condition and all evidence of senility. Rate separately every disability found. Comply fully with appropriate paragraphs, Book of Instructions.[81]

During the same month, Shields presented himself as a competent and respectable manager in hosting a visit from New Jersey's governor, Woodrow Wilson. Shortly thereafter, the pension authorities responded with their judgment. As exasperated as he had been with pension bureaucrats and doctors when denied an increase, Shields probably read with disbelief their new view that his thigh wound now merited an increase—but he was not going to receive it: "Your above entitled claim for increase of pension . . . is rejected on the ground that the evidence fails to show that a rate in excess of $24.00 per month is warranted for the degree of disability from . . . gunshot wound of neck. The claim for additional pension, based on gunshot wound of right thigh has been allowed, but the combined rate not to exceed $24.00 per month, which you have been receiving."

Every time Shields claimed an increase and underwent an examination, doctors responded according to each claimed disability in turn. The physician took appropriate measurements or made qualitative judgments, and the summary medical view supported a disability based on a constellation of mutually related phenomena. Oddly, the thigh wound entered the picture late because Shields's earliest pension applications focused solely on the neck. The late appearance of the thigh injury in pension claims elicited skepticism. Pain eluded firm categorization and therefore pension rating: it was variable, transitory, not amenable to measurement, and idiosyncratic. Although the Mitchells were very interested in pain phenomena because of the associated nerve damage, the pension authorities still had no gauge for pain.[82]

The pension office directed the examining physicians' attention to the "Book of Instructions." Examiners appeared to narrate their findings in ways intelligible to themselves and their colleagues, not to pension bureaucrats. They certainly read the instructions but still retained a professional language characterized by the case study, a narrative about the patient circumscribing his or her physiognomy in an era before genetic analysis was possible. Mitchell's case studies, for instance, identified a patient's age and sex, profession, perhaps something about ethnicity, and appropriate medical and treatment history. Like a legal brief, Mitchell outlined the relevant issues, results of the examination and diagnosis, and concluded with treatments applied and anticipated. That physicians did not write their observations in pension code was no accident. Physicians avoided instructions from bureaucrats on how they were to write reports.

Shields turned his attention to the needs of the Vineland home in the following years, apparently having determined the pointlessness of inundating pension authorities with more examinations and affidavits of disability. A new building was added to the soldiers' home, which was by this time a small precinct. The fire escape was installed, and more furniture was purchased. The board of managers increased Shields's salary and that of executive staff for good reason: in only a few years, the resident population had grown by 70 percent. Despite the vagaries of the state budget process, Shields was able to make new improvements each year. The board approved funds for headstones for the graves of widows. The cemetery was expanded and beautified with new plantings. Given the rate by which Civil War veterans were disappearing, the GAR post at the home conducted the most significant event for residents except for Christmas: Memorial Day ceremonies. Each grave received a red geranium and a flag for this occasion. "Here the membership of the Home assembles with their friends, patriotic groups, and addresses are heard, the roll of deceased since last year called, the Home's firing squad salutes the dead and the flag, which has been at half staff all morning, is run to the top of the flagpole." Shields took great care to make the occasion meaningful, heartfelt, and grand.[83]

Shields decided on a new approach with the pension office: a claim for *total* disability. To that end, in 1912, he filed another "declaration for pension," this time, listing his occupation as "machinist" and citing support from the newest congressional adjustment to the pension scheme, an Act of May 12, 1912. The Civil War Division of the pension office replied that it required statements of two credible witnesses "showing whether you are unfit to perform manual labor by reason of disability on account of gunshot wound of neck and . . . thigh alone. The affiants should describe the disability and state the extent to which you are disabled thereby." Dr. Halsey examined Shields anew and swore to his incapacity to perform any manual labor. "He is unable to dress himself without the aid of an attendant. In the act of drinking—the right hand holding cup or glass must be steadied by the left hand. He is unable to use right hand in cutting his meat at table and any exertion of right arm causes very marked tremor. He is unable to turn head toward the right side owing to injury of muscles. The wound in thigh makes it very difficult for him to assume a stooping position and still more difficult to assume the upright positions from a stooping position."[84]

Shields's adjutant at Vineland, Edward P. Southwick, and Samuel Weaver, age sixty-nine and a resident of the Vineland home, provided supporting affidavits as credible witnesses. Both men, who claimed acquaintance with Shields for twenty-two and twenty-five years, respectively, stated that they were "well aware that the said John Shields is not fit to perform manual labor on account of wounds received while in the [war]." A form filed a week later by a pension authority confirmed an increase to thirty dollars[85] per month.[86]

Shields's pension file includes memoranda exchanged between pension authorities that reveal problems in interpreting the pension laws in relation to the maladies claimed by Dr. Halsey. In response to a recommendation to reject the claim, another official stated, "If the conclusion of the [medical referee] is to be followed it is not a simple matter to see what he has done and reject the claim giving no heed . . . to additional evidence. Our instructions are to carefully weigh and consider the new evidence." Another internal memorandum observed, "The evidence filed shows soldier very seriously disabled—unable to dress himself without aid. He is clearly entitled to the maximum rate for disability under pending claim."[87]

In 1915, the Vineland home opened a new hospital. As the institution's population grew, however, so did complaints. In 1914, the board of managers met to investigate charges made by some residents (still referred to as "inmates" in institutional records) against Shields. The meeting aired complaints, but no further action was taken. Later, Shields recommended the expulsion of a resident from the home because of "his gross, offensive, unmanly and repeated violation of the rules and regulations. He has threatened bodily harm to employees and grossly insulted the female diet cook." Just as in the army, when one malcontent soldier endangered group morale, the army moved quickly to remove the cancer. Shields requested expulsion of the veteran "if good order is to be maintained in future." Alluding to a persistent problem now apparently on the wane, Shields wrote in his annual report that drunkenness was "almost a thing of the past."[88]

Shields's health had deteriorated to the extent that he could not perform his duties, so Edward Southwick became the acting commandant in early 1916. The board of managers granted Shields a month "to recuperate from long illness," and the next year, the governor appointed a commission to examine the home. It was time to invigorate the institution; it was time for Company E to receive a new captain, expand recruiting, and be organized under a new brigade. In 1918, two years after Southwick's temporary appointment, Shields resigned at age seventy-nine due to his health. The pension office approved an increase to forty dollars[89] monthly. This time, he had not even asked for it.[90]

Two days after the armistice that ended World War I, in Elkton, Maryland, a Catholic priest married Shields to Lydia Bontecou of Trenton, age forty-eight, a spinster living in Vineland. A friend of the Southwicks for decades, she may have been an employee of the home. There is no reason to presume a lack of affection by either party, but the marriage gave Shields the in-home assistance the pension authorities had refused. In return, she would be eligible for a widow's pension.[91]

Jobless and without outside income, in 1919, Shields appealed once again to the pension office. In a letter, he stated, "I am a pensioner but have been growing more helpless lately. I cannot dress myself or go anywhere without an attendant. I think I ought to have a 100.00 per month." He recited his military record, claiming to have participated in all battles of the Second Corps until his wounding at Gettysburg and "was never off duty except when wounded." He stated that he had been receiving forty dollars per month but "would like your advice on how to proceed on this matter." A few weeks later, he wrote to the pension office again to relay a change of address and added, "I wrote you a short time ago for information about getting an increase of Pension, but have not received an answer yet. May I hope for an early reply."[92]

The pension office responded within a week. Their letter recognized Shields's disability "as to require the frequent and periodical aid and attendance of another person, [therefore] you are at liberty to file a declaration for the re-issue and increase of your pension under the general laws." The sender thought to include a blank form for the purpose. Shields continued his urgent efforts to receive a favorable decision from the pension authorities. He wrote again, "Pardon me for being somewhat anxious about my increase of Pension, but in May I will be 80 years old, and I have to have a constant attendant, which makes it expensive. Any thing you can do to facilitate matters will be greatly appreciated by me." The Civil War Division responded quickly saying that "sworn medical testimony" was required to support the claim for aid from a caregiver.[93]

Dr. Halsey immediately supplied the requested medical affidavit. He wrote that he had known Shields for eleven years—the duration of the Vineland home—and had attended to his medical needs during that time. Halsey described Shields's bodily limitations: "He is unable to put on stockings, shoes, pants or underwear. He is unable to stoop over [or] take a bath. He has to make great physical exertion to keep his person cleanly . . . he is unable to arrange his collar, necktie, or shirt . . . he is unable to walk except with cane and has greatest difficulty sitting in a chair or arising therefrom." Despite Halsey's statement, the pension office rejected Shields's claim because "the evidence on file fails to ascribe a degree of disability from former pensioned causes" that would require the personal aid. "Your condition is due in part to rheumatism, disease of heart and the infirmities of age," not war wounds. The letter also stated that Halsey's sworn statement was unnecessary.[94]

Shields appealed to a legislator to write the pension office on his behalf. E. C. Hutchinson, Fourth District, New Jersey House of Representatives, asked, "I shall appreciate your advising me if there is any authority for you to grant an increase, and if not, what the maximum is that such men are allowed by special legislation?" The pension office responded with the same explanation of rejection as it had given Shields and ignored the special legislation question.[95]

By 1920, Shields and his wife owned their home in Clayton, New Jersey. The census recorded no one else living with them. Congress amended the pension legislation that year, so Shields submitted another pension increase request, this time asserting that he could not "see so as to distinguish Almost Blind has to have personal attendance." Shields submitted another statement, sworn before a notary, in which he admitted to being blind and that he required the constant, personal attendance of his wife "to undress and dress [him] + lead him wherever he goes." Lydia also contributed a sworn statement that confirmed the same issues but also mentioned bladder problems, noting that a local Dr. Fisler had attended Shields, and identified two other witnesses to her husband's condition.[96]

Charles F. Fisler, MD, submitted a letter to the pension office. He cited the familiar litany of wounds, adding "arterio-sclerosis" and stressing the need for assistance with stark language. Shields "is almost helpless, cannot walk without assistance, cannot read on account of eyesight being almost gone, being dependent on his wife when needed to urinate or when his bowels are to be moved." He described the bladder difficulties arising from "enlargement of the prostate" and concluded, "Altogether he is very feeble, and liable to suffer a stroke of apoplexy at any time, which condition I have looked for months past, and which almost surely happen soon."[97]

Another legislator, US senator Walter E. Edge, wrote to the bureau requesting a pension increase to seventy dollars. "Captain Shields is nearly blind, has serious kidney trouble, and must have care both day and night. . . . Will you not kindly give this matter your early attention, with a view to favorable action upon his application, which, I am informed, has been previously filed?" Shields's notary, J. Ellis Paulin, wrote that he had submitted Fisler's statement and asked the board whether he needed to return to Fisler for further documentation as "John Shields is so nearly helpless he has to [have] personal aid & attendance all of the time. . . . Kindly answer." This time, the pension office raised Shields's monthly allowance to seventy-two dollars.[98]

Based on Shields's last request for an increase, the pension office ordered yet another physical examination, this time by one physician only, Ralph R. Charlesworth, MD, in Millville. The doctor found Shields at age eighty-one to weigh 180 pounds. Unsurprisingly, he confirmed the partial paralysis of the right shoulder and arm, evidence of arteriosclerosis, and bladder difficulties and incontinence, and he concluded that these findings "require an attendant." While Charlesworth's surgeon's certificate was passing through the appropriate channels, notary Paulin wrote again to the pension office, "Is there any further evidence needed to complete his case so as he can draw his full claim that is due him."[99]

Paulin's letter was only days too late. On August 27, 1923, after another two years of uncertainty about a pension increase and, perhaps, by this point, indifference, Shields died at his home, age eighty-four. Attending physician Dr. Fisler stated on the death certificate that he had cared for Shields since the previous March and judged the death due to "Arterio Sclerosis" and "Enlarged

Prostrate" coupled with "Chronic Cystitis." No autopsy was deemed necessary.[100]

The obituaries dutifully recounted Shields's immigration to the United States, wartime service and injuries, railroad contracting, and administration of the Vineland home. Some accounts differed on the number and names of surviving children or Shields's hometown in Ireland. The lead obituary in the *Camden Post-Telegram* stated that following his neck injury, Shields was "forced to wear a silver tube in his windpipe for years." Although the metal stent was removed following his tracheotomy in 1863, Shields might have told friends and family that the stent was a wartime artifact as much as the fugitive bullet under the scapula, objects the mere mention of which reminded both Shields and his audience that for his body, the war remained ever in progress. If he experienced self-conscious public moments when his speaking was strained or his right arm and leg did not obey his will, announcing the embedded artifacts as causative would have sufficed to explain and justify his odd behaviors to an accepting audience. Employing these artifacts in his presentation of self-conveyed dignity to his sacrifice of personal health. Knowing about these artifacts and their lasting effects on Shields's body heightened the respect of the GAR, Vineland home residents, and fellow business partners and bank directors.[101]

Shields's civic body was dead, but his pension body was not. Lydia promptly pursued her widow's pension, applying only four days after her husband's death to obtain the final pension payment due him for the period of August fourth to the twenty-seventh. She then applied for her own pension. The commissioner of pensions explained to Lydia the proof she would need to earn her pension in a letter identical to the one Janey Dawson had received. As Janey had experienced, the pension office required evidence that the first Mrs. Shields had died and affidavits from credible people that Lydia and Anna Curran Shields had not been married previously. Lydia produced sworn statements from two longtime friends who attested to her wedding to Shields and their subsequent cohabitation and swore that Lydia had not been previously married. The Southwicks also swore that they had known Lydia for fifteen years and attested to the wedding and her cohabitation with Shields. Lydia received her pension.[102]

Shields was buried at the family plot at Prospect Hill Cemetery in Flemington, alongside Anna Curran Shields and their daughter, Anna Shields Golden. Lydia was buried with her parents at Siloam Cemetery in Vineland. She passed away in 1939 at age sixty-nine, having only been married to Shields for a period of less than five years. She shares a tombstone with her parents, George B. and Margaret D. Bontecou, who predeceased her marriage. The name on the stone is Lydia Bontecou Shields.

CONCLUSION: MUTED IDENTITY

Shields's frequent medical examinations can be seen as persistent acts of defiance in asserting his physical identity, despite the reluctance of the pension office to recognize the totality of his bodily suffering. He presented a challenge to pension authorities, medical examiners, and his business and social peers in that his body did not *appear* unusual. When speaking, Shields was hoarse or coughed, symptoms that did not indicate to others that he had sustained injuries during the war. Although his two injuries did not cause visible disfigurement, he suffered not only physical pain but also the progressive decrease in functionality throughout his postwar life. Only in his final employment as a manager of a veterans' home did his bodily failings become obvious and public. At the Vineland home, Shields worked in an environment of support and understanding, surrounded as he was by fellow Union veterans and their widows.

For decades, Shields presented a continuum of increasing debility by identifying his health problems holistically as a progressively worsening cluster of difficulties. At each examination following Shields's submission of a claim, physicians deconstructed his ailments into allowable pension categories, thus negating a holistic appraisal. Some doctors, however, appeared to resist formulaic responses to veterans' claims and left it to authorities at the pension office to rate medical problems in monetary terms. Only the Mitchells engaged Shields in a dialogue about his body that constituted a mutual, open-ended exploration. They appreciated Shields's view of his injuries as dynamic phenomena, not as static moments of compensable damage, forever anchored in the war.

Worried about his own financial future, Shields sympathized with Vineland residents of limited means and social connections whose descent into poverty created a public presumption that moral backsliding or sheer laziness accompanied their condition. The repeated resistance from the pension office, his changing domestic circumstances, and his physical degeneration led Shields to stop arguing a model of progressive disability based on his two original wounds. By fully embracing a medical model in the twentieth century, Shields's final plea meant dependence or, in the eyes of some, "harboring undeserving dependency on others."[103]

Through his business affairs, Shields was aware of increased postwar industrialization, the broader move to standardize factories and categories of workers by the actuarial practice of insurers, and the corresponding tension with social causes from child labor to old-age pensions. As an administrator at the Vineland home, he stridently defended the needy veteran from politicians who would group the veteran with the insane or destitute. He carried the banner for the perennial honor of the soldiers who saved the Union and the corresponding obligation of society to respect those veterans. His pension examinations were exercises in counternarrative: he seemed to say,

> Look at me. I am an honorable, working gentleman but I live every day with war wounds that create misery that I must endure as my sacrifice to

> my country. I demand your attention to my body as it changes through time, and the interdependence of the phenomena I exhibit; I demand that you recognize that my body cannot be compartmentalized into numerical ratings; I demand that you not see me as a static relic; I demand that you recognize my pain; I demand that you recognize me as a living embodiment of a war that is daily becoming more distant from the lives of most Americans.

By seeing Shields as he demanded to be seen, pension doctors—and, he hoped, pension officials—would understand that his inability to perform manual labor, the criterion for awarding a pension, was ultimately meaningless. Pension attorneys told their veteran clients to list on their pension applications some kind of manual labor they had once performed, a fiction that Shields tried at least once but abandoned later only to return to it just before he died. The implicit meaning of disability was an inability to create a different criterion that Shields and many of his peers did not meet. And yet, Shields *created* two construction businesses and supervised a veterans' home, clear evidence of his ability to build, contribute, and generate despite his waning health. He wanted to be seen as a man still recovering from severe wounds and not as a "social fugitive, a prisoner of expectations molded by a society that he makes uncomfortable by his very presence." His experience challenged people's understanding of disability and the prerogatives of the disabled in society. His experience also tells us that disabled veterans' expressions of masculinity were far more elastic and accommodating than those within "normal" society.[104]

The medical trap that challenged physicians in placing wounded veterans within a masculine universe was the presumption that the ideal featured self-control as a component of moral rectitude. A veteran unable to control his bowels without help veered in the direction of the "vicious habits" that physicians were required to address in physical examinations. Doctors and the pension bureaucrats to whom they reported applied the label *disabled* within a working environment of rapidly evolving meanings despite the pension office's attempt to fix them to a static system.[105]

Shields's resistance to the pension ratings system might have been partly due to his fierce allegiance to GAR ideology. While disabled veterans relied on the GAR to affirm their wartime identities and lobby for pensions within an unchanging view of 1860s Republicanism, employment opportunities in the United States became progressively more mechanized. Workers' bodies became standardized, a process that excluded the amputee or sightless veteran. Healthy factory workers, for example, were replaceable and interchangeable, and their lives and productivity could be transmuted into data, as was demonstrated in the lists, graphs, and tables of *The Medical and Surgical History of the War of the Rebellion*. Shields's role in the GAR and his directorship of the Vineland home with its military administrative structure, its own GAR post, and the ritual affirmation of identity on Decoration Day and other occasions, militated against the national focus on growth and expansion. Resisting this focus came at the expense of creating a national vision emanating from the meaning of the Civil War. In maintaining one foot in the world of railroad construction and the other in a disabled veterans' home, Shields was doubtless aware of broad national trends in employment and the increasing distance between the worldview of the Civil War and the early twentieth century. He nevertheless sought help from the Vineland resident physician to claim pension increases, and he doubtless supported many resident veterans and their widows to argue their claims as he did.[106]

Vineland was part of an emerging network of national homes—asylums—for disabled soldiers, at first as a haven for those without family support and later primarily for those impoverished by life circumstances. The establishment of homes resembled the trends in pensions. Evolving criteria for the award of pensions for disabilities paralleled the rules for admittance to homes like Vineland. The homes were administered like military institutions, but after the 1920s, they gradually metamorphosed into social service institutions under hospital-like management. Shields did not live long enough to see his Vineland home undergo a philosophical change in management, but he did live through the Spanish-American War and World War I. His fervent faith in the Civil War veteran as an exemplar of the highest calling of a citizen in time of national peril was evident in the pride he took in sacrificing his health for a cause greater than himself. He died with a bullet still lodged in his shoulder, an injury that endured throughout his life. He died with a severely damaged larynx after repeatedly presenting himself to doctors as a man with evolving wounds, effectively communicating to his examiners the "indeterminacy" of his body and his refusal to be coded as some monthly rate of payment.[107]

In 1862, Sergeant John Wilson, a soldier in Shields's Company E, wrote a letter that appeared in the *Mauch Chunk Gazette*: "[My] company has the fullest confidence in [Shields's] ability to lead us through the coming struggle. He is an officer who takes care that his men are well treated, and they love and respect him, and all pray that a kind Providence will guide him safely through the campaign." Shields would have been pleased if the newspaper obituary recalled these words that also reflected his devotion to veterans at the end of his life.[108]

EIGHT

THOMAS R. HAWKINS (1840–1870)[1]

THE WIDTH OF A CLERK'S DESK

For the last few months in the lingering Virginia summer heat, Sergeant Major Thomas R. Hawkins had become accustomed to boarding steamboats and gunboats up and down the James and Appomattox Rivers. His regiment, the Sixth United States Colored Infantry, had challenged rebel troops at various points along the vast trench works protecting the Confederate capital, Richmond, Virginia, and Petersburg, the closest city and railroad to the southern and western routes providing supplies and manpower. For much of Hawkins's time on the river, a green wall of trees overhung the shore, blocking the view inland. Occasionally, his transport barge passed cultivated land, plantations, and small settlements.

It was disconcerting to find Confederate soldiers in almost any direction, despite the secure supply depots and small forts created by the Union army as bases for forays into the interior. Hawkins was no passive observer. As the only sergeant major of his regiment, he was the highest-ranking noncommissioned officer, and he represented the division between the rank and file and the commissioned officers. He may not have understood the strategy of the moment, but he knew more than any other enlisted soldier. Something about Hawkins impressed his white officers in August 1863, when he enlisted as a private in Philadelphia, a substitute for a draftee seaman. Those officers appointed Hawkins as sergeant major within a few weeks of his enlistment when he entered Camp William Penn near Philadelphia—the same camp at which Presley Dorsey/Dawson would later train. In this role, he mastered army regulations, served as the arbiter of discipline, transmitted orders accurately and comprehensively, and ensured that orders were obeyed. At twenty-three, he had worked as a plasterer and mason before the war. His obvious intelligence, maturity, and self-possession led to his promotion from private.

Near dusk on September 28, 1864, as his boat steamed down the James River from Dutch Gap, Hawkins surveyed the soldiers in his charge, anticipating what was to come. His regiment belonged to the Army of the James under Major General Benjamin F. Butler, a lawyer and politician whose political connections earned him the appointment despite his lack of military background. In collaboration with General Grant, Butler planned an offensive that was to begin the next day.[2]

Hawkins had seen the elephant, the common reference among soldiers to experiencing combat. Three months earlier, the Sixth had participated in an attack on Confederate defenses a few miles from Richmond that required Hawkins to lead soldiers through thick woods, uneven terrain muddied by endless creeks, and finally into the open before a rebel fort. In the fury of combat—the first time the Sixth came under fire—Hawkins was shot in the right arm just below the elbow and was forced to leave the field. As he did so, he observed with disgust the flag bearer toss down the colors and crawl to the rear. Hospitalized for several weeks after the bullet was "excised near bend of elbow," Hawkins returned to the regiment in time to join the expedition to Deep Bottom, an embankment on the north side of the James River south of Richmond where federal troops had established a small garrison, a toehold in uncertain territory. He recalled the difficulty at Dutch Gap of maintaining order when his men advanced in the dark through thick undergrowth and stumbling over concealed ditches, mud, and fallen trees while being pummeled by rebel artillery.[3]

At Deep Bottom, Hawkins supervised the debarkation of his regiment around dusk. Soldiers quickly set up campfires and prepared their meals but did not pitch their tents. They knew they would be roused in the dark to march into rebel country. A friendly face lightened the mood, that of Hawkins's friend and counterpart Sergeant Major Christian A. Fleetwood of the Fourth United States Colored Infantry, also a veteran of the same fight of the previous June. Fleetwood later wrote that "a strong, deep feeling of friendship" grew up between them as they "often shar[ed] the same blanket, haversack, and canteen on the toilsome march—fighting side by side in action, or sharing the relaxation of life in camp."[4]

Hawkins might have managed a short nap, but a few hours into the morning's dark, the troops roused themselves and prepared for the day. They had been ordered to leave most of their gear at the depot and travel with three days' cooked rations in their haversacks, a rolled blanket, and sixty cartridges. The Fourth and Sixth marched in close order in the morning's humid air and creeping fog two miles to their destination.

As sunrise approached around 5:30 a.m., the fog became luminous in morning light just as both regiments emerged from the woods onto an open field. As the sun rose, Hawkins saw that the ground gently sloped down to a creek and then uphill to the rebel fortification. Soldiers were to attack parallel to a branch of a larger stream, Four Mile Creek. Hawkins understood the difficulty of moving two regiments over challenging terrain with no cover. General Butler rode up to where the soldiers were forming lines and yelled, "Those works must be taken by the weight of your column; not a shot must be fired." Hawkins understood that the attack would have to be made swiftly if it had any hope of success. Individual soldiers stopping to load rifles, aim, fire, and then reload would cause a confused human mass under intense gunfire. Butler also ordered soldiers to remove the percussion caps from their rifles: without them in place, the guns could not fire. Soldiers were expected to capture the rebel redoubt at the point of their bayonets. Butler roused them to give the cry on attack: "Remember Fort Pillow!" The previous April, the namesake Union garrison on the Mississippi River in Tennessee surrendered to rebels under Major General Nathan Bedford Forrest. Confederate soldiers massacred surrendering black soldiers, killing approximately three hundred. Hawkins and every other man in his regiment were aware of this.[5]

Hawkins worked to keep order in the line as troops descended a mild decline before heading uphill to the rebel trench line. Several officers called out to their companies, "Forward." With a collective yell—and as rebel soldiers began firing at them—Hawkins and his men crossed "a sluggish stream with slimy banks and mossy bottom, about four yards wide" and stepped into a marsh, as recollected by Lieutenant Nathan Edgerton. The soldiers marched in close columns "at right shoulder shift" [rifle resting on right shoulder], a posture adopted on the parade ground, but fog, terrain, timing, and rebel fire resulted in disorganization and confusion. Behind the advancing troops, their brigade commander, Colonel Samuel A. Duncan, saw them "disappear, as they entered the fog that enwrapped them like a mantle of death." The two regiments numbered about 750 men, the entrenched rebels about three times that, and those immediately in front of Hawkins were the battle-sharpened Texas Brigade.[6]

Presenting an attacking front "not wider than a clerk's desk," as Butler later recollected, the column of black soldiers relied on fog cover and a rapid advance to overwhelm their enemies, but the rebels' intense firing from behind earthworks prevented any kind of orderly attack. After slowing at the creek, Hawkins and his men negotiated a line of abatis—trees felled in the direction of the attackers, which presented a chaotic mesh of branches and sharpened logs, their stumps challenging soldiers to climb over or around them. While troops stalled to cut paths through the branches, punishing rebel fire rained down on many of the officers. No sooner had soldiers cleared the abatis when Hawkins and other sergeants tried to re-form the line to get beyond the next obstacle, the *chevaux de frise,* a line of logs bristling with attached sharpened stakes. Hawkins noticed that the planned simultaneous attacks on the rebel line to his east and west were not happening. His and Fleetwood's regiments were alone.

Hawkins saw the color guard at the head of the column shot down. Those immediately retrieving and raising the colors soon fell as well. The officer who picked up the national colors was likewise killed. Lieutenant Edgerton removed the colors from the dead man's hand and held the flag forward, but he suddenly reeled and fell. As he tried to arise, he discovered that a bullet had passed through both the flagstaff and his wrist. As Edgerton struggled, First Sergeant Alexander Kelly took the colors and waved them to rally the men. Meanwhile, Hawkins helped Edgerton to stand and picked up the regimental colors. In the Fourth regiment at the same time, Fleetwood was trying to keep order and replace the color guard. "Keep on, boys," he urged his men. He later wrote, "It was a deadly hailstorm of bullets, sweeping man down as hailstones sweep the leaves from the trees." Hawkins held the fraying regimental colors high, waving the flag from side to side to embolden the advancing men and to defy the enemy's bullets.[7]

Three months before, Hawkins had realized that in battle, he was not only a participant but an observer as well. He gave orders and labored to keep troops advancing in formation, but at the same time, he registered the violent deaths and wounding of comrades. On this day, once again, he observed with an odd detachment other men reacting to the moment and its random violence.

Some men appeared calm and determined. Others trembled with fear, clutching the earth, desperately trying to form a barrier of dirt in front of their prone bodies. Others yelled curses in a rage. Some lost control of their bowels. Hawkins disconnected from his own physical sensations to focus on the imperative to move forward and dislodge the enemy. "The matters of food, water, and comfort were forgotten, and one Northerner described what almost appeared to be an out-of-body experience."[8]

The two flags—and the commitment to prevent their capture—were crucial. Soldiers drew inspiration from the colors; their morale and will to fight depended on the visibility. The banners moved, fluttered, changed direction in the wind, and showed exuberance and life. When the din of battle prevented the troops from hearing the shouted orders and the inevitable confusion turned their courageous fighting into disordered, panicky flight, the position and attitude of the flags let soldiers where they were supposed to be and where their leaders were. The national colors motivated them to do their duty and anchored their allegiance to their country, the national body. The regimental colors anchored them to home and comradeship, the community body. By the time Edgerton faltered with the national colors, both flags had been shot to ribbons.

Local citizens sponsored the design and fabrication of regimental colors. The Sixth received its flag in a ceremony before departing Camp William Penn. Designed by a Philadelphia African American artist, David Bustill Bowser, the Sixth's flag depicted the figure of Columbia bestowing a blessing on a black soldier, as a woman in the blue background pressed her palms together in prayer or joy at the soldier's commitment. "Freedom for All" read the banner over the scene. The opposite side depicted "the American eagle in front, over it the words 'Presented by Colored Citizens of Philadelphia'" and the 1863 date. In a ceremony at Camp William Penn, community leader, abolitionist, and recruiter Robert E. Purvis formally presented the colors to the Sixth. He addressed the audience as one "of those who have procured for you this beautiful banner, to transfer it unto your charge, and on their behalf this splendid guidon, this glorious emblem of freedom, I present . . . to you. You will prove yourselves worthy of the gift; you will see that the flag of your country suffers no dishonor at your hands." When Hawkins saw that the colors were in danger of being destroyed or seized, he had no choice but to risk his life to save them. The capture of his regimental flag would mean emasculation, cowardice, loss of dignity, and shame.[9]

Before the two flags were recovered, the thinning ranks of soldiers advanced to within several dozen yards of their enemy. Although the fog had begun to burn off, the smoke from artillery and rifle fire obscured much of the action. Rebels shouted insults and taunts: "Come on, darkies, we want your muskets!" Reluctantly, the remaining federal officers judged their situation as hopeless. An officer in Fleetwood's regiment, Lieutenant James H. Wilkes, watched as "the whole line seemed to wilt down under the fearful fire which was then poured into us. The line was growing too weak and thin to make an assault. It began to waiver." The order came to withdraw. Emboldened, rebel soldiers stood on the embankment, shooting down at Hawkins and his retreating comrades. Captain John McMurray of the Sixth later wrote, "That was perhaps the most trying five minutes or ten minutes we endured in all our army life."[10]

At about the time Hawkins was rescuing the regimental colors, a bullet struck him in the upper third of his right thigh. Within minutes, a second bullet entered the upper third of his right humerus, splintering the bone. A third bullet penetrated the big toe of his right foot. As he led his men in retreat while holding the colors in his left hand, he collapsed close to the creek beyond the abatis, where, according to Fleetwood, he remained for three hours until he was rescued and taken to the hospital tents at Deep Bottom. Fleetwood wrote, "His recovery from these fearful wounds was deemed hopeless, but his strong constitution with God's blessing again placed him on his feet though crippled for life."[11]

The retreat was as orderly as the two regiments could manage. The regimental and national colors were saved as rebels left their trenches to continue firing at the retreating black soldiers. Several of Hawkins's comrades surrendered, and wounded others were murdered. The two shattered regiments regrouped and retreated as other units attacked the rebel line in two waves around 7:30 and 8:30 a.m., ultimately driving off the Confederates.

A decade later, General Butler revisited the battlefield and recalled the scene:

> There, in a space not wider than a clerk's desk, and three hundred yards long, lay the dead bodies of five hundred and forty-three of my Colored comrades, slain in the defence of their country, who had laid down their lives to uphold its flag and its honor as a willing sacrifice . . . and as I looked upon their bronzed faces upturned in the shining sun as if in mute appeal against the wrongs of the country for which they had given their lives . . . feeling I had wronged them in the past, and believing what was the future of my country to them—among my dead comrades I swore to myself a solemn oath: "May my right hand forget its cunning, and my tongue cleave to the roof of my mouth, if I ever fail to defend the rights of those men who have given their blood for me and my country this day and for their race forever;" and, God helping me, I will keep that oath.[12]

Back in Deep Bottom, the remnants of the two regiments attended to their wounds and took muster of the remaining troops. The Sixth entered the attack with 367 soldiers and ended with 210 of that number as casualties. Company D lost 87 percent of its soldiers, the highest number of fatalities reported during the war involving one company in one battle.

Hawkins's comrades set him on the ground next to other injured men. A hospital steward inspected his wounds, determined they were not life-threatening, and decided he could wait for the transfer by steamboat to Portsmouth, Virginia. The steward applied lint—compressed strands of linen—to the wounds and

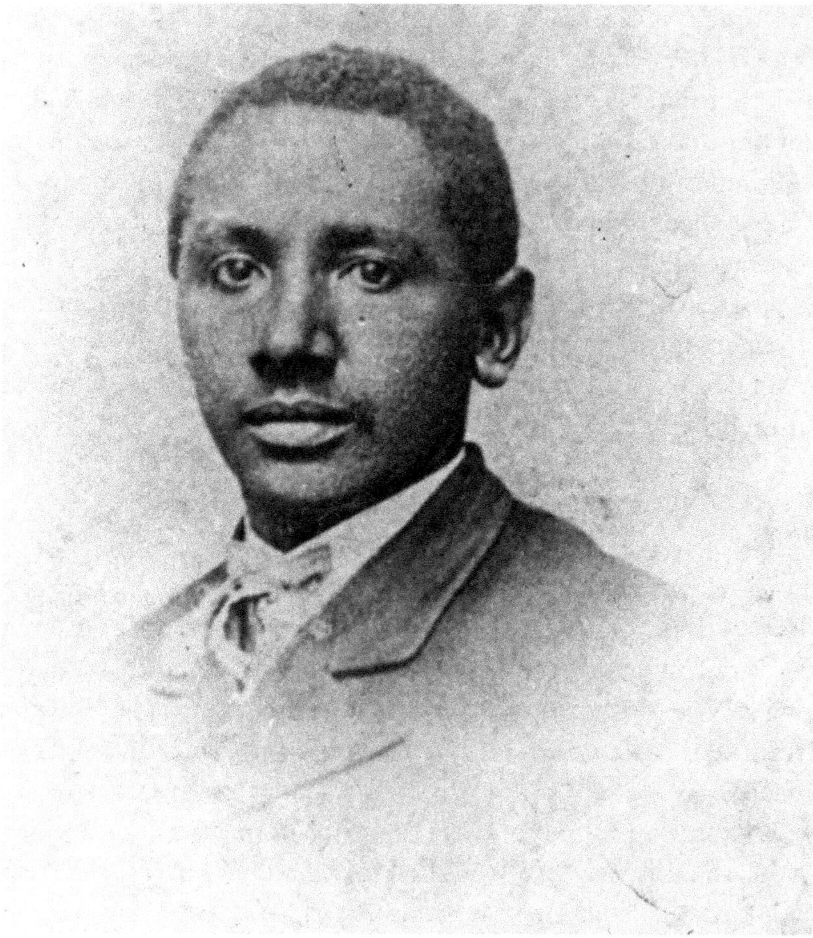

The only known image of Thomas R. Hawkins, 1860s. *Credit: Library of Congress (LC-DIG-cph.3c18559).*

bandaged his foot, shoulder, and thigh as best as conditions allowed.

The survivors felt cheated. Their blood was up, and they asked to return to the fight. Their wish was granted, but not at New Market Heights. The two regiments marched about five miles to Fort Harrison, another rebel garrison defending Richmond, occupied by Union troops following an attack that morning. The soldiers of the Sixth and Fourth arrived in time to engage in another fierce battle and drive the Confederates away. General Butler noted that "a few more such charges, and to command colored troops will be the post of honor in the American armies. The colored soldiers, by coolness, steadiness, and determined courage and dash, have silenced every cavil of doubters of their soldierly capacity, and have drawn tokens of admiration from their enemies."[13]

Hawkins exhibited all of these characteristics, but, sadly, his military career had just ended.

WOUNDED MANHOOD

After Hawkins was shot in the arm in June 1864, the army sent him to Balfour General Hospital in Portsmouth. He resumed duty on August 13, so his recovery was interrupted by the fighting at New Market Heights. After the September battle, Hawkins returned to the hospital, which by that time had reached its capacity. Several days after the battle, Balfour assistant surgeon J. H. Franz appealed to a higher authority that without notification, an additional 150 wounded men had just arrived, some of whom came from Deep Bottom. Franz asked for permission to house some of the men at the local Baptist or Episcopal church. To further complicate matters, Franz had to arrange for segregated wards.[14]

Surgeons examined and attended to Hawkins's wounds. First, they tried to place Hawkins in the same posture he had been in when he was struck by bullets. According to one of the most influential texts on gunshot wounds by British physician Thomas Longmore, "In almost every instance the examination will be facilitated by attention to this precept. Occasionally it will at once indicate the probable injury to vessels or other important structures, in cases where the mutual relations of the wounds of entrance and exit, in the erect or horizontal posture of the body, would lead to no such information." Doctors looked for entrance and exit wounds to assess the damage in between and to determine what projectiles remained in the body. At this time, both armies used rifles that fired minié balls. This potent bullet "seems to derive its chief importance in surgery from the conical end possessing the mechanical characteristic of a wedge, while the [round lead ball] acted simply as an obtuse body. . . . The wedge-like quality of the conical bullet is rendered particularly obvious on its being driven into the shafts of the long bones of the extremities."[15]

Probing the wound tissues revealed that the bullet that had struck Hawkins's toe had exited through his foot. Doctors likely recovered a bullet while removing spicules (sharp fragments) of bone from the upper arm, but the bullet in the thigh remained. The doctor cautiously inserted a finger into the wound in the arm, hoping it would come into contact with the bullet, thereby indicating its path and position. According to Longmore, this method causes the least damage to tissues. "If bones are fractured, the number, shape, length, position, and degree of looseness of the fragments may be more readily observed." Failing this, the surgeon inserted a Nélaton probe, a segment of wire capped with white porcelain tips. Bent to accommodate the size and shape of the wound, the wire was carefully inserted. If the porcelain tip lodged against a barrier, the doctor rotated it; if upon removal the tip was discolored by the lead bullet, then the projectile and its location were known.[16]

Examination of the thigh wound did not reveal the location of the bullet, which would remain in Hawkins's body for the rest of his life. Of the thigh and upper-arm wounds, the former was regarded as the biggest challenge. "Gunshot wounds of the lower extremity vary much more greatly in the gravity of their results, as well as in the treatment to be adopted, according to the part of the limb injured, than happens in those of the upper extremity."

The surgeons took a very conservative approach by treating the visible wound and leaving the bullet in the body; if they noticed a dislocation of the femoral head, they did not consider a surgical or therapeutic option to repair the problem. Hawkins's chief postwar difficulty was lameness in the right leg.[17]

Hawkins did not regard his wounds as serious enough to warrant discharge, so he planned to return to duty and resume his status as sergeant major. Hospitalization meant helplessness and lack of independence. When he left his regiment, his colleagues were clamoring to return to the fight and defeat the rebels. Their "fighting rage," described by some historians as "combat narcosis," was still intense after the previous fight and did not diminish as they marched to another one at Fort Harrison. Hawkins might have felt that fervor as he recovered and longed to reexperience it with his men. In gauging a soldier's morale, it is important to "[recognize] emotion as having agency in shaping perceptions and actions."[18]

On the battlefield, Hawkins was both warrior and observer, but as a wounded man in the hospital, he must have felt disoriented and grasped for a temporary identity that signified his authority as a leader and demonstrated his dignity as he underwent treatment, serving as a model to his ward mates. To Hawkins, doctors in uniform were just officers in a different context, and he would have been subject to their orders. Doctors, orderlies, and nurses, however, would not have given Hawkins's rank any special consideration—he was just another body in the ward, feminized by his imposed inaction and dependence. Hawkins might also have felt that, as a black man, his participation in the war betokened a higher calling, a holy mission as emblazoned on the regimental standard "Freedom for All."

Hawkins's self-perception as a military leader who came through battle with honor and courage must have seemed ironic given the circumstances of being in the army in the first place: he was not drafted, nor did he volunteer. Hawkins agreed to serve as a paid substitute for Passmore Henry, a single African American man about five years older than Hawkins, a Philadelphian described in the census as both a waterman and a seaman. Standing in for another man was not an automatic process. Henry was first drafted and then examined before an enrollment board that accepted his substitution. Once Henry paid Hawkins $300, the substitute officially took the place of the draftee. Despite complaints that the draft protected the rich and penalized the poor, army regulations took a relaxed attitude: "It is obviously impossible to frame a conscription act which shall bear equally" on the soldier who fights for a cause or principle while to another man "it becomes an expenditure of substance and treasure."[19]

Army service meant immunity against some of the hazards of being black in Northern society. Soldiers still endured catcalls, taunts, and even violent behavior from resentful white people, but a group of black soldiers could sometimes intimidate their attackers enough to avoid violence, and occasionally, their officers would support them. Throughout Hawkins's adult civilian life, he was aware of the possibility of being kidnapped into slavery. In the hospital, Hawkins's treatment was conditioned by racist assumptions about his body; for example, the black body's supposed resilience to pain or susceptibility to tropical diseases.

On the steamer to Portsmouth from Deep Bottom, Hawkins saw many soldiers like himself, wounded, conscious, or semiconscious, all trying manfully to face their destination with quiet resolve. He also watched them die. Walt Whitman observed the death of a Wisconsin officer, the circumstances of which were certainly familiar to Hawkins. "Notice that water-pail by the side of the bed, with a quantity of blood and bloody pieces of muslin—nearly full; that tells the story." Hawkins may not have become inured to the deathbed intimacy of dying soldiers' final words, gestures, and expressions coupled with indifference as ordinary life went on. Whitman wrote, "The poor young man is lying panting, struggling painfully for breath, his great dark eyes with a glaze already upon them, and the choking faint but audible in his throat. . . . He will die here in an hour or two. . . . Meantime the ordinary chat and business of the Ward a little way off goes on indifferently. Some of the inmates are laughing and joking, others are playing checkers or cards, others are reading, &c."[20]

In his segregated area of the hospital, with no white soldiers looking on, Hawkins developed supportive ward friendships. These relationships were a temporary comfort for loneliness. There is no record of any extant correspondence between Hawkins and his friends or family. A sergeant with the Third United States Colored Infantry, Tillman Valentine, wrote to his wife from the field, "I look up at the stars and ask god to bless you and take care of you." An unmarried man, Hawkins doubtless prayed the same for his family.

Hawkins may have been visited by the regimental chaplain of the Sixth, the Reverend Jeremiah Asher, a man who radiated strength and confidence and promoted the cause of the black soldier as a sacred duty. As attentive as the white doctors were, their cultural background and medical training reinforced the implication of the biological inferiority of black bodies. Hawkins could never have overcome this view. Doctors had invented the concept of race as encompassing inherited characteristics, a view that "resolve[d] the contradiction between slavery and liberty." The Sixth's motto of "Freedom for All" implied freedom from physical enslavement but also an ideological freedom from racialist theory.[21]

In the hospital, Hawkins had plenty of time to think about damaged bodies. He probably did not yet think of his body as disabled, but he must have recalled the images of the dead and dying from New Market Heights. The photographs of dead soldiers—or wounded ones in hospitals—that were published as early as 1862 did not include any depictions of black soldiers. Their ultimate sacrifice would not be witnessed by a curious public.[22] The heroism of black soldiers was pictured in woodblock prints for newspapers that expressed hackneyed, theatrical poses and expressions. These images had little emotional impact on their audience: "White artists and audiences resisted visualizing the disabled [or dead] black body." To exhibit dead black soldiers would place their sacrifices as equal to those of dead white soldiers in publicly viewed images. Further, viewers of images of dead or disfigured white soldiers challenged assumptions about male anatomy, stimulating improved hygienic practices within regiments, "popularizing the metaphor of purification, and so avoiding the fact of putrefaction." The lack of images of wounded black soldiers for public consumption removed black bodies from these discussions. Most white citizens gave them little thought.[23]

Hawkins must have revisited the sights and smells of his dead comrades near Petersburg and New Market Heights. He was aware that rebels sometimes took the body parts of dead black soldiers as trophies or otherwise mutilated their bodies. Taking trophies from slain enemies is a practice as old as war, a ritual of the hunt that "shifted into the domain of human relations, and made to serve there as a model for violence between social groups." Taking and exhibiting trophies of mutilation in the case of black bodies affirmed a collective identity to rebel soldiers, "as material evidence of the naturalness of racial hierarchy and the permanence of differences."[24]

Fearful of trophy hunting and out of respect, Hawkins wanted to recover so that he could bury his comrades. Knowing that they lay unburied or remained undiscovered must have caused him great distress. Shorn of their manhood and will, slain soldiers were rendered feminine in their "vulnerability to dishonour and a need for protection by their kinsmen." Most black soldiers believed that their part in saving the Union demonstrated to a hesitant country that their courage and resilience merited citizenship. Their sacrifice of life represented the full democratization of the state. Black and white corpses mingled on the battlefield as a testament to this ideal. Walt Whitman endeavored to document the names and lives of dying Union soldiers, haunted as he was by imagining the anonymity of soldiers' graves. Soldiers' deaths "eclipse all other consequences, as though the entire war was waged upon [damaged organs and bones retained for medical study, as detritus of the battlefield, or as trophies of the enemy] as an 'emblem' of the democratic body."[25]

Hawkins would later find that racism affected access to pensions. Black men as federal soldiers entered the war in 1863—two years after many white men—and some of their infantry regiments saw limited battlefield action as they mainly served for garrison or fatigue duty—building roads, clearing forests, creating fortifications—all while receiving pay at a laborer's and not a soldier's wage. Hawkins had been spared garrison duty in the South—as Prestley Dorsey/Dawson had endured in Texas—within communities of resentful white citizens. An armed black man in a military uniform implicitly threatened white manhood. As sergeant major, Hawkins likely harbored resentments due to discriminatory pay, but he could not have expressed this attitude to anyone other than fellow sergeants major such as Christian Fleetwood.[26]

Hawkins might have speculated about the role of his physiognomy in his promotion to sergeant major. His only surviving photograph shows a face with a narrow nose, thin lips, high cheekbones, and light skin color. In one government document, he is described as a mulatto. About 40 percent of noncommissioned officers in black regiments were mulatto, which was defined at the time as mixed white and black. In comparison, on average, one-fourth of all soldiers in black regiments were mulatto. The percentage of black and white privates who were promoted to noncommissioned ranks (sergeants) was about the same, around 17 percent. Hawkins's dedication to his role and regiment is evident in the fact that he achieved and did not later resign his promotion, as some did. While Hawkins sought a pension as a veteran, he must have reflected on the significance of his disability and the army's classification of his body for the rest of his life, despite his role as a leader and the severe injuries he had sustained.[27]

TWO-THIRDS DISABLED AND A MARRIAGE

Following months in the hospital, Hawkins was furloughed until the end of December. At the end of April 1865, he returned to his regiment, which was encamped in Wilmington, North Carolina, after the surrender at Appomattox. Hawkins's foot wound caused a pronounced limp, and it became obvious to his regimental officers and surgeon that he must be discharged. Fleetwood later recalled, "He still refused to leave the service his whole heart and soul being in the cause for which he fought, and rejoined us after the fall of Fort Fisher and Wilmington, while we were at the latter place. Ordered shortly afterward into the interior to operate against the Confederate General Johnston, he was unable to march, and left at Wilmington whence he was honorably discharged for disability on account of wounds received in action." When Hawkins returned to his regiment, he found that General Butler had issued a medal to commemorate the Petersburg siege to the black soldiers who participated in the campaign. He also discovered that Lieutenant Edgerton had been promoted to captain and Fleetwood and Kelly had received the Medal of Honor for rescuing the colors, although he had not been so honored.[28]

Hawkins's rudimentary physical data in the military record listed him as being five foot four and a half inches tall, with a light complexion, black hair, and brown eyes. To these basic statistics were added the very specific descriptions of his wounds. The certificate of disability, countersigned by multiple medical authorities, states that Hawkins could no longer perform his duties due to "wounds received in action. He was wounded with bullet passing close to elbow joint on 15th June 1864 and was also on 29th September wounded in three different places with bullets in upper third of humerus injuring the bone in that several pieces were taken out; in the upper third of the thigh, the ball being lodged in the limb causing permanent lameness [and another] in the great toe." Before the surgeon recommended that Hawkins's disability receive a two-thirds rating, the doctor documented his prewar profession as mason, which was intended to help the pension office imagine how manual labor could be accomplished without the other one-third of a body.[29]

Once discharged, Hawkins traveled to Philadelphia, where he stayed with friends or relatives on Lombard Street. He engaged a pension agent in that city, Joseph E. Devitt & Co., Military and Naval Agency, who submitted Hawkins's initial pension application. The claim provided additional information to that of the discharge certificate, stating that the elbow wound "fractured bone" and that the combined shoulder and elbow wounds "partially destroyed the use of the arm." The application noted the presence of the bullet in the thigh, which "prevent[ed] him from walking any distance and from performing manual labor." Two witnesses (of two years' acquaintance) swore to Hawkins's inability to perform his prewar trade.[30]

Within a month, Hawkins had received his pension certificate that duly awarded him a two-thirds disability at the monthly amount of $5.33 1/3.[31] The record over the next two years is incomplete regarding Hawkins's whereabouts. After a stay in Philadelphia, he moved to Washington, DC, where he was hired as a messenger for the internal revenue branch of the Treasury Department in 1866. Committed to his wartime vow, General Butler arranged the job for Hawkins.[32]

On May 2, 1867, at the Fifteenth Street Presbyterian Church in Washington, DC, Hawkins married Julia B. Landre, a nineteen-year-old schoolteacher from Poughkeepsie, New York, described as mulatto in the 1870 federal census. Established in 1841 as the first black Presbyterian church in the capital, Fifteenth Street Presbyterian was a vital nexus of African American society.

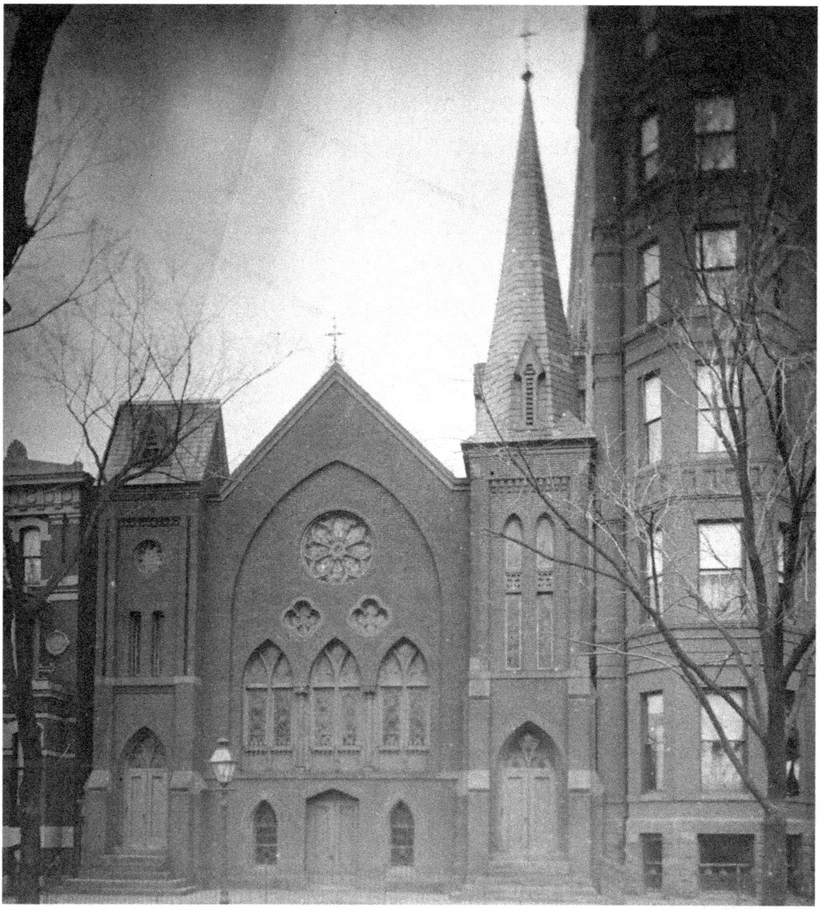

Fifteenth Street Presbyterian Church, Washington, DC, c. 1899.
Credit: Library of Congress (LC-DIG-ds-07872).

Abolition and civil rights advocate Rev. Henry Highland Garnet served as pastor from 1864 to 1866. Parishioners included William Slade, Abraham Lincoln's valet; Elizabeth Keckly, Mary Todd Lincoln's dressmaker; and two particularly conspicuous men in uniform, Alexander T. Augusta, MD, and Anderson R. Abbott, MD, Canadian-trained physicians who offered their services to the Union and received appointments as officers.[33]

The Fifteenth Street Presbyterian Church served the same wartime goals as Hawkins, embodied his goals and beliefs, and might have been where he met his wife. The Reverend John C. Smith, pastor at the church after Garnett, performed the marriage. Smith, a Scotch Irish pioneer in establishing a presbyterian presence in Washington, was acquainted with Lincoln and was appointed as chaplain to the army in 1862. He was proud of his pastoral work at Judiciary Square Hospital, claiming to have helped a total of eleven thousand men. In fact, the Fifteenth Street Presbyterian Church aggressively organized to recruit black soldiers when Hawkins entered Camp William Penn. Smith was well connected not only with the black elite of the city but also with the white political powerbrokers. He might have found work for Julia in one of the church-affiliated schools or drawn attention to Hawkins as a distinguished parishioner who had performed heroic war service.[34]

Julia gave birth to her first child, Thomas V., on October 24, 1867. At around this time, the Hawkins family lived in a townhouse at 1307 Rhode Island Avenue (which is still standing in what is today northwest Washington). Located a few blocks from the Presbyterian church (which thrives today), the Hawkins household was close to the Freedmen's Hospital and Asylum, established near the intersection of Thirteenth and R Streets, an institution that in 1862 served disabled and elder African Americans but later was absorbed into the Howard University campus. After the war, black soldiers looking for employment, medical treatment, spiritual guidance, or other assistance traveled through the Hawkins neighborhood. Some were students: the church housed the first high school for black students in the nation.

The Hawkins family was on the ascendant; in addition to his pension, Thomas worked for the government helping veterans, and Julia was a teacher. They had started a family. Their community, centered around the Fifteenth Street Presbyterian Church, provided them with social, economic, spiritual, and medical connections. Hawkins's health, however, was becoming progressively worse. He claimed that he was unable to perform manual labor and pursued a reclassification as being completely disabled. The year after his child's birth, he applied for a pension increase, claiming total disability because of the progressive immobility of his wounded limbs and the attendant pain.

Navigating a white medical establishment, Hawkins must have learned that his military service and willingness to risk his life for the Union were his chief attributes among white physicians. Despite all that he had endured in battle, however, he met examining physicians who held racist notions about black bodies. In an essay written after the war, Dr. Sanford Hunt, acknowledged by his white peers as an expert on the black military body, found the prototypical African American man to be inherently passive, "his simple mind filled with the grand metaphors of Holy Writ, and his doubts all silenced by an implicit faith that in the Lord's good time his deliverance would come." Writing after the war, Hunt asserted that "in no instance did [the black soldier] assume leadership, in no instance did he organize to strike a blow for his own liberty."

The idea that the black soldier was biologically incapable of embracing "the profession of the soldier [as] too noble and manly for this pariah of the land" had profound implications for medicalizing the black body. In particular, Hunt cited numerous unexplained hospital deaths among black people and surmised that some were caused by "the superstition of 'fetichism.'" Hunt's monograph dealt only with black soldiers' health; the numberless migrating black people during the war and after, those escaping enslavement and trying to find new lives were deprived of narratives about their health. Their starvation, diseases, exposure, and privation were hardly documented because they did "not fit into the patriotic narratives" of the war. For Hawkins, however, the fact of military sacrifice seemed to attract white doctors' attention, and he eventually succeeded in obtaining a higher pension.[35]

In his application for a pension increase, Hawkins argued that the bullet wound in his right thigh caused the dislocation of the femur from the pelvis, thus creating an artificial socket for the proximal head of the femur. This dislocation effectively gave him a longer right than left leg. In addition, the bullet wound to his right shoulder had reduced his movement and use of the arm. The application was accompanied by the endorsements of two men who swore that Hawkins was the man he presented himself to be. Dr. Phillips, an examining surgeon who supported a claim for total disability, endorsed Hawkins's application. Phillips stated that Hawkins had "lost the usual power of the shoulder and cannot completely flex the forearm." Philips also noted that the thigh wound continued to suppurate.[36]

The following January, Hawkins subjected himself to another medical examination. Dr. W. W. Potter confirmed the claim of total disability although he confused right with left: he described Hawkins's various wounds but flipped them to the left side of the body. He noted the "perforation of left [right] great toe," the consequence of which, in combination with the thigh wound and dislocation of the femur, impaired "progressive locomotion + caus[ed] lameness." Potter added that the bullet that caused the thigh wound had remained embedded "near the hip joint." In Potter's estimation, the thigh wound coupled with the dislocation and lameness constituted Hawkins's chief justification for the total disability rating. "These two examinations won Hawkins a pension increase to eight dollars per month, to be sent to him via his place of work, the Internal Revenue Office." This first increase in pension amount, however, proved insufficient. By the summer, Hawkins had filed new paperwork and was awarded a monthly pension of eighteen dollars,[37] effective from November 14, 1868.[38]

Hawkins would not have been alone among disabled veterans in feeling emasculated by his condition. Many of the same writers who lauded the black soldier in the African American press "avoid[ed] referencing the disabled black body immediately following the war." Worse, disabled black bodies became a subject of parody on "racially pejorative sheet music." Hawkins likely would have avoided the taint of passivity and emasculation of his wounded condition by working: he continued as a government messenger until his death.[39]

MEDAL OF HONOR

The first years of Reconstruction and the creation of the Freedmen's Bureau presented circumstances that supported the expansion of black middle-class families. Black veterans justifiably developed self-confidence and pride, which mirrored in their communities' expectations of their leadership. A Freedmen's Bureau employee observed that "no negro who has ever been a soldier can be again imposed upon; they have learnt what it is to be free and they will infuse their feelings into others." Although black veterans were more likely to be unemployed than their white counterparts, they provided more capital in their communities than other black workers. As veterans combined their political will via the Grand Army of the Republic, black veterans tried to keep their wartime service in the public eye despite the emerging national narrative—the Lost Cause myth—that denied recognition of their service. From the late 1800s well into the next century, competing memories of how the war should be defined created a "contest over who exercised the power to make some historical narratives possible and to silence others."[40]

Hawkins must have wondered why he had not received the Medal of Honor for his participation in the same event and activity that earned the award for his comrades. Soon after the war, he appealed to Major General Joseph B. Kiddoo, who submitted a nomination to the War Department on his behalf. Kiddoo had been a colonel of black troops who participated in the New

Market Heights battle and knew of Hawkins's eligibility. On February 8, 1870, Hawkins was awarded the Medal of Honor, receiving vindication that his continued suffering was worth the sacrifice. His manhood should now be unassailable by both black and white people.

Hawkins died eight days after receiving his medal. The attending physician certified that he died "of Phthisis Pulmonalis [tuberculosis or consumption][41] and in his opinion [Hawkins's] disease was the result of the combined effect of gunshot injuries and exposures in the field."[42]

Hawkins's civic death was followed by a predictable sequence of documents pertaining to his surviving pension body: pension claims by his widow and affidavits concerning the circumstances of his death. Julia was pregnant with her second child and swiftly applied for a widow's pension and a dependent's pension for her first son and the coming child. Edwin H. Grant, MD, presented a sworn statement that he had been acquainted with Hawkins for years, confirmed that Hawkins had been employed as a government messenger until death, and added:

> And I further certify that said Hawkins frequently conversed with me, knowing that I was a physician and formerly an assistant surgeon in the Army, relative to his health. He constantly complained of suffering from the wounds that he had received as a soldier during the late war, and was enfeebled by them, in my opinion, during the entire period of my acquaintance with him . . . I did not attend him as a physician during his last illness but I very well remember conversing with him about a week before he died and he then told me that his wounds were very painful and rendering him unfit to perform his duties as a messenger.[43]

Hawkins's pension applications and supporting documents address immobility and lack of functionality but not pain. Pain was present to a disabling degree, but its lack of specific and visible physical causes fell outside the scope of pension claims and ratings. The government physicians, constrained by pension laws, could not judge Hawkins's pain as relevant. They therefore conducted no tests to ascertain the presence or intensity of pain in specific parts of Hawkins's body. His pain remained an unpredictable private matter.

In 1870, the Hawkins household included Julia; Sarah Landre, her mother; Edward Landre, one of her three brothers; and Thomas V, her son. She wasted no time in completing and submitting the requisite paperwork to receive a pension that was awarded effective one day following her husband's death, eight dollars per month plus two dollars[44] for every dependent child (to be received until the child's sixteenth birthday). In August, Julia gave birth to William H., her second son, delivered by Dr. Augusta, who provided a sworn statement to the effect. William died the following spring.[45]

Julia was punctilious in her correspondence with the pension office to retain her good standing and that of her son. As was the case with veterans, their surviving spouses also inhabited the shadow pension body of their husbands until they remarried or died. At Washington's First Presbyterian Church in 1874, Julia married Henry Fleetwood Grant of Washington, DC, a barber who was described in the census as mulatto. She and Grant had two children, and Julia took legal steps to assume guardianship of son Thomas V., paying a $300 bond to ensure performance of guardianship. The record does not indicate why she took this step. It is possible that doing so ensured her son's legal standing for a pension. Julia notified the pension office of her new status, and her pension was immediately suspended, although she continued to receive the two-dollar pension for her son Thomas until he turned sixteen. Christian A. Fleetwood provided one of two sworn statements confirming the identities of Julia's children, the fatherhood of Thomas V., and his years-long acquaintance with the Hawkins family.[46]

In 1904, Julia's second husband, Henry F. Grant, died of heart disease at age sixty, his death certificate listing his occupation as music teacher. Years later, Julia decided to reactivate her pension as Hawkins's widow. Her correspondence with the pension office guided her reapplication with proper notarization. Just as the pension authorities required a thorough documentary history of Prestley Dorsey/Dawson's marriages from his claimant second wife, Janey, the pension office requested similar data from Julia. Subsequent paperwork required the pension office to gather all of Hawkins's military and medical records for review, including the documentation of his four bullet wounds and associated circumstances.

Julia's documents indicate that her two other brothers, Charles and William, also came to live with her, along with her mother, after Grant's death. E. D. Willison, MD, the family doctor in 1917, and the family's pastor, Francis J. Grimké, both District of Columbia residents, attested to Julia's two marriages and their issue and her eligibility for a pension.[47]

Julia received a monthly pension of twelve dollars[48] effective in late 1916. She died in Washington in June 1919. By the time she had applied for the resumption of her pension, Thomas R. Hawkins's civic body was disappearing from public view. A portion of his pension record had been destroyed by a fire in the Washington office, requiring an auditor from the interior department to approve the pension.[49]

CONCLUSION: FULLY RECOGNIZED AS EQUALS

Hawkins might have experienced nervous shock or neurasthenia to a degree that left him damaged but functional. If doctors had noticed these conditions, they could have diagnosed insanity and ordered that Hawkins be placed in an asylum. He endured prolonged depressive states, periods of memory loss, atypically nervous responses to loud noises, and insomnia. Just as doctors could not rate the existence of pain for pension purposes, they were suspicious of these symptoms. Asylum managers were also skeptical about such symptoms because the war "did not even have the potential to affect the sanity of Billy Yank." A recent study has shown that Civil War soldiers' most traumatic stimuli included "intimate violence" and the "exposure of war atrocities." The study considered many "predictor variables" including family history, past trauma, economic background, evidence of postwar disease, and age at death. Each veteran in the study had at least one physical examination for pension purposes. Soldiers who were young at enlistment (Hawkins was twenty-three) appeared to be at higher risk for postwar medical issues and were especially "likely to receive diagnosis of cardiovascular disease, greater risk of showing comorbid physical and nervous diseases."[50]

Hawkins likely experienced recurring visions of the dead, eviscerated bodies of his comrades that led to feelings of isolation, even as he was surrounded by well-meaning friends and family who could never understand his thoughts and emotions. He may have, as many veterans did, transformed stories of personal trauma into entertaining adventures to tell children or retell them infused with patriotic purpose to conform with the structure of romantic tales of heroism. Nevertheless, in private, he was constantly aware of his scars and dislocated bones, revisiting painful moments or affirming the miracle of healing, marveling at how time reshapes human bodies. This meditation on his body extended to empathy with the suffering of his comrades in an increasingly distant war. In the privacy of his home, Hawkins could still hold communion with the Sixth.

The Sixth mustered out in Philadelphia months after the war ended in 1865. Living in Philadelphia at the time, Hawkins likely joined them for a farewell. Soldiers would have exchanged handshakes and good wishes. The white officers held their own farewell dinner and over glasses of port toasted the black men they led, none of whom would have been present. The conversation among them led to a written resolution of their collective views and praise of their soldiers:

> 1. Resolved, that, in our intercourse with [black soldiers] during the past two years, they have shown themselves to be brave, reliable, and efficient as soldiers; patient to endure, and prompt to execute.
> 2. That, being satisfied with their conduct in the high position of soldiers of the United States, we see no reason why they should not be fully recognized as equals, honorable and responsible citizens of the same.[51]

However Hawkins appraised his suffering body, his service to the Union, and his dedication to his family, one artifact of his military service—his signature—reveals an unfulfilled ambition. Although his reading ability was sufficient for him to function as a sergeant major, his penmanship did not indicate a formal education. Hawkins's signature on official documents is striking because it shows not a trained and habituated hand but a slow, unsteady, and unsure movement. Each letter was formed with deliberation and care as if the appearance of his signature was a vital statement on his character. During his campfire conversations with Christian Fleetwood, he confessed to a longing for a formal education. Fleetwood wrote that Hawkins "proved himself a prompt capable and efficient officer, though suffering a little, as he frequently expressed with great regret, under the disadvantages of a neglected education, which he could not but feel in the duties of his position." Lamenting young Hawkins's death, Fleetwood acknowledged his "remarkable ability and talent, the exercise of which was hampered by his imperfect education."[52]

NINE

HENRY SHIPPEN HUIDEKOPER
(1839–1918)

FIRST DAY

On June 30, 1863, Henry Shippen Huidekoper, lieutenant colonel of the 150th Pennsylvania Volunteer Infantry, had a premonition that he would be wounded in the next fight. He told the commanding officer, Colonel Langhorne Wister, and the next senior officer, Major Thomas Chamberlin, that all three of them would be wounded by gunfire. Huidekoper asked the regimental surgeon to make him a tourniquet to keep with him on the battlefield for the inevitable wound. "I expected to lose a leg or an arm and I hoped it would be a leg," Huidekoper recalled later.[1]

The 150th had been on the march north from Virginia for several weeks. Once the regiment was on home ground, soldiers were eager to confront Robert E. Lee's forces. On the morning of July 1, Huidekoper and his comrades awoke to the sound of distant guns. As the soldiers rolled up their blankets and refilled their canteens, a short rain shower left the air "sultry beyond measure," causing the soldiers to perspire heavily as they moved about in their woolen uniforms. Huidekoper breakfasted on a cup of coffee and a piece of hardtack because the supply wagons had not yet arrived. There was little or no breakfast.[2]

Soon, with the sounds of cannon fire still in the distance, the regiment resumed its march toward the crossroads town of Gettysburg. Despite the air of urgency and tension, Huidekoper admired the "long stretches of golden grain and luxuriant growths of corn [that] looked beautiful in the sunlight." He quickly returned to vigilance when a messenger rode up and asked the regiment to move up the road at the double quick, an army command to run in formation. As he headed toward the sound of battle, Huidekoper passed fleeing townspeople and farmers driving cattle. He stared at a little girl and boy riding to safety on the family horse, both children crying.[3]

Huidekoper and his troops stopped briefly in the shadow of the Lutheran seminary on a ridge west of the town where General Abner Doubleday, the new division commander for the past two hours, spoke to the soldiers, "reminding them that they were upon their own soil, that the eye of the commonwealth was upon them, and that there was every reason to believe they would do their duty to the uttermost in defence of their State." Huidekoper learned from several officers hurrying about that their former division commander, the highly regarded General John Reynolds, was dead, felled by a rebel bullet to his head just a few hours earlier. Colonel Wister ordered the men to unsling and stack their knapsacks and, "with colors unfurled and full battalion front, the 150th moved rapidly westward," to take up position at McPherson's farm just east of a wood occupied by another brigade. The farm was bounded by a fence fronting the north and extending to the east before turning ninety degrees at Chambersburg Turnpike to front east, toward Seminary Ridge.[4]

At the McPherson farm, the 150th created a line of soldiers behind the fence facing north, while the other two regiments in Huidekoper's brigade, the 143rd and 149th Pennsylvania, faced east along the fence bordering the turnpike and waited. In their "eagerness for the fray, some of the men indulged in hilarious exclamations which would have sounded strangely enough an hour or two later." Huidekoper and Chamberlin surveyed their troops and in the apparent lull began talking together when an elderly man approached, "tall and bony," carrying a rifle, and dressed in "a blue swallow-tail coat, with brass buttons, dark trousers and a high hat, from which the nap had long since disappeared." He asked the officers, "Can I fight with your regiment?" Before Huidekoper or Chamberlin could answer, Colonel Wister strode up and demanded impatiently, "Well, old man, what do you want?" "I want a chance to fight with your regiment," the volunteer answered. "You do? Well, where is your ammunition?" "Right here," the man replied and slapped his pocket bulging with cartridges. "Good, I wish there were more like you." Wister told him to join the adjacent regiment in the woods. The civilian, John Burns, a veteran of the War of 1812, fought throughout the day. Although wounded, he survived to become a local celebrity after the battle.[5]

Shortly after 1:00 p.m., Huidekoper saw the approach of the huge Confederate army and noticed how they were deploying themselves for battle. His line of soldiers and that of the adjacent regiments appeared skeletal compared with this fully fleshed, mobile mass. To Huidekoper's eyes, the rebel army, which extended as far as he could see, presented "a beautiful spectacle" that did not panic his soldiers because they were confident that Union reinforcements were on the way. Suddenly, rebel cannon fire pounded the brigade. Some of the troops facing east hurried to join their fellows facing north as their rifle fire slowed the double line of Confederate battalions advancing obliquely to Huidekoper's line. Additional rebel cannons had come into action, pummeling the east-facing troops. A rebel force, concealed in the deep railroad cut to the east, suddenly rose into view and attacked the line of 149th soldiers, taking their regimental colors. Seeing this, Colonel Wister immediately drew his sword, climbed over the fence, and ordered his soldiers to follow him. His sudden attack drove back the rebel soldiers and recovered the colors.[6]

Casualties in Huidekoper's brigade mounted quickly. Brigade commander Colonel Roy Stone was shot in the hip and arm and was moved to the McPherson barn, now an aid station. Wister took brigade command until a bullet through his mouth forced him to relinquish it to Colonel Edmund L. Dana of the 143rd. Huidekoper now commanded the 150th. Rebel troops pressed hard on the brigade, and Huidekoper ordered a "change of front" to meet the challenge, a military movement executed with skill and promptness. Virtually all the other officers in the field had either been wounded or killed when Huidekoper was shot in his leg by a rifle.[7] "I dropped to the ground and I felt as if my whole leg was gone. But it wasn't." The bullet had nicked the bone but exited the body. Huidekoper took stock of his wound, determined that it was not disabling, rose, and continued to direct his soldiers. He saw his friend, Major Chamberlin, fall and remain on the ground. The commander of an adjacent regiment, the 116th Pennsylvania, St. Clair Mulholland, later recalled, "Never in the history of wars did men stand up under like conditions and make such a defence. There they were, one thin line, without a man in reserve, meeting charge after charge, and seeing beyond, as far as the eye could reach, other lines of fresh troops, ready to take the places of those repulsed. Every field officer in the brigade, save one, was shot, and many of them several times."[8]

For the next two hours, the diminishing Union brigade continued to exchange volley after volley of gunfire with the rebels, who "drew closer and closer, firing and loading as [they] advanced, but [were] met by a resistance which time and again staggered [them], though it could not shake [them] off." The expected reinforcements never materialized. Gradually, the men of the 150th moved back, overwhelmed by the oppressive enemy tide. To raise his soldiers' spirits, Huidekoper ordered Sergeant John Peiffer, "a man of large stature and boundless courage," to advance with the colors. Under "galling fire," he did so, and the regiment followed. After Peiffer was shot dead, another soldier, already wounded, recovered the colors. Shells from the rebel batteries continued to rip through Union lines but with more intensity than earlier. A moment after Peiffer fell, Huidekoper "felt his right arm shattered by another missile, and was forced to visit the barn to obtain aid in bandaging his wounds." Desperate to return to the fence line, he drew his tourniquet from his pocket and wrapped it around his upper arm, the surgeon being engaged with other injured men. He tried to avoid looking at the shreds of bloody tissue and bone that dangled from what remained of his elbow. Once his tourniquet was applied and his arm bandaged, Huidekoper hurried outside to resume command in time to see the adjutant shot through the shoulder.[9]

In pain and experiencing shock, Huidekoper was driven by duty to keep directing his soldiers. He felt moments of faintness coupled with fatigue. His senses were distorted due to intermittent semiconsciousness. His bandage had become a purple-red bulge on his sleeve, and the skin above the tourniquet swelled with increasing sensitivity and pain. About a half hour after he returned to the firing line, a reserve force finally arrived, and he was able to leave his position. By this time, about half of his regiment had fallen. At about four o'clock, Huidekoper turned to the east and walked uphill to the seminary where Union troops were preparing a firing line. His mouth was parched, his uniform saturated with sweat, and the haze of smoke from rifle and cannon fire made him hoarse in gasping for breath. Just as he began his journey to the field hospital in town over a mile away, his brigade was given the order to withdraw to the seminary grounds.[10]

Although dazed and disoriented, Huidekoper remained on the ridge to help Colonel Wister organize the retreating soldiers, "although prevented by the lacerated and swollen condition of his mouth and face from again taking active command, [Wister] had remained on the field, doing what he could by his presence and example to animate the men." Weakening, Huidekoper continued his progress to the makeshift division field hospital at Saint Francis Xavier's Catholic Church on West High Street. He was amazed to find that he could make his way into the town unmolested. In the regiment's retreat from Seminary Ridge to Cemetery Ridge just south of town, the bearer of the 150th regimental colors had stopped to rest, and the rebels had made off with the flag. Confederate troops walked along streets, as dazed or confused Union soldiers departed. Dead and wounded bodies were everywhere. Huidekoper arrived at the church at around 5:00 p.m. and saw one of the two regimental surgeons and his assistants attending to a wounded soldier on a makeshift operating table on the church porch. A hospital orderly directed Huidekoper to wait inside, so he entered the opened doors and found an unoccupied pew. He sat down, removed his belt with scabbard and pistol, and "asked some men to tear the pew-door off its hinges and place it crosswise on the back and front of the pew. On this [he] placed [his] swollen arm and got some relief from the intense pain, then called for some whiskey and got and swallowed the largest drink [he] ever took in [his] life."[11]

After about an hour, an orderly called for him. Dr. Philip A. Quinan examined Huidekoper's arm and saw that the bullet had passed across the widening of the humerus at the elbow, from the medial to the lateral epicondyles. The knot of ligaments connecting the humerus to the ulna and radius—the forearm—was shredded by the blow. Huidekoper thus lost most of the control over his forearm. The tourniquet might have saved his life because the supporting muscles were also torn and the brachial artery almost severed. His elbow was beyond repair; amputation was the only remedy. Huidekoper later recounted: "I went to the [operating] table and got onto it with my head toward the west. I took some chloroform but not enough, for I distinctly remember having said, 'Oh, don't saw the bone until I have had more chloroform.' What I next remember was my saying, 'You took my arm off, did you, Doctor . . . I thought you were only going to examine and dress it; well, when we next march through Maryland, I will have to salute with my left hand.'"[12]

During Huidekoper's surgery, frantic, battle-mad rebels entered the church and inspected the wounded. Some hovered around Huidekoper to observe the surgery. The rebels inside ordered those soldiers with apparently mild wounds to leave the church and line up in the street. They were told to relinquish their shoes and, as prisoners, laden with captured weapons, they marched to the Confederate rear. After his surgery, Huidekoper arose unaided and walked back into the church, looking for a place to rest. The number of soldiers recuperating within now exceeded perhaps a few hundred. Finding no space for himself, Huidekoper ascended the stairs to the gallery, spied a nook near the organ, and lay down there, his head to the west. As evening came on, he fell asleep but awoke intermittently throughout the night: "The night was a horrible one. All night long I heard from downstairs moans, groans, shrieks, and yells from the wounded and suffering soldiers."[13]

KICK HIM DOWNSTAIRS

The next day, Confederate lieutenant general Richard S. Ewell and several staff officers entered the church. They ascended to the cupola for a broad view of the battle, except for Ewell, who had only one leg and thus remained in the gallery sitting on a bench. The officers occasionally called down to Ewell, who responded with questions. He evidently ignored the Union wounded. Huidekoper, who lay only feet away from the general, studied his Confederate enemy, noting "the gorgeous gold lace which adorned the sleeves, collar, and front of his gray coat." As Huidekoper languished in the church on July 2, he saw Catholic nuns, the Daughters of the Charity of Saint Vincent de Paul from nearby Emmitsburg, Maryland, who had come to help. Distinctive in their black robes and elaborate white cornettes, their "charitable and valued work" could not have been more needed. "Oh how tender and welcome were their services to the poor suffering boys, to whom a gentle hand was everything in their wretchedness!" Meanwhile, gun and cannon fire were everywhere, and Huidekoper wondered how his regiment had fared. Still in progress, the battle's outcome remained unpredictable. He was a Confederate prisoner. Whatever worry he experienced over medical attention—his amputation not being "complete"; that is, suppuration of the amputation site necessitating changes of bandages—was somewhat eased by neighborhood women acting as nurses and the Catholic sisters proving themselves a priceless boon. Once again, soldiers, feminized in their dependency, were rescued by women.[14]

Sometime during the day, two young women made their way among the wounded in the church and approached Huidekoper. One asked, "Are you badly wounded? Can we do anything for you?" In response, he opened his blanket to reveal his amputation and said, "I have had nothing to eat since daylight yesterday and I do want a bite." The women left but returned minutes later. The older of the two who spoke, Elizabeth Salome "Sally" Meyers, a schoolteacher on summer vacation whose parents lived a few houses west of the church, brought Huidekoper "a glass of homemade wine and one cracker, which [she] had to carry under her shawl lest she might encounter some hungry rebel." Later during the day, Meyers and the other woman helped him get up and walk the short distance to the Meyer house, where he was taken to a room with a bed. To Huidekoper's surprise, Major Chamberlin, twice wounded by bullets but alive, occupied the other bed.[15]

Huidekoper and Chamberlin recuperated in the Meyers's home until July 9. They wondered at the lull in fighting during the morning of July 3, but shortly after noon, hundreds of cannons on both sides opened fire as a prelude to Lee's final attempt to break the Union line. Huidekoper and Chamberlin must have speculated on what was happening, learning that a charge of thousands of Confederates across over a mile of open field was in progress. By July 4, all was quiet until some neighbors called out that the rebels were leaving. Aware that Union doctors and their stewards and orderlies were attending to the wounded with very limited resources, Huidekoper decided to obtain civilian medical help to care for his and his companion's wounds. He asked his volunteer nurses to find a civilian doctor in town and summon him with the promise of pay. The doctor soon appeared and visited the two men for the final four or five days of their stay. After the doctor finished, "he asked me for $20.00 for what he did, and opening my pocket-book with one hand I handed him the money. Major Chamberlin . . . exclaim[ed], 'Why don't you kick him down stairs?'"[16]

During his days of confinement in Gettysburg, Huidekoper assessed his military behavior and the loss of his arm to reaffirm his motivations for participating in a war to save his country. Huidekoper did not believe that his injury and amputation signified the end of his career. As a student at Harvard University, he had read books on military tactics and organized a company of students to drill in anticipation of military service. He could not recall a time when he did not shape his future in terms of bodily sacrifice to his country. Also, he could not recall a time when he did not have abolitionist views. As a child, his grandfather had taken him by the hand and walked to the road to witness an exodus of exhausted black families traveling to Canada to escape enslavement. "I not then knowing why he pressed silver money into the hands of these refugees, and thus showed them that the whole world was not against them."[17]

Huidekoper's military fervor accelerated when he was an undergraduate at Harvard as the secession crisis intensified. During the election campaign of 1860, after reading Lincoln's "house divided" speech, he said to his brother Frederic that until that moment he had not heard of Abraham Lincoln, "but that there was in his words just what the North had been yearning for, and that the speech would make him the next President of the United States. The doctrine he taught—Lincoln's *first* mission, as it were—that a 'house divided against itself could not stand, and that this government could not exist with one-half slave and the other half free, that it would become all slave or all free'—touched a responsive chord in every patriotic heart," especially his own.[18]

Military circumstances introduced Huidekoper to Abraham Lincoln in the fall of 1862. Huidekoper detached a company of 150th soldiers to Lincoln's summer residence, the Soldier's Home. Lincoln became so fond of these men that he employed them as his special White House guard for most of the war. Huidekoper later wrote that his own "youthfulness and small stature must have struck the good man" because Lincoln remarked that he expected a tall, corpulent commander. Then Lincoln turned serious and commented on Huidekoper's Dutch background: "Mr. Lincoln laid his huge hand on my shoulder, and, in the most serious manner, said, 'Will you answer me a question which I asked the captain, and which he said *he* could not answer?' I replied in some cautious way, and he then said, 'When the captain told me about your family and its Dutch origin, I asked where the difference lay between an *Amster*-dam Dutchman and any other damn Dutchman?' It was thus I first met the greatest man of the age."[19]

Huidekoper became friends with Lincoln and visited him often when the regiment was quartered in Washington.

When Huidekoper was well enough to leave the Meyers home, he found the town suffused with an intensifying stench of rotting animal and human corpses in the summer heat. Thousands of casualties received treatment at both makeshift hospitals and large medical compounds with tents to protect operating theaters and recovering soldiers. Burial details of soldiers and civilians were omnipresent. He was proud that in the events leading to his amputation and after, he never lost the ability to walk on his own. On July 10, he walked several blocks to the Continental Hotel where

Dr. Hunt rebandaged his arm, and then he boarded a train to Baltimore and a military hospital. At the depot, Huidekoper and Chamberlin boarded a freight car that had transported ice to Gettysburg. In the car, they were forced to lie "on the damp floor with little straw under us and suffered much from the jolting during the twelve hours to Baltimore over a wretched roadbed." They were accompanied by Brigadier General Joshua T. Owens, whose medical problem was "a severe attack of rheumatism." During the long and unpleasant train trip, Owens "sat on the head of a barrel and entertained us by telling us funny stories until we laughed ourselves sore."[20]

After a period of hospitalization in Baltimore, Huidekoper went to Philadelphia at the end of July where he obtained a medical certificate in which the physician, following a careful examination, stated that Huidekoper's arm was amputated "and in consequence thereof, he is in my opinion, unfit for duty." The doctor stated further that the colonel would not be able to resume his duties in under twenty days. Huidekoper forwarded the certificate with a letter to the adjutant general of the army in Washington, saying, "Particularly desirous of returning to my regiment, I ask further indulgence of time." Leaving Philadelphia, Huidekoper went home to Meadville, Pennsylvania, to recuperate further. By mid-August, his medical leave had expired, and Huidekoper underwent another examination and was pronounced unfit for duty for another twenty days.[21]

After about three months of convalescence and medical exams, Huidekoper wanted to return to duty. In September, he decided to go to the War Department in Washington and request a light-duty assignment until he felt well enough to return to his regiment. Accordingly, he visited the one friend who might be able to help him. He called on President Lincoln, who asked what he could do for him. Huidekoper said that he hoped that the War Department would agree to his plan for light duty. Lincoln responded, "Oh, let me fix that" and wrote a request to the War

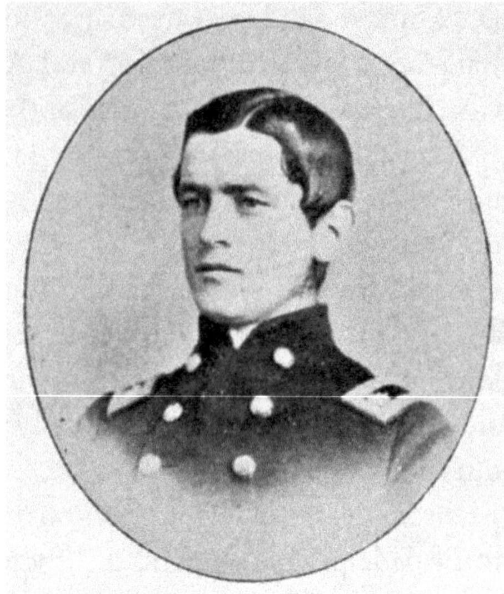

Lieutenant Colonel Henry S. Huidekoper, c. 1863. *Credit: Thomas Chamberlin,* History of the One Hundred and Fiftieth Regiment Pennsylvania Volunteers. *Philadelphia, PA, 1895.*

Department to grant Huidekoper any request. His request for light duty was approved. In October, he traveled to Philadelphia to an army depot for draftees, there "to receive conscripts assigned to his regiment" and take them to Virginia where the 150th was encamped.[22]

In mid-December, after further conscript duty, Huidekoper returned to the 150th with his "empty sleeve pinned across his breast . . . a pleasurable event to his immediate command and to his many friends." With new conscripts in the ranks, Huidekoper returned to maintaining military discipline and appearance within the ranks. "He had hardly reached the camp before he was in his 'working harness,' and when Sunday dawned, an added polish to arms and accoutrements bore witness in advance to the thoroughness of his anticipated inspection, and to the desire of the men to maintain their old-time reputation."[23]

Perhaps Huidekoper expected too much of his body. In January 1864, he requested a ten-day leave of absence. The reason was not noted, but the unexpected leave might have been due to a slow recovery. Meanwhile, Colonel Wister retired, and Huidekoper was promoted to colonel and commander of the regiment in February. Because the regiment was under strength, per army regulations, however, he could not muster in as colonel and was forced to resign because his arm had not healed completely and was still quite painful. "The loss of his arm proved so serious a disability that, despite his devotion to the cause and his natural fondness for military things, he deemed it only the part of wisdom to return to civil life." On March 2, he submitted his resignation, "and three days later he took leave of the regiment, to the great regret not merely of his own command, but of the many officers . . . who recognized in him one of the ablest tacticians of his rank and one of the best disciplinarians in the army."[24]

PHANTOM MANHOOD

Historians have generalized about the post–Civil War adaptability of veterans. These generalizations characterize public perceptions of disabled soldiers as weak, lazy, morally vacant, and ill adapted to the business-oriented work ethic. Some historians have observed that military service weakened veterans' lives in ways that "hinder[ed] the development of manhood." The veteran could overcome these deficiencies by the "constant application of genius and energy," the sure method of achieving success and happiness. Perseverance in business and the pathway upward through visible echelons of financial success marked the Gilded Age visions of manhood. War veterans also maintained visibility as a political cohort through the Grand Army of the Republic despite the pressure of industrialization and the transmutation of the American worker into interchangeable economic units.[25]

Many historians have argued that veterans needed to maintain their status and visibility in American culture by reframing public notions of disability. For example, a popular Left-Handed Penmanship Competition attracted many amputee veterans who, through their essays, presented "the amputee as a man of action and self-control who has already illustrated his manliness through injury and recovery." The visible evidence of amputation proved privation and sacrifice in the national interest as if no other statement of manhood was necessary.[26]

Some veterans saw their visible disability of a lost limb as a rebirth of personal citizenship, an avenue for a renewed dynamic life. The soldiers profiled in this book did not think of themselves as underachievers whose soldierly experience encouraged lax moral habits. None of them retreated from public view or waved sentimental banners to elicit pity. All expected their due from the government and were especially aggressive in securing it when the government was unresponsive. None offered self-pitying pleas to doctors or government agents to secure pensions.

Veterans who had lost limbs occupied a subcategory of disabled veterans. One characteristic of this subcategory was the veteran's relationship to the severed limb. Some amputees worried about the continued existence of those limbs, attributing to them some peculiar agency or consciousness. Some referred to their missing limbs as "a lost family member or a departed and sadly mourned 'best friend.'" Among most amputees, however, the lost limb continued to haunt the body as a phantom limb, a term coined by S. Weir Mitchell. Huidekoper adjusted to the challenges of living with one physical arm and one intangible and sometimes unpredictable arm. The manifestation of a lost limb brought about pain and frustration due to the inability to subdue or control it. Mitchell estimated that about 95 percent of amputees experienced the phantom sensation. He wrote, "A person in this condition is haunted . . . by a constant or inconstant fractional phantom of so much of himself as has been lopped away. . . . There is something almost tragical, something ghastly, in the notion of these thousands of spirit limbs haunting as many good soldiers."[27]

Amputee veterans who moved through life with a phantom limb threatened public order. Some people worried that these veterans could not be trusted. In an "appearance-driven American culture: were Civil War amputees who they appeared to be?" If their bodies had been physically reduced, were the veterans complete men? Were their identities altered? When Huidekoper returned to his regiment for duty, soldiers trusted him no less and paid him greater respect for his obvious sacrifice in a contest in which all participated. Enlisted soldiers were not permitted to return to the ranks following an amputation, but for officers, the loss of an arm was acceptable. Esteemed as gentlemen in civil society, officer amputees were accorded a social exemption not available to other disabled men. An officer who lost a hand, arm, or part of a leg or a foot was still socially accepted. Partial amputations or disfigurement, especially of the face, however, resulted in a deformity that meant social ostracism. Deformity had no honor in appearance and disrupted social conformity more than a cleanly severed limb.[28]

Huidekoper's appearance elicited different reactions among those he encountered in civil life. His phantom sensations were not constant: they diminished, disappeared, or altered in configuration or location in the body. Pension examiners had no way to categorize this bodily misbehavior, much less award it a pension value. Only Mitchell recognized the phenomenon as a distinct pain response of his body, not measurable but activated by electrization. He marveled, "How remarkable must be the sense of the existence of the part lost is to be gathered from the fact that even after twenty or thirty years men are sometimes deceived by this sensation into acts which are founded on a moment of deception as to the real presence of the limb." Mitchell noted that phantom limb sufferers reassessed their self-image daily. One of his patients said, "Every morning I have to learn anew that my leg is enriching a Virginia wheat crop or ornamenting some horrible museum."[29]

GEORGE DEDLOW, MD, AND HIS PHANTOM LIMBS

Not only soldiers but physicians were wounded by gunfire, and some became their own experiments in phantom limbs and associated pain. At the end of his first year of study at Philadelphia's Jefferson Medical College, George Dedlow became an assistant surgeon in the Seventy-Ninth Indiana Volunteers and was posted along the Cumberland River near Nashville, Tennessee. Sent alone to obtain supplies through hostile territory, Dedlow was ambushed, shot in the right arm, and captured. When Dedlow regained consciousness, he explored the condition of his right hand with his left. The bullet had passed through the biceps and right arm and exited below the shoulder. Shortly after being wounded, his "right hand and forearm were cold and perfectly insensible." As the Confederates placed him in a cart and took him away, a burning pain developed in his right arm and gradually intensified. "The pain became absolutely unendurable." By the time he saw a surgeon, Dedlow was desperate to do anything to stop the pain. The surgeon ordered the amputation of the arm, which was performed without anesthesia because the rebels had exhausted their supply. The pain of the operation was less than that of the burning sensation of the impaired nerves. "I made no more of losing the limb than of parting with a tooth on account of toothache." Once Dedlow's arm had been removed from the shoulder joint, the burning sensation vanished. Dedlow turned his head, saw his detached arm, and thought, "There is the pain, and here am I."[30]

Later, Dedlow participated in an exchange of prisoners. Once he recovered his health, he returned to his regiment, this time at the 1863 battle of Chickamauga in Tennessee. His regiment advanced under fire when, suddenly, rebels began firing at the soldiers from the left. Dedlow felt a "horrible shock," which knocked him unconscious. He awoke in a makeshift field hospital in the open under a tree and learned that he had been shot in both thighs and that shell fragments had lacerated his legs beyond repair. A flying projectile had torn the flesh of his remaining arm. Orderlies carried Dedlow to the operating table where chloroform was administered. He came to a tent and felt an itch in his left leg. Unable to reach it with his remaining hand, he asked an orderly to scratch his left calf. The attendant replied that Dedlow no longer had legs and then removed the blanket to reveal the remaining stumps. Both legs had been removed at the upper third of the femur. Dedlow was transferred to a Nashville hospital to recuperate.[31]

But Dedlow's anguish was far from over. An outbreak of gangrene ravaged the hospital wards, and the disease took hold in Dedlow's still-suppurating left arm. "The usual remedy, bromine, was used locally, but the main artery opened, was tied, bled again and again, and at last, as a final resort, the remaining arm was amputated at the shoulder joint." To his surprise, Dedlow recovered from this surgery only to find "himself a useless torso, more like some strange larval creature than anything of human shape." At an army hospital in Philadelphia, Dedlow had time to study other patients and their responses to lost limbs. He continued to feel painful phantom sensations and considered their cause. "When the part is cut off, the nerve-trunks which led to it and from it, remaining capable of being impressed by irritation, are made to convey to the brain from the stump impressions which are as usual referred by the brain to the lost parts, to which these nerve-threads belonged. In other words, the nerve is like a bell-wire."[32]

Dedlow found that phantom sensations did not mimic the entire contour of the limb in question. "Where the leg, for instance, has been lost, they feel as if the foot was, but as though the leg were shortened. If the thigh has been taken off, there seems . . .

to be a foot at the knee; if the arm, a hand seems to be at the elbow, or attached to the stump itself." Dedlow suffered from causalgia, the burning sensation in the extremities, for which he received small injections of morphia. But among his fellow patients, Dedlow witnessed "the horrible variety of suffering," including a man who could walk only sideways or another with no sense of smell. Over time, Dedlow discovered that he was transforming into another kind of human: reduced of his four limbs, he ate and slept less and his heartbeat slowed. Even more strangely, he became "less conscious of [himself], of [his] own existence." "I felt like asking some one [*sic*] constantly if I were really George Dedlow or not." He reasoned that consciousness of self and identity diminished in proportion to his loss of physical self. "Thus one half of me was absent or functionally dead . . . I thus reached the conclusion that a man is not his brain, or any one part of it, but all of his economy, and that to lose any part must lessen this sense of his own existence."[33]

Written by Mitchell but published anonymously in the *Atlantic Monthly* the year after the war, Dedlow's first-person account so impressed readers that they sent gifts and money to the hospital identified in the story. The story, however, was fiction. George Dedlow did not exist. Mitchell had invented him and attributed to his body all the major nerve injuries of clinical interest. He derived Dedlow's wounds and symptoms of nerve damage from his own case notes. He wrote that the intent of publishing the fictional saga was to highlight the psychological aspects of limb loss and associated nerve phenomena. "By creating literary stories which paralleled but remained separate from his case histories, [Mitchell] delimited the boundaries of the space within which his critical interrogation of military medicine would take place." As such, the Dedlow story reveals Mitchell's conception of a male body—and anxieties about his own body in relation to the suffering he treated in others—in reflecting on the importance of bodily wholeness as a precondition to male identity.

Mitchell's choice of fiction to describe Dedlow and his afflictions constituted Mitchell's first published narrative of the phantom limb syndrome. By focusing on the psychology of limb loss, in the words of a suffering army assistant surgeon, "Mitchell gave visibility and voice to human pain, attempting to transcend its mastery of the body."[34]

Like Huidekoper, Dedlow shunned prostheses. The use of prosthetic limbs to render the body useful for manual labor presents an ambiguity. Such limbs have no nerves and hence no sensation and therefore constitute bodily fakery. Many artists of the war era portrayed "maimed Civil War veterans as aberrant bodies." To many people, dismembered bodies represented a loss of personality, hence their suspicion and lack of trust in those afflicted. Mitchell conceived of the human body holistically: nerve impulses traveled throughout the body and intertwined with skin, muscle, bone, and brain, creating a wholeness of self. Mitchell's concern, as reflected in the story's theme, is the question: Can parts of a man be physically subtracted while he retains the essence of manly identity? As Dedlow said, "I have so little surety of being myself, that I doubt my own honesty in drawing my pension, and feel absolved from gratitude to those who are kind to a being who is uncertain of being enough himself to be conscientiously responsible." Did this concern occur to other amputees—Henry Kircher and Richard Dunphy? They—and Huidekoper—appear to have retained a resilient identity and sense of manhood despite their losses. If they thought that others saw them as feminized, it apparently did not matter. Huidekoper not only maintained his prominent pinned-up sleeve as public evidence of his loss; his display of his physically reduced body also perpetuated an ongoing Gettysburg battle. His amputation remained in the present tense.[35]

As Mitchell's projection of self, Dedlow is the protagonist of a story that has "horrifying open-endedness." Dedlow is skeptical of spiritualism but agrees to attend a séance at which a spiritual being communicates to the medium a combination of numbers and letters: "United States Army Medical Museum Nos. 3486, 3487." Skepticism set aside, Dedlow recognizes the accession numbers of his limbs in the collection of the Army Medical Museum in Washington, DC. At this recognition, the phantom legs resume their original place on Dedlow's body. He rises and walks a few steps, but the legs fade, and he sinks to the floor. The story ends with Dedlow's future unknown. "I am not a happy fraction of a man." As he awaits death, Dedlow is the ultimate feminized patient.[36]

Ironically, although Mitchell jokingly uses spiritualism as a way for Dedlow to acquire the sense of bodily wholeness through illusion, Mitchell's work shares certain similarities with a spiritualist movement of his time, mesmerism. The mesmerist and the subject (or patient) merge bodies in a sense and are thus "*en rapport* [as] they both became conductors of the magnetic fluid" characteristic of the essence of animal magnetism. The magnetic fluid is electricity, a process demonstrated by physician Franz Mesmer, who discovered the phenomenon of mesmerism. Especially relevant to Mitchell's work, some modes of electrization require a circuit connecting the electricity source, the patient, and the person administering treatment.[37]

Many public amputees exhibited "fraudulent body language" due to the contradiction between their appearance and self-image. Huidekoper's postwar career attested to Victorian America's expectations of male health, the vigorous, adaptable body with "a correspondingly strong spirit and providing that spirit with a vital means of material expression." If he had read the Dedlow story, he would have found his phantom limb pain described as he experienced it. The story also would have enriched his knowledge of and insight into the spectrum of pain responses of other amputees. The story, then, possibly informed his later advocacy for disabled veterans.[38]

TRUE REPUBLICAN PRINCIPLES

Within two months of his discharge, Huidekoper had contacted the pension office. By May 1864, the office sent him a questionnaire to establish baseline data and told him that his file contained no evidence of disability. Huidekoper lost no time in filing his claim for a pension with the requisite supporting documents: a surgeon's certificate attesting to the Gettysburg wound, a disability certificate, and confirmation of his service record from the adjutant general's office. Swiftly, the pension authorities granted his pension of thirty dollars[39] per month for "total disability." As with Dunphy and Kircher, pension authorities waived any requirement for Huidekoper to be subjected to a medical examination every other year. The lack of a forearm was apparently sufficient to approve a pension. The pension authorities mistakenly believed that there was no need to assess amputees every year, assuming that their bodies would remain static for the rest of their lives.[40]

Four months later, Huidekoper married Emma Gertrude Evans in Germantown, just outside of Philadelphia. In response to a pension office questionnaire about the date and place of his marriage, he mentioned the clergyman who solemnized the vows, the Reverend John Rodney. The marriage must have taken place at St. Luke's Church in Germantown where Rodney had served as rector since 1825. This new church had been organized in 1819 to promote "the doctrine, discipline, and worship" of Protestant Episcopalianism. It is unknown whether the decision to marry at St. Luke's was made by the husband, the wife, or both. If worship in this parish was important to Huidekoper, the surviving records of his life do not say. The details of his spiritual life are vague.[41]

The newlyweds moved to Meadville and settled into the family businesses. According to the census, Huidekoper's father, Edgar, had been a "land agent" and "land booker"—similar to a real estate broker—who died the year his son Henry went to war in 1862. Edgar had married a member of the local elite, Francis Shippen, whose surname indicated a genealogical connection with the upper ranks of Philadelphia powerbrokers. Both parents were prominent local citizens. At the beginning of the war, the Meadville household included Francis and siblings Henry, Frederic, Herman, Gertrude, Elizabeth, Rush, Frank, Edgar, one French seamstress, and three "domestics," one of whom was German. If the newlyweds made their first home in Meadville at the family mansion, Pomona, their first child, Gertrude, was born there in October 1865. Just weeks later, Henry and his brother Frederic, co-owners of a new business in a woolen mill, suffered a disaster. A fire broke out one night in November 1865, and "in less than a half hour the building was a sheet of flame" so intense that the firemen were forced to retreat. While no workers lost their lives, the business was a shambles with the loss of a building, stock, and "splendid machinery, which cannot promptly be replaced." Worse, as many as thirty families of employees were left homeless, the fire having extended to nearby homes. Henry and Frederic planned to rebuild.[42]

Huidekoper proudly displayed his pinned-up sleeve as he headed the household as oldest son and war veteran. Almost immediately after the war ended, he became politically involved with the Republican Party by organizing a constituency to petition a Mr. Pettis to run for Congress because of his "long and faithful services in behalf of true Republican principles." Huidekoper remained politically active for the rest of his life but never held office himself. His activism embraced lobbying for expanded pensions for veterans. He also waved a Gettysburg banner to ensure that public memory continued to celebrate and honor the sacrifices of soldiers like him whose bodies bore the scars from a battle now viewed as the high watermark and the beginning of the end of the Confederacy. His empty sleeve evoked

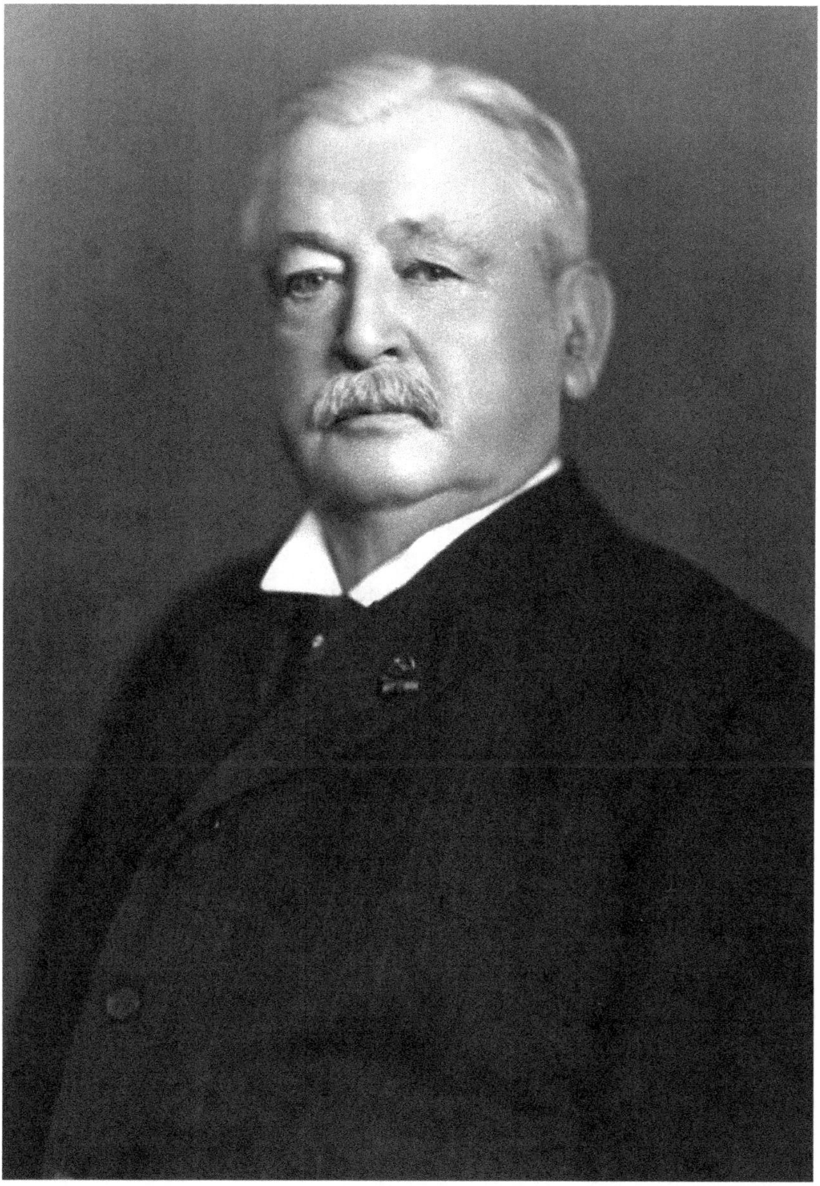

Henry S. Huidekoper, c. 1915. *Credit: Courtesy of the Union League Legacy Foundation, Philadelphia, PA.*

the memory of the war and its meaning, renewed constantly as a "Won Cause," as opposed to the growing Lost Cause ideology of the South, which, by 1900, had become the predominant national narrative about two honorable contestants, North and South, the former prevailing only because of superior numbers and industrial might, the South withdrawing into its distinctive culture. White veterans sidelined or dismissed their black brethren, and "states' rights" became the mantra of Southern politicians. The enslavement of millions became irrelevant to the causes of the war. Huidekoper and his fellow veterans—particularly those who returned from war minus limbs—"not only self-identified as the symbolic emblems of the war's consequences; they self-positioned themselves as the rightful referees of the war's causes."[43]

In the next decade, Huidekoper acquired a uniform and military responsibilities for the first time since the war. In 1870, he and his young family (with a son, Thomas Wallis, born the same year) continued to live in Meadville. Thirty-one-year-old Huidekoper identified himself as a "manufacturer" for the 1870 census and lived with his wife, daughter, son, nurse, housekeeper, and one domestic servant. The same year, the governor commissioned him major general in the National Guard of Pennsylvania. A few years later, he published a *Manual of Service* for the use of the guard.[44]

In July 1877, Pittsburgh witnessed a railway workers' strike that caused sufficient commotion, vandalism, and violence to warrant mobilization of the National Guard. Huidekoper's firm hand provided military order. He received high marks for his ability to negotiate and his reluctance to punish working people. Pittsburgh was most affected by the railroad strike, along with Scranton and Reading. Across the country, similar strikes and labor grievances erupted over reduced wages and increased work. Kircher's community in Illinois was similarly afflicted. Pittsburgh, however, achieved notoriety because of the casualties—at least sixty people killed—and millions of dollars in damage to railroads and locomotives. Many politicians recognized a link between the civil unrest and the Panic of 1873 and the consequent closure of businesses, loss of jobs, and reduced manufacturing. Further, troops arriving in Pittsburgh and many local police were sympathetic to the strikers and refused to suppress the crowds with force. The crux of the confrontation was a standoff between troops and citizens at which the soldiers fired into the crowd, killing and wounding dozens. Aside from organizing and deploying troops to guard facilities and railroad property, Huidekoper reputedly "went alone and in civilian's dress . . . and did much efficient work in putting down the disturbances, during which many attempts were made upon his life." Most of the praise for Huidekoper's handling of the civil disorder appeared in his obituaries.[45]

To promote his vision of Gettysburg's legacy, Huidekoper gave talks such as "Gettysburg" at the Society of Inquiry of the Meadville Theological School in 1873, for which he served as trustee from 1864 to 1908. Soon, he gained a wider platform. He moved his family to Philadelphia where his military and family business reputation secured him prestigious appointments. The 1880 census found him at forty-one, living with his wife, son, daughter, and two Irish immigrant women who were household servants. Appointed postmaster of Philadelphia, Huidekoper served in the role for five years, during which time he received credit for various administrative and managerial improvements. Of course, the job served as a social nexus, particularly among war veterans who occupied important government and business positions. He resigned his commission in the National Guard the following year.[46]

Philadelphians saw Huidekoper as a community leader, one who stood for the rights of veterans and kept alive the memory of the war. Veterans worried that a new generation of citizens had reached adulthood with no memory of the conflict. Their children would, of course, have no direct link to the sacrifices of their parents. Huidekoper collaborated with GAR. Ellis Post Number

6 to erect a statue to the Union veteran at the market square in Germantown, which still stands. A stone sentinel resting at arms surmounts a column fixed to a base of granite from the Devil's Den, a cluster of boulders at Gettysburg and the site of a fierce contest. Bronze plates on each side of the base remind the viewer of the essential facts. One side shows the GAR emblem and the motto "Fraternity, Charity, Loyalty" with an inscription by Byron, "They never fail who die in a great cause." Accompanying the arms of Pennsylvania on another side is the statement "Liberty without Obedience is Confusion, and Obedience without Liberty is Slavery." The third panel displays the arms of the city, and the fourth shows the national emblem and the inscription "Liberty and Union, now and forever, one and inseparable." The overall construction towers at thirty feet and commands the attention of the square. A huge audience turned out for the July 4, 1883, dedication and parade led by General Huidekoper as marshal of the event. He represented the ideals and sentiments expressed by the monument. With other veterans present, many who bore the scars of battle, he looked on with pride as his body with the pinned-up sleeve presented a living monument—a soldier effigy—to correspond with the ageless bronze and granite public aide memoire to recall the war's sacrifices.[47]

If an ex-Union officer of the Civil War wanted to socialize with other like-minded veterans in Philadelphia who held Republican ideals, two organizations in the city met that need and provided a venue where healed wounds and amputation stumps were regarded as living saints' relics: the Union League and the Military Order of the Loyal Legion of the United States (MOLLUS), both of which are still thriving today. Founded in 1862, the Union League aimed to support the Union and President Lincoln's prosecution of the war. Similarly, MOLLUS was founded on the day of Lincoln's assassination by Philadelphia Union army officers to defend against threats of conspiracy to overthrow the national government, to aid widows and children of members,

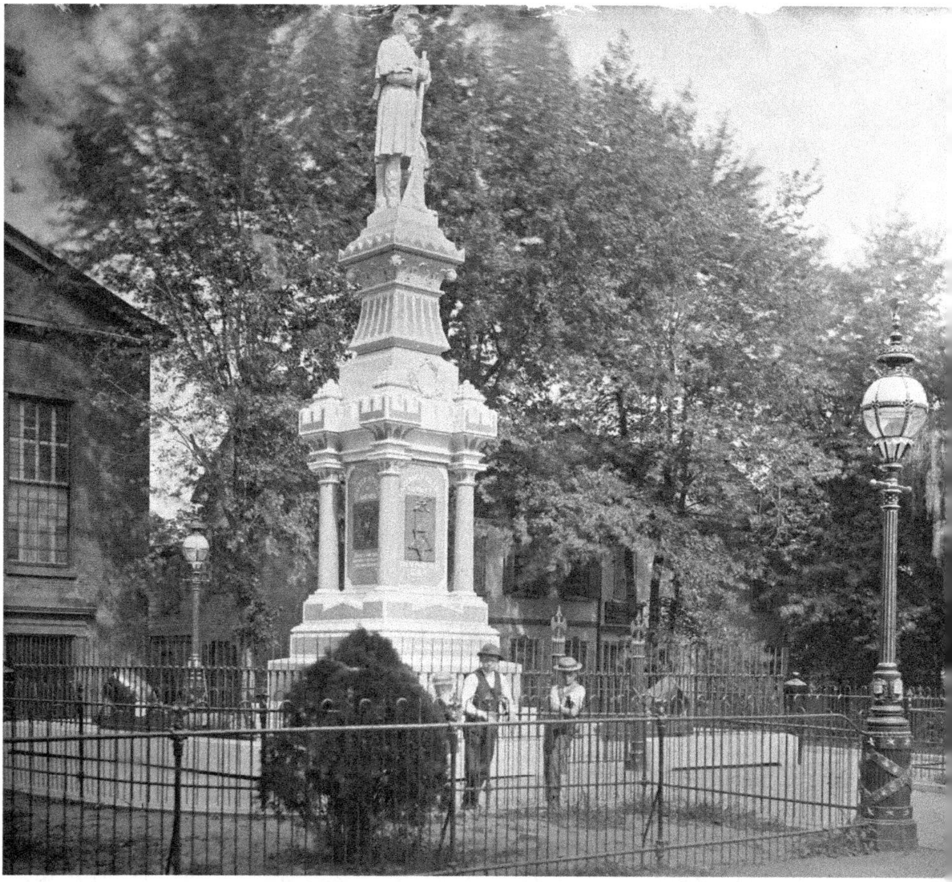

Civil War soldiers' monument, Germantown, PA, erected 1883.
Photograph taken by Marriott Canby Morris same year.
Credit: Library Company of Philadelphia.

and to promote camaraderie among veterans. Several founding members of both organizations were alive and active when Huidekoper came to Philadelphia. In 1883, Huidekoper became a Companion of the First Class (a title reserved for those who had fought in the Civil War).[48]

These organizations and the GAR rallied to Huidekoper's aid when President Grover Cleveland replaced him as postmaster in

1885 at his patronage's discretion. Meade Post Number 1, GAR in Philadelphia, organized a protest that included a formal petition to Cleveland presented by a retired general. The petition argued that Huidekoper was removed without just cause and offered arguments about the president's public vow to support veterans when they perform their offices honestly and competently. The final argument asked the president to consider "whether the removal of our comrade without charges or cause in opposition to an almost unanimous business or non-partisan sentiment and in the midst of great usefulness is not detrimental to the public service." Cleveland's appointment prevailed. The issue remained troublesome for veterans who felt that patronage appointments of their comrades should be honored above other considerations. Cleveland's replacement for Huidekoper was not a veteran.[49]

STUMP REDIVIVUS

Huidekoper's thirty-dollar monthly pension had remained fixed for decades since it was first awarded. In 1887, the pension office ordered a medical examination "to determine the point of amputation." According to the medical examination report, Huidekoper had requested a pension review due to a congressional act of August 4, 1886. The stated purpose of the examination concerned whether he could wear a prosthetic arm: the answer determined the three examiners' recommendation. At his examination, Huidekoper presented as "a healthy looking man" at age fifty-two, five feet eight inches tall, 145 pounds, normal temperature, pulse 72, heart and lungs normal. His right arm showed a stump nine inches long "from acromion"[50] and six inches from the middle of the axilla (armpit.) The accompanying diagram in the examiners' report showed that the amputation was made about two inches above the distal end of the humerus. Measuring nine inches in circumference, the stump displayed a healthy cicatrix and was "not adherent to bone." Although Huidekoper told the doctors that he sometimes wore a prosthesis for "dress occasions," doing so caused significant pain, so he removed it. Examination revealed a large neuroma[51] on the inside of the stump about an inch up, the size of a walnut and "quite sensitive to pressure and no doubt causes the pain alleged." The examiners recommended a pension increase to forty-five dollars[52] monthly, which the office promptly granted "for Ampu Right Arm near Shoulder Joint as to prevent use of artificial limb."[53]

In veterans' circles, particularly at the Union League and MOLLUS, the manifestation of physical deformities and loss of limbs became such a symbol of patriotic manhood that veterans often laughed at the absurd and potentially embarrassing social situations they were forced to negotiate. Huidekoper had become friendly with another amputee Union soldier, Pennsylvania state senator Francis A. Osbourn, also a MOLLUS member, whose left arm had been removed. Over several years, they developed the habit of sharing new pairs of gloves. "Whenever the general purchased a new pair, he invariably sent the right glove to the senator, and when the senator invested the general would get the left glove."[54]

At the same time, veterans throughout the country were commissioning monuments in large numbers for placement at Gettysburg and other battlefields, many of which supported sculpted or cast life-size soldiers. Even if these figures were presented in attitudes of fatigue or distress as if wounded or slain, they were unblemished, no limbs torn, no splints or bandages evident. Only in the latter twentieth century have new statues depicting Civil War soldiers shown evidence of bodily suffering as opposed to manly resolution. The wars of the twentieth century, most with unimaginable casualties, have been memorialized in the form of symbolic monoliths, effigies of soldiers whose expressions seem melancholic or fearful but resolute.

In 1887, Huidekoper took on his final professional role (1897–1913), in which he led the expansion of new communications technology as "Vice-President and General Manager of the Metropolitan Telephone and Telegraph Company." The company evolved as quickly as its technology, later becoming the Metropolitan Telephone & Telegraph Company, then the New York Telephone Company, and, finally, the American Bell Telephone Company, for which Huidekoper acted as agent. In this public role, he appeared before citizens' groups, institutional boards, and legislative committees, and not always in a friendly capacity. The demand for telephones outstripped the infrastructure that supported them, especially telephone exchanges. At this same time, Huidekoper's alma mater asked him to serve as an overseer, an honorific role he held until about 1910.[55]

By the end of the 1880s and into the 1890s, Huidekoper became more politically active in advocating for veterans' pensions and the memorialization of their wartime deeds. In 1890, he and others with the Maimed Soldiers' League in Washington, DC, met before the pension committees of both houses of Congress to argue for one-hundred-dollar monthly pensions to any soldier who lost hands, feet, the sight of one or both eyes, or any combination thereof, and increased pensions for sufferers of multiple disabilities. Veterans' claims and petitions frequently received a sympathetic hearing in Congress, but the public was not uniformly supportive. As veterans aged, their health needs increased, and soon the federal budget's largest expense was pensions.[56]

HIGHLY MERITORIOUS AND DESERVING

Gettysburg still drove Huidekoper's campaign to memorialize the battle and perpetuate its importance in the public memory. For the lifetime of veterans, the new monuments furnished a prop, a backdrop to their political activities and consciousness-raising about their physical sacrifices decades earlier. A committee of veterans from the North and the South labored to create a national military park by raising funds and securing national legislative authority. Thus began the reshaping of the battlefield to its 1860's appearance with key milestones inscribed on bronze plaques and placed along roads for tourists. In 1894, Huidekoper, likely an event organizer, gave a speech to veterans of his regiment at Gettysburg. The veterans walked around the battlefield and visited two monuments to their regiment, the original having been placed near McPherson's farm in 1888 and later moved to Cemetery Ridge (where the regiment fought on July 2–3, 1863). The larger monument with a relief sculpture showing a panoply of arms was placed near the farm in 1889. In 1899, Huidekoper presided at the dedication of a statue of Major General John Reynolds, whose death early in the Gettysburg battle emboldened the men of the 150th as they marched into combat.

As the principal speechmaker, Huidekoper emphasized the significance of Gettysburg, observing that from the moment of Lincoln's Gettysburg Address and the dedication of the national cemetery, "the world has set Gettysburg apart, above all other battlefields, in ancient or modern times, to represent patriotism, honor, bravery, and loyalty." At the event highlighted by music performed by the Carlisle Indian School Band and an artillery salute, a grandnephew of Reynolds unveiled the equestrian statue accompanied by retired generals reading tributes. Surveying the audience, Huidekoper quoted from Lincoln's address and added, "It seems fitting, as we meet here now, with renewal of the pledges of a comradeship cemented by the marches, battles, and prisons of four long years, that we should tell our sons now battling, as we did before them, but in foreign lands [the Philippines and Cuba], that a grateful country will thus, in due time, lay laurels and drop tears in remembrance of their glorious deeds." The loyal fight to preserve the Union and promote liberty remained in progress. The wounds of Civil War veterans remained fresh. Huidekoper probably presided in his National Guard general's uniform (with pinned-up sleeve) that he was authorized to wear on state occasions.[57]

On these occasions—dedications of monuments, parades, funerals—veterans marched in military order, their civilian clothes bedecked with GAR pins and medals and wearing military hats. The veteran needed to display not only his physical body but the corporate body as well. In these processions, despite the infirmities of aging, veterans evoked the self-image of uniformed soldiers marching home after a brutal campaign. In 1864, Walt Whitman observed a parade of battle-hardened soldiers returning from war. His description reflects that self-image: "It was a curious sight to see these ranks after rank . . . march by, worn and sunburnt and sweaty, with well-worn clothes and thin bundles, and knapsacks, tin cups, and some with frying pans strapt over their backs, all dirty and sweaty, nothing real neat about them except their muskets; but they were all as clean and bright as silver. . . . They are all so gay, too. Poor fellows, nothing dampens their spirits."[58]

In 1900, Huidekoper lived in Philadelphia with his wife, son (now an insurance agent), and two servants, both Irish immigrants. He continued his work as an agent for the telephone company and found a new way to perpetuate the memory of Gettysburg: he made and sold miniature versions of Gettysburg. After years of conducting extensive research into the Gettysburg battle and reading official reports and reminiscences by participants and interviewing veterans, he created a relief map of the town and environs that he sold with a booklet, the three-foot, eight-inch-by-two-foot, four-inch map designed for students or anyone with an interest, but especially for veterans. The advertisement published in veterans' periodicals stated that the relief map depicted the Gettysburg battle of 1863, "designed and modeled by Gen. H. S. Huidekoper from Data Furnished for the Purpose, by the Gettysburg National Park Commission." The advertising brochure featured endorsements by two Confederate and two Union generals, among others, and was favorably reviewed in several military-interest periodicals.[59]

The primary objective of the Spanish-American War (1898), like the Mexican War (1846–1848) a half-century earlier, was to establish a United States empire and compete with European empires, a goal that was not accepted by all Americans. Mindful that his country had committed troops abroad under the dubious premise of promoting democracy, Huidekoper took the conservative approach and supported his country's military drive to preeminence among nations. Many veterans from both the North and South viewed the new war as a final reconciliation of the two sides of the Civil War as officers from the older war helped to lead the new. Huidekoper, along with many veterans, disparaged the old European empires and was furious when Americans appeared to defer to them. He spoke on the matter at the Union League in response to reports that Americans had kissed the hand of the newly enthroned King Edward VII of England. Although the news was shown to be false, Huidekoper railed, "I have no use for such toadies . . . Americans inherit at birth a love of liberty and a spirit of democracy, both of which have no place in Great Britain. It makes my blood boil to hear that American citizens have gone over to England and made cheap flunkies of themselves. . . . This fawning over the King—this senseless servility to glittering royalty—is sickening absurdity." Huidekoper reminded listeners that during the Civil War, Britain supported the Confederacy.[60]

The speeches, dedications, and relief map gave Huidekoper a way to continuously renew public consciousness of the wartime sacrifice of a disappearing generation, but his own sacrificial limb required a new definition, one that would transcend his lifetime and perpetuate his wounding and amputation as an immortal act. Through his participation in Union League, MOLLUS, and GAR activities, Huidekoper stayed in contact with officers who had served at Gettysburg. In 1902, he asked them to nominate him for the Medal of Honor. Accordingly, Roy Stone, who commanded Huidekoper's brigade at Gettysburg, wrote to the War Department:

> Colonel Huidekoper, after his elbow joint was shattered (which resulted in an amputation) came into the McPherson barn, where I lay wounded, and had a rough tourniquet applied . . . and then, disregarding the danger to his life by further exertion, returned to his regiment, which was then without a field officer, and while the brigade was holding, as he then thought and as was afterward officially confirmed, the key of the position of the First Day. The battle continued all about the barn and I know that Colonel Huidekoper did return to his regiment and did further duty there until exhaustion compelled his retirement. I consider [his] action in this particular exception and highly meritorious, and deserving, even at this late day, of recognition by the Department, and to that end, I do hereby recommend that he shall be awarded a Medal of Honor.[61]

Major General Oliver O. Howard wrote a similar letter and endorsed the Medal of Honor request.[62]

While the medal correspondence was pending, Huidekoper decided to ask for a pension increase to fifty-five dollars[63] per month. A medical examiner endorsed the request because of the stump's "diseased condition as to prevent the use of an artificial limb." Presumably, the neuroma was still present, possibly even larger than at the last examination. The legal examiner agreed that the stump would not permit the use of a prosthesis. In a very short time, Huidekoper was granted the increase.[64]

Huidekoper achieved the increase before the secretary of war responded to the Medal of Honor nomination. Addressed to Major General Howard, the letter stated that the attorney general had agreed with the secretary that "a medal of honor cannot be awarded to a person not in the military service of the United States unless an application or recommendation for the award of a medal to him was made while he was in military service." Huidekoper and his sponsors were doubtless disappointed but resolved not to end the matter there. Over the next year, Huidekoper's friend, fellow veteran, and chair of the commission to establish the Gettysburg National Military Park, Colonel John P. Nicholson, pressured his contacts at the secretariat of war and MOLLUS to get the medal. Huidekoper received a letter copied to Nicholson in his role as recorder for the Pennsylvania Commandery, MOLLUS: "I have the honor to advise you that, by direction of the President . . . a Congressional medal of honor has been awarded to you for most distinguished gallantry in action at Gettysburg, Pennsylvania, July 1, 1863, the following being a statement of the particular service rendered in that action: On this occasion Colonel Huidekoper received a severe wound of the right arm while engaged in repelling an attack of the enemy, but instead of retiring he remained at the front in command of the regiment."[65]

In a personal note to Nicholson, Huidekoper wrote, "But for your influence and assistance, I fear I should not have been thus favored, and I thank you sincerely for your efforts, and am grateful for your friendship." From this point on, Huidekoper's pension documents were stamped "Medal of Honor" in red, which privileged his administrative records in some way and might have influenced the awarding of future pensions.[66]

IN HIS DREAMS

Huidekoper did not receive a questionnaire from the Mitchells in the 1890s, but he met S. Weir Mitchell socially and told him about his wartime experience and the challenges he experienced because of his amputated right arm. Referring to a past conversation with Mitchell about "the loss of a limb," in 1906, Huidekoper set his thoughts down in a letter (that he typed) and gave Mitchell permission to use the account provided that Huidekoper's name did not appear in print. In the letter, Huidekoper set the scene at Gettysburg on July 1, 1863, and described the injury to his elbow at around 4:00 p.m. "A cord with a noose at the end of it, which I carried for the purpose, was used a ligature [tourniquet], and, walking a mile and a quarter, had my arm amputated, about six oclock [*sic*], never quite loosing consciousness." The bandages remained in place until July 10 when Dr. Hunt applied "the first dressing" at the Continental Hotel in Gettysburg. Following this intervention, his "arm healed up directly. Never was I unable to walk about from the time of wounding, to the time of healing."[67]

Shortly after Huidekoper's arm stump healed, "an opening appeared on the side of the stump [possibly where the neuroma later developed] and it was not until eight months and four days after wounding, that suppuration stopped and the opening commenced to close." Huidekoper compared his situation with Britain's most famous naval hero, Admiral Horatio Nelson, who also endured an amputation of the right arm below the shoulder. Huidekoper observed that "Lord Nelson's arm troubled him in the same way, although the ligature came away in six months."[68]

Huidekoper described the beginning of his phantom pains. He described himself driving an open carriage when "a gust of wind would make it possible that my straw hat would blow off," whereupon he instinctively raised his phantom right hand to grasp it. Gradually, however, he trained himself to substitute his left hand, as he was forced to do with penmanship. "This feeling of the possibility of using the right hand gradually grew less, until it entirely disappeared, and now, I never think of my right hand with any thought of using it. The fingers, however, remain in a half closed condition, and never have I been able to feel them extended or fully closed, no matter what force I apply to the imagined tendons. Of course, as with everybody else who has lost a limb, the fingers are distinctly felt, and pains occur oftentimes to various parts of them, lasting, in my case, from one or ten seconds."

Huidekoper's remarkable letter must have impressed Mitchell—the prose stylist—with its specificity, concision, and acuity of self-awareness. Even more remarkable was what followed:

> Now for the curious part. I was 24 years old when I lost my arm, and am now 67. Almost two-thirds of my life has passed without thought of the possible use of my right arm, and yet never have I dreamed once, that I was not without two arms, and only last night I dreamt that I was holding a paper with my two hands. When I ride, or drive, or cling to limb on the trees, or write, in my dreams, I always have the use of both hands.
>
> I am now fond of writing with a pen, fond of the mechanical skill which writing requires, and I write often in my dreams, but always with the right hand I used over forty years ago. To do this, I attempt to use the tendons which would hold and guide the pen, and this is done with so much fatigue in attempting to control the hand and move the pen, that I suffer great pain in my finger tendons, even to wakening me up from the most profound sleep because of the pain in the lost hand.[69]

By the time Mitchell had received the letter, he and his son, John, had already published all they would have to say about phantom limbs. Huidekoper must have presented an astonishing case study of how a recurring dream evoked phantom pain, a connection absent from the Mitchells' published studies of nerves. Huidekoper likely never communicated the same intimate narrative of hidden suffering to anyone else but a physician with a specific interest in nerve phenomena. Huidekoper's dream returned his body to its prewar wholeness in an era of peace, but while it caused phantom pain that awakened him, the awakening was also traumatic, as he was instantly transported to his wartime wounding and the death of his comrades, creating a link between mourning and phantom sensations. Mitchell would have been interested in pursuing Huidekoper's description of his dream because he had investigated a sleeper's control of dreams: "Can one initiate lucid dreams by visualizing certain objects or scenes in the period before falling asleep?" For two-thirds of Huidekoper's life, his carefully and circumspectly managed daytime public persona was challenged during nighttime dreams in which he struggled to assert control over his youthful body. In dreams, his prewar body claimed mastery over his identity, but doing so aroused and awoke the postwar body into pain. He concluded his letter to Mitchell: "Thus, in my dreams, I remain a man with a perfect frame, but while awake, I never think of myself otherwise than a one-handed being."[70]

As a mild apology for misleading readers of the Dedlow story into believing that it was true and that the paraplegic doctor lived in a Philadelphia hospital, Mitchell wrote an essay (not anonymous this time) to explore the phantom limb phenomenon. He acknowledged that there was a great deal of ignorance regarding the topic, noting that there was no precise record of the number of wartime amputation survivors and that until recently "no careful scientific study has been made of the physiological conditions which arise in persons who have been so unhappy as to lose limbs." He, however, was not the only investigator to explore the phenomenon. Stimulated by Mitchell's work, in the 1870s, William James, then assistant professor of philosophy at Harvard, surveyed by letter 185 amputees, including war veterans. His study, however, failed "to explain the causes of the enumerated differences." The differences included the fact that some people continued to feel the presence of the severed part, while others did not; some experienced the phantom as "always in one fixed position," and some felt that the phantom migrated; and some felt that the position of the phantom could be changed by force of will, while in others, the position changed with no such effort.[71]

Mitchell introduced the idea that phantom sensations deceived the sufferer. He, like James, found it difficult to create a system to classify phantom sensations in a way that would enable physicians, as if consulting a chart of medicines matched with symptoms, to treat or at least ease the pain that accompanied phantoms. For instance, James observed that "the consciousness of the lost limb varies from acute pain, pricking, itching, burning, cramp, uneasiness, numbness, etc., in the toes, heel, or other place, to feelings which are hardly perceptible, or which become perceptible only after a good deal of 'thinking.' The feeling was not due to the condition of the stump, for in both painful and healthy stumps it may be either present or absent." James concluded that "neither the state of the stump nor the place of the amputation absolutely determined the differences of consciousness which different individuals show" but speculated, in the absence of discovering clear rules about how phantom sensations come and go, that perhaps one ought to "invert the popular way of looking at the problem" and consider why some people do *not* experience phantoms. James could "throw no new light of a positive sort on those individual differences, the explanation of which was the aim of my inquiry," so he left the matter in Mitchell's hands. Had Mitchell examined Huidekoper, he might have concluded that the neuroma was the source of the phantom pain because of the then-common belief that neuromas somehow forced the severed nerves to send false signals to the brain and central nervous system.[72]

However Huidekoper and his fellow amputees managed their postwar lives, they must have been aware that others saw their bodies as feminized due to varying degrees of helplessness or disability. Advertisers of prosthetic limbs emphasized their lifelike qualities, implying their ability to restore manly completeness to the body because the prosthesis "enabl[ed] the amputee to regain his role as productive citizen and to fend off accusations of dependency, emasculation, and radical impairment." Huidekoper and many of his comrades continued to experience the fugitive pain that accompanied phantom sensations—variously described as burning, pricking, tickling, or akin to an electrical current. Thus a malady thought specific to females, hysteria, now became associated with veterans, embedded within a spectrum of odd pains and symptoms. As we have seen, Mitchell applied hysteria to the behavior of veterans afflicted by causalgia.[73]

Perhaps Huidekoper and other amputees considered that part of their identity had been lost with the severed limb. Perhaps, too, hearing Huidekoper's many speeches reminding people of the war and its casualties, veterans mourned anew not only for fallen comrades but also for their vanished limbs. The pinned-up sleeve was a form of perpetual mourning for the loss, and the phantom sensations forced a physical recall of the conditions and moment of loss. As a form of mourning, phantom sensations were "inscribed upon the body. The past returns as physical sensation: sight, smell, and sound." Wearing the prosthesis, however, brought on different sensations and emotions: if properly fitted, the limb might satisfy the wearer in presenting the self as a whole person, but the limb might also compound or confuse phantom sensations. "The reality of the phantom is also enhanced by wearing an artificial arm or leg; the phantom usually fills the prosthesis as a hand fits a glove."[74]

The consensus among physicians today is that the phantom sensation is not a replicate of a missing limb. Indeed, a trickster is at work. "Phantoms are today conceived as parts not accountable to gravity, symmetry, time, or the principles of human morphology, not answerable to the laws that had always governed the physiology of human bodies." Like Civil War veterans, the majority of those who reported pain in a recent study described it as analogous to electrical shocks, pricking of needles, or knife stabs. Physicians have not yet come to a consensus on a definitive explanation for phantom sensations, and so the amputee veteran today who reports phantom phenomena remains a sidebar curiosity, as during Mitchell's era. Effective treatments remain elusive, but mirror therapy has proven beneficial to many. Just as the Dedlow story ended with a ghostly return of his legs via a séance, some amputees find relief in placing a mirror where the amputated leg would have been, facing the remaining leg. Looking down at his legs, the patient views the good leg and its reflection while the brain registers a complete body. The pain fades. The body must summon a phantom to control a phantom.[75]

GODDESS OF VICTORY

At the beginning of 1910, Huidekoper lived in Philadelphia with his wife and three Irish servants and told the census taker his occupation was "director, telephone co." His children had left the household. His mother died in 1897, the same year as his elder brother John. His brothers Herman John, Frank Calhoun, and Rush Shippen died in 1868, 1890, and 1901, respectively. His brother and business partner Frederic Walters died in 1908. Huidekoper was survived only by his two children, his two sisters, and his only living brother, Edgar.[76]

Huidekoper's last great enterprise was the erection of the largest monument at Gettysburg today, the Pennsylvania Memorial, originally conceived as five-acre Pennsylvania Park with an appropriation of $150,000 by the state legislature. He headed a commission of nine veterans to plan the memorial. With a deadline of October 1910 for completion, the proposal required "four triumphal granite arches surmounted by a dome, capped with a colossal bronze 'Victory.' There will be four large panels of bas-reliefs showing incidents of the great battle. Smaller panels will contain the names of all the corps, divisions, and brigade commanders, together with 69 bronze panels, one for each of the 69 regiments and batteries from Pennsylvania, on which will be the names of all the soldiers of Pennsylvania who took part in any of the three days' fighting."

The memorial occupies a section of the Union line near where Pickett's Charge was met and repelled. The structure incorporates the names of all the soldiers who fought: Each regiment received its own bronze panel listing officers and enlisted ranks, together with notations denoting those killed. Veterans returned to this memorial to find their names and regiments and contemplate the sacrifice and victory of their collective body.[77]

Thousands gathered for the dedication of the new memorial on Tuesday afternoon, September 27, 1910. "The crowd was as large as any that ever visited the town since the battle was fought . . . the crowd present was an immense one, but it was orderly, good natured, and was well handled." Visitors shielded their eyes from the sun to examine the winged female embodiment of victory

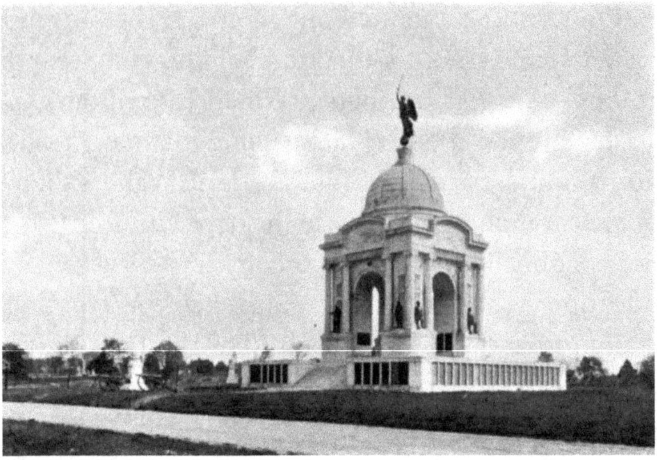

Dedicated in 1910, this view shows the Pennsylvania Memorial at Gettysburg with the statue of Winged Victory facing the west. *Credit: Pennsylvania at Gettysburg, vol. 3. Harrisburg: William Stanley Ray, 1914. Via Wikimedia Commons.*

110 feet up, a statue made of melted-down Civil War cannons. A constant stream of spectators walked around the memorial to appreciate its entirety, some stopping to identify friends or family listed on the bronze tablets under their regiments. Veterans of the 150th Pennsylvania studied the frieze above the west portal, which depicts their stand at the McPherson farm on July 1, 1863. Huidekoper's name appears in two places on the monument: on the bronze tablet listing the soldiers in his regiment and on a tablet inside the monument naming the commissioners who steered the project to completion.[78]

Chaplain M. B. Biddle of Pittsburgh opened the ceremony with a prayer. Huidekoper followed and began his oration by reminding the audience that Pennsylvanians commanded many "divisions and brigades" at Gettysburg and one Pennsylvanian commanded the entire army. "They are now gone," he said but added, "I must tell you of the shouts for joy that went up, in our march northward, as each Pennsylvania regiment crossed the State line six miles from here, and the men once more breathed the pure air of their native State." He recounted several highlights of Pennsylvanians' contributions to the Gettysburg battle, by this time prominently portrayed by Huidekoper and others as the war's turning point. The wounded and dead were described as supreme martyrs, members of a secular sainthood. To Governor Edwin S. Stuart, sitting near the podium, Huidekoper cited the new memorial as "a sacred focus of pilgrimage" and "an inspiration to each successive generation of youth, firing their patriotism," thus ensuring that young men of the future would yield their bodies to national salvation in times of crisis.[79]

Huidekoper concluded his speech with a formal presentation of the memorial to the governor. He spoke as if he were offering an infant in swaddling clothes to a trusted friend, with delicacy and care: "I tender you this Memorial and beg acceptance of it." He suggested that the veterans present would be rejuvenated if the governor provided the appropriate encouragement: "If you will address them, and give them the title they hold dear above all others—'Soldiers of the Army of the Potomac'—you will see their bent forms straighten up . . . you will see their eyes, dimmed by age, sparkle a little yet with fire, and the blood will flow through their veins with quickened impulse, as their step was quickened, when, half a century ago, they marched to the sound of the guns on yonder hills which opened up one of the greatest battles of the world." Turning to the memorial in its red, white, and blue bunting, Huidekoper described the building as a body "made of everlasting granite of exquisite texture, and of enduring bronze . . . planned and built as well as we knew how, and, aloft, the beautiful Goddess of Victory and Peace."[80]

Over the next few years, Huidekoper traveled between Philadelphia and his hometown of Meadville, where his brother Edgar managed a household. At his own expense, Huidekoper commissioned a "splendid and appropriate memorial tablet" in bronze that listed all the soldiers who served in the 150th, to be placed in the local courthouse. In 1912, he hosted a 150th reunion dinner at a local hotel "to commemorate the 50th anniversary of the departure for war of the four companies from Crawford county." A few weeks after the dinner, Huidekoper's wife, Emma, died.[81]

Gettysburg never relinquished its hold on Huidekoper. He helped to organize a fiftieth-anniversary reunion of Gettysburg veterans from both the North and South that included days-long lectures and tours. In 1914, still chair of the Pennsylvania Gettysburg Monuments Commission, he returned to Gettysburg to facilitate the placement at the memorial of bronze statues of three Union generals who distinguished themselves in the battle. The commission anticipated unveiling the figures on the fiftieth anniversary of the Confederate surrender at Appomattox Courthouse in 1915. That year, Huidekoper supervised the first repairs to the memorial to "rectify some faults that resulted in the original construction work." He continued to remain active in speechmaking. In Philadelphia in 1915, "he presided at the meeting in the Academy of Music in Philadelphia on the Fiftieth Anniversary of the founding of [MOLLUS]."[82]

The pension office had not forgotten about Huidekoper. In 1915, it sent him a questionnaire to verify key details about his life, particularly about the status of his marriage and offspring. His daughter lived in New York City at this time, and his son in Montana. As always, Huidekoper dutifully and promptly answered the pension office. The questionnaire also served to verify that Medal of Honor awardee Huidekoper was still alive. A few months after Huidekoper returned the questionnaire, his pension record reflected an increase in pension to sixty-five dollars[83] per month. Residing for the summer of 1916 in York Harbor, Maine, Huidekoper wrote to the office, asserting that his pension should not be subject to income tax (citing "the Medal of Honor act") and pointing out that the act "clearly exempts the pension named." Annoyed, he asked, "Can you advise me as to this disregard for the provisions of the act? Looks like a german 'SCRAP OF PAPER.'"[84] The office responded that no such exemption existed and that "the annual value of pension must be reported on income tax return."[85]

On November 9, 1918, Huidekoper died in the hospital of "Uraemia" (a buildup of toxins in the blood) in Philadelphia, two days before the eleventh hour of the eleventh day of the eleventh month when World War I came to an end. He lay in state at the Union League and was returned home by train to Meadville. There his coffin was displayed in the parlor of his brother Edgar's house, and a service was conducted with a solo singing performance. Veterans from Company K, 150th Pennsylvania, served as pallbearers to Greendale Cemetery where the local GAR post gave military honors: "With the sounding of taps the solemn rites were concluded." A newspaper obituary understated that Huidekoper's "empty sleeve, as well as history, bear testimony to the fact that he was no holiday soldier."[86]

CONCLUSION: NO HOLIDAY SOLDIER

A recent study of Union army veterans observed that they constituted "fictive kin" who worked strenuously to keep the memory of the war in the public consciousness. To oppose the gradual disintegration of the patriotic fervor of the war, veterans frequently and publicly took firm moral stands against views that threatened a conservative and fixed vision of the nation. To neglect to honor the memory of the war meant that its "unresolved political, social, and racial business would render [the veterans'] injuries meaningless." They remained keenly aware of the rise of the Lost Cause ideology, which implied a moral equivalence between the North and South and avoided the issue of slavery. As a veteran and spokesperson, Huidekoper shared their sentiments about the sacred memory of their common experience. He sympathized with their desire to prevent the country from being "condemned to an indeterminate future of grappling with what *their* rebellion accomplished—and left unfinished."[87]

The existing documentation on Huidekoper's life reveals the nightly combat between his prewar and postwar bodies only in his letter to Mitchell. Perhaps he decided that his evanescent but permanent phantom pain was a necessary physical prompt to his efforts to memorialize the war and his regiment's sacrifices. It may also have strengthened his desire to obtain a Medal of Honor. But he did not share the pain with the examination panel that inspected his body for a pension adjustment. Unlike John Shields, he never mentioned the pain to the pension office in hopes of securing a higher allowance. At the forefront of twentieth-century news were American soldiers lost in Cuba, the Philippines, and, at the time of Huidekoper's death, in France. More than ever, citizens were aware that "the preservation of national unity required the mutual destruction of its citizen-soldiery." The national mantra about making the world safe for democracy had become increasingly challenging to demonstrate as the bodies piled up.[88]

Against a backdrop of patriotic suffering in recent wars, Huidekoper increasingly tried to rally fellow veterans and inspire new generations to maintain the vision of an ongoing battle to champion unity and democracy while European empires were on the ascendant. In addition to creating monuments and asserting their importance to posterity, Huidekoper published short pieces such as the "Historic Church" leaflet that he wrote for visitors to Saint Xavier Catholic Church in Gettysburg. The leaflet outlined how the war had transformed the church into a temporary hospital and prompted the reader with "A Patriotic Suggestion." The text noted that the leaflet had been produced for church visitors by battle survivors "for information and favorable consideration of all patriotic citizens," and its authors hoped that the leaflet constituted "a permanent object lesson to posterity for all time, as a part of the records of heroic achievement and historical incidents of '*Pennsylvania at Gettysburg*.'"[89]

Huidekoper would have shared his most intimate thoughts about soldierly manhood only with his fellow veterans of the 150th. In 1896, his comrade, Brevet Major R. L. Ashhurst, disclosed his private thoughts to his regimental comrades about what they meant to each other and the nation. Ashhurst recalled that the most "eventful years" of the war "seem to have been the prime of our life." He observed, "Superfluous lags the veteran on the stage." Solidarity among veterans competed with the dissolution of memory in time. "We find growing up around us a spirit which is impatient of any return to the thoughts and feelings of those glorious days. . . . What unity has there been in our lives like military unity?" The essence of the soldier, Ashurst, Huidekoper, and their comrades agreed, "is unselfishness—the abrogation of self; the devotion of life and all that makes life dear to country and nation." Achievement of this quality requires a purging of egotism to bring forth "out of the crucible of toil and suffering the type of perfected manhood," a view that informed Huidekoper's dedicatory speeches and writings. More so than the other former soldiers profiled in this book, Huidekoper's veteran body was guided by a distinct ideology on public display through commemorative events. Despite Huidekoper's public words to audiences at these events, people did not see that body shifted between phantom and corporeal selves, young and old, antagonistic and complementary, until his death. As Lindsay Tuggle wrote, "I never left the house / I just took the door with me."[90]

At the start of 1919, the pension office closed its record on Huidekoper. The last record for him cited the date and amount of his final pension payment, and, next to an earlier stamp, "Medal of Honor," another stamp read in large black, bold letters: DEAD, DROPPED 2/6/19. A week before, Commissioner G. M. Saltzgaber of the pension office sent a form for endorsement to

J. H. Devine, a pension officer in Philadelphia, requesting permission to close Huidekoper's file. Devine approved and added a handwritten note at the bottom of the form: "The General died November 9, 1918, in the Polytechnic Hospital. I was with him about 7 weeks on an average of 5 nights each week. He received his November check ok, it was found by his Daughter who is one of the executors of his Estate." Thus ended Huidekoper's veteran, civic, and pension bodies.

Huidekoper's postwar civic life ushered in new technologies as he strove to anchor the memory and legacy of the Civil War for future generations. His pension life was rounded with a sleep, sealed by that final form in the file. The new generation performs the funeral obsequies as life goes on. On the form, pension officer Devine added a personal note to his friend and colleague Saltzberger: "How are you and your family? Best wishes for the New Year."[91]

TEN

THE WIND OF THEIR PLACE AND TIME

Woe for the homes of the North,
And woe for the seats of the South:
All who felt life's spring in prime,
And were swept by the wind of their place and time—

Herman Melville[1]

BEWILDERMENT

The examination of these seven cases—one physician and six soldiers—reveals complex body narratives. A history of the body requires us to hear another's music, attend church services, peer over the shoulders of attending physicians, preside at business meetings, plow a farm field, create models of landscapes, march in parades, give speeches, bury wartime companions, and listen to dreams. This history observes the body as it breathes, moves, thinks, and acts. With heavy reliance on service and pension records, we obtain moments of clarity. The bodies of our subjects are dynamic and draw our interest.

Despite our best efforts to engage with the past, veterans' interior lives can, at best, be glimpsed and heard only from a distance. "Union veterans belonged to an era with its own terms and conditions, which should be respected rather than subordinated to the present." The men profiled here, despite the debility of their bodies, exercised agency over their civic, pension, and veteran lives. Our physician—S. Weir Mitchell—labored to help veterans increase their agency despite the degradation of his own health in the process. In this study, physicians are identified if possible. In most cases, little is known about them, but merely supplying names provides them with a modicum of personality.[2]

Our six soldiers inhabited and displayed three bodies or personae after the war: one was shared exclusively with other veterans, the second with pension officials, and the third (civic) with family and community. Among their fellow veterans, their wounds were acknowledged and celebrated. These injuries were organic medals, testaments to the republican ideals for which soldiers fought. In the company of veterans, camaraderie and approval were ensured. Veterans rallied around disadvantaged brothers, particularly those left behind by the new industrialization driving the country. With pension officials, veterans hid their achievements when claiming complete or partial disability from their war injuries or illnesses.

All six soldiers championed a vision of a resilient American democracy because of the assumption that an innate quality of manliness drove men to enlist, fight, die, or live diminished lives with disabilities, injuries, or diseases that persisted until death. Prestley Dorsey/Dawson was the least engaged with the fraternal organizations of war veterans, and yet his only surviving relic is his veteran's badge, doubtless obtained at a convention or gathering of black veterans. Henry Huidekoper, John Shields, Richard Dunphy, and possibly Henry Kircher attached themselves to the Grand Army of the Republic in various ways, and within this or other veterans' organizations, their disfigurements were welcomed and honored. No stigma was attached to their veteranhood. As a corporate body, the GAR was critical during the late nineteenth century in maintaining the public visibility of the veterans of a fast-receding war and their increasing need for help in maintaining their aging bodies. At the same time, veterans projected themselves as superpatriots and were in the vanguard of flag-waving for the Spanish-American War and World War I.

Projecting their veteran bodies, "Northern men pieced together their manly identities in a bewildering variety of ways." Those ways have been generalized to include extremes from violence born of a rigid sense of honor and moral purpose or rough fraternization, to gentlemen of refined habits, feminized through education and cultural achievements such as the patronage of the arts. Of the seven men profiled, only Mitchell continued his prewar profession except for Huidekoper's service in the Pennsylvania militia. The *ur*-masculine profession at the time, already sentimentalized by the war era, was farming. Success in farming exhibited ideal manhood: subduing nature to one's will by taming beasts and growing crops, the farmer was an independent economic agent in the honest and Bible-affirmed work of living off the land. Of the six soldiers, only Dorsey/Dawson (and Shields, briefly) pursued farming after the war, the only likely route to financial independence for a nonliterate black veteran. He achieved success with land transactions that solidified the family's presence in rural Maryland.

All profiled soldiers lived into the twentieth century except for Hawkins, who died only five years after the war. The GAR was no help to him, as it had not yet achieved the stature and influence it would enjoy from the 1880s to the turn of the century. Nevertheless, the veterans in this study, even if partially disabled, relied on the government to help restore their manhood. Dunphy and Hawkins both worked as government messengers, a job created for disabled veterans for whom other manual labor was not possible. Huidekoper and Kircher prospered with help from fellow veterans, although Shields experienced a setback of bankruptcy, requiring assistance from fellow veterans and placement in a quasimilitary environment as commandant of a veterans' home.[3]

All six soldiers exploited all legal avenues to get pensions and argued for their expansion over the course of their lives. All regarded pensions as their legal due, government recognition of their service in the war, whether pension income was vital to them or not. The soldiers who applied for pensions entered a contradictory universe in which the funds awarded were intended to compensate for debilitating bodily sacrifices that made it impossible to perform manual labor, yet they concealed their white-collar employment and swore to their inability to profit by the manly endeavor of manual labor. Veterans might be bank managers, professors, salesmen, or accountants, but what really mattered was whether they could harness oxen to a plow, shoe a horse, build a fence, or perform on a factory assembly line. The manual labor requirement was meaningless to the veterans discussed here.

The government's rules also enforced a moral order: examiners were ever alert to discovering "vicious habits" that would have doomed a pension award. Nevertheless, pension officers sometimes turned a blind eye to evidence of moral backsliding. The evidence for Dunphy's excessive drinking never rose to a pension denial, and the reviewing pension officer was adamant in explaining that he would not deny a pension to a veteran who suffered the consequence of being armless. For surviving spouses eligible for pensions, the government imposed a moral mandate: if they remarried, they lost their pensions.

In projecting their civic bodies with their communities and families, veterans managed their abnormalities to be socially accepted. Amputations might be acceptable and accommodated in some work environments, but disfiguring scars, burns, or poorly healed lacerations led to ostracism and a perception of moral weakness. Huidekoper's pinned sleeve was accepted by both veterans and the public. Dawson's lameness was not disfiguring. His upper-body strength compensated for his limp, a comparatively common public sight in any setting. Hawkins and Shields, without such visible scars, elicited sympathy for their pain among fellow veterans, but it made social situations challenging.

The civic body threatened public order owing to disfigured bodies in public venues. Veterans wore prostheses for practicality but also to disguise the damaged or missing parts of their bodies that, if apparent, might invite inquiry, joking, or exclusion. Kircher displayed his pinned sleeve but concealed his missing leg with a trousered prosthesis. By wearing the prosthesis, his civic body avoided confusing, scaring, or otherwise disturbing people, whereas his missing arm was acceptable and nonthreatening. While he tailored his public appearances to avoid unwelcome public scrutiny, his continual arguments to pension authorities to recognize the totality of his loss ended with his sarcastic suggestion that in future wars, the government should limit amputations to one limb per soldier. Huidekoper's pinned-up sleeve (instead of a prosthesis) did not threaten his community; in fact, his use of it to signify an unending Gettysburg battle turned it into a badge of republicanism.

Dunphy wore a cape in public to conceal his arm stumps, yet in one social venue—saloons—he became a performing armless marvel, bending over a glass to secure it between his lips and then emptying it down his throat as he stood up. His missing arms created severe cognitive dissonance among pension authorities, although publicly Dunphy promoted himself as a respectable patriarch of a middle-class family. Losing one limb could be regarded as a misfortune to be borne honorably through a folded sleeve, but losing two limbs looked like carelessness or worse.

Shields bore little visible sign of disability, but his advancing pain and decreasing mobility over the years confused pension authorities because the pain seemed to be disproportionate to the apparent wound. The solution, albeit temporary, to reconcile his need to make a living with a fragile and deteriorating body was rescue: the veteran's body fused with the civic one when, with the GAR's help, he was appointed as commandant of a home for veterans. Had Hawkins lived longer, he would have experienced a similar situation: to outward appearances, he was "whole," yet he experienced advancing pain that rendered most physical labor impossible. Dawson's wartime injury remained evident in his limp, but his malaria was dormant most of the time except for a recurring cluster of symptoms that removed him from physical labor on occasion. Dorsey/Dawson was able to ignore painful symptoms to remain active and working without anyone knowing about his difficulties. His motivation for this behavior is speculative at best: the impulse to work for his own benefit—and not that of a slave owner—may have pushed him to succeed as a farmer.

Kircher's, Huidekoper's, and Dunphy's visible missing appendages alternately disturbed onlookers, confused some, and caused others to look away with pretended courtesy and discomfort. Community and familial respect were clearly important to all six soldiers. Properly concealed or diminished in some way, an arm amputation or a public display of strength (Dawson) received public approval and respect. We are left to guess at the small measures these men took daily to adjust their public bodies to project their manly, capable selves when their very appearance could disturb, embarrass, or terrify others.

A NEW WORLD

> The scene was, indeed, an impressive one. The men lying up and down the hospital, in their cots, (some badly wounded . . . some never to rise thence,) the cots themselves, with their drapery of white curtains, and the shadows down the lower and upper parts of the Ward; then the silence of the men, and the attitudes they took . . . the whole was a sight to look around upon again and again.[4]
>
> Walt Whitman

Hospitals were transformative environments. The soldiers whose anesthesia hallucinations are recounted in the first chapter emerged with altered bodies in the confrontation with their subconscious, regardless of their medical treatment. The medical infrastructure of the Union war effort was complex. The wounded soldier made a short detour within the medical tent or hospital followed by recovery and a return to civil life or military duty. A longer detour would have meant hospitalization until the war's end, whereupon the soldier was sent home to recuperate. Hospitals were not assembly lines driven by faceless technicians in bloodstained aprons. The conventional perception of Civil War hospitals as places of suffering, unsanitary conditions, and primitive medical practices fails to withstand critical examination when considering the men profiled in this book. The field hospitals, like those in Vietnam or World War II, practiced triage to prioritize patients based on their likelihood of survival. Once transferred to remote general hospitals, soldiers encountered a different world. Many soldiers recalled their hospitalizations later with fondness. Walt Whitman, who had an intimate understanding of how these hospitals operated, found the hospital not "the repulsive place of sores and fevers" but instead "a new world . . . full of its separate action, play, suggestiveness—surely a medium world, advanced between our well-known practiced one of body and of mind." In general hospitals, soldiers formed intimate partnerships with the physicians assigned to heal them and enjoyed a period of focused introspection about their bodies that re-created their perception of manhood into a more subtle, complex form.[5]

The hospital was a "borderland between the familiar, physical world of the body and the afterlife of the soul." It was a borderland between conventional manhood turned upside down by grievous bodily damage and the invention of a modified or new identity borne of the soldier's healing partnership with doctors and his observations of healing and dying comrades. An acute observer of soldiers' behavior in hospitals, Whitman wrote that "everything [was] bent to save a life from the very grip of the destroyer. . . . Not a bit of sentimentalism or whining have I seen about a single death-bed in hospital or on the field, but impassive indifference. All is over." Veterans learned how precarious their bodies were and recognized with "providential pragmatism" the spectrum of phenomena spawned by their wounds and diseases. They resolved to negotiate their lives despite occasional or chronic pain or other ailments that interfered with raising families and enjoying careers, at least until the pain subverted expected manifestations of manhood. The idiosyncratic pains experienced by veterans confounded pension authorities by defying the rational language of pension laws, and it accompanied veterans' daily activities as demons existing in the shadows of their bodies, within the habitual motions of sinew and nerve. Every veteran negotiated these fugitive pains differently.[6]

These soldiers learned more about their physical selves than they would have imagined possible and became sensitive to minute phenomena, particularly the evanescent pains of healing. They married after the war, determined to create a new benchmark for their futures. From the beginning of their married relationships, they assessed their bodies' abilities to be husbands and fathers and had frank discussions with their brides about their hopes and ambitions regarding the behavior of their bodies. Some considered this dialogue to be unhealthy self-centrism and self-indulgence, behaviors perceived by many as feminine. That their marriages happened at all testifies to discussions of manhood that would not have happened between unwounded courting adults.[7]

S. Weir Mitchell saw firsthand the trampled and bloodied field of war, a vision that haunted him for the rest of his life. His arrival at the fresh battlefield of Gettysburg and his relentless work both as a physician in private practice and as a contract assistant surgeon placed him in intimate and long-term interaction with scores of soldiers during the war and with veterans to the end of his life. He deserves equivalence with our six soldiers as a fellow veteran. His notions of manhood were rooted in white American men, his ideal unrealized by some of his soldier-patients. An astute observer of the bodies of his patients, he held them to his conservative, antebellum notions of white manhood.

Although his case records ended once patients recovered sufficiently to return to duty or to their homes as civilians, Mitchell's curiosity about long-term health outcomes led him to circulate his unique questionnaire to a list of white soldiers he compiled with the War Department. Following his postbattle stint at Gettysburg, Mitchell did not have to amputate limbs or stanch bloody wounds; his Turner's Lane Hospital ward was devoted to long-term recovery and a reintegration of the body. This reintegration necessitated the use of electricity as a kind of inner bandage to reconnect and reactivate a disordered nervous system. The intimacy of contact via electrical devices required new medical terms to denote unprecedented bodily interventions. Those patients who exhibited the American masculinity Mitchell praised discussed their bodies, adopted the vocabulary of treatment, and left the hospital with their powers of introspection expanded to consider the nature of their nervous system and how it could be managed to improve their health.

The men profiled in this book suffered some of the postwar phenomena listed in the *Diagnostic and Statistical Manual of Mental Disorders*. That does not mean that they would receive a clinical diagnosis of posttraumatic stress disorder (PTSD) today. All of them, however, found ways to create productive lives. "Indeed, scores of men suffered with invisible injuries after the war, such as attacks of anxiety and depression with frightening nightmares and hallucinations. But these walking wounded were able to cope and carry on, leading mostly healthy and well-adjusted lives."[8]

Mitchell's questionnaires were recently examined for descriptions of the physical manifestations of psychological stress that are linked to PTSD symptoms. The study notes that the surveys "did not include direct questions that measured current PTSD criteria (such as intrusive symptoms, avoidance of trauma-related stimuli, negative changes in mood and thought, or increased arousal and hyperactivity)." Rather, the questionnaire highlighted symptoms of phantom limbs and associated pain, the phenomena of particular interest to Mitchell and his son.

Mitchell did not extend his study of soldiers' bodies to African American veterans. Hawkins was an exception in that his postwar recovery took place in an environment of literate and socially mobile black professionals. He was attended by both black and white physicians; one of the latter, because of their shared military experience, served Hawkins well during his last days. Most white doctors, however, and possibly Mitchell as well, viewed black bodies as "inherently abnormal" and assumed various defects including insensitivity to pain, an ability to thrive in tropical environments, and a lack of delicacy in features. Indeed, many doctors agreed with slavery's apologists that "African-American bodies inherently existed in an inertia of disability from which they could not extricate themselves; indeed . . . disability itself came to symbolize stasis and perpetual dependence during this period in opposition to 'traditional' American ideals of independence."[9]

Racist assumptions continued to influence the understanding of black soldiers' postwar health. A study of pension records claims that the experience of combat created a higher probability of mental illness among black soldiers than white. Skepticism about health claims by pension officials resulted in a diminished motivation to seek their consultation, so both mental and physical maladies may not have been addressed, much less documented. Among black soldiers, postwar suicide rates were lower than those of white soldiers, although some physicians attributed the difference to the perception that black soldiers had less anxiety than white soldiers due to their so-called simple minds. Many doctors and some slavery apologists believed that with their newfound freedom, black men gave into licentious behavior and sabotaged their bodies, leading to early death and increased diagnoses of insanity.[10]

THE BODY AS DATA

> A new, maturing generation has swept in, obliterating with oceanic currents the worst reminiscences of the War; and the passage of time has heal'd over at least its deepest scars. Already, the events of 1861–65 . . . have lost their direct personal impression, and the living heat and excitement of their own time, and are being marshall'd for casting, or getting ready to be cast, into the cold and bloodless electrotype plates of History.
>
> Walt Whitman[11]

Because of the government's belief that the war would end the enslavement of African Americans and that city-based industrial work would expand at the expense of rural occupations, policymakers decided that guidelines for occupational insurance should be formulated. Chapter 6 includes a discussion of two studies sponsored by the US Sanitary Commission in 1864 that required army doctors to conduct anthropometric measurements of black and white soldiers. Our six soldiers and one physician thus contributed bodily data to these massive studies. The studies, published in 1869 and 1875, reached different conclusions, but the former may have had the most influence on subsequent anthropometric studies in normalizing white males as the baseline standard of health in its arrays of numerical data. The 1869 study found inferior physical performance among black soldiers in comparison with white soldiers, and the study methods, much praised at the time for scientific rigor, enabled an institutional view of black people as a subordinate race with measurable shortfalls in physical abilities. When bodily phenomena translate into tabulated numbers, the data acquire authority and truthfulness. Comparable anthropometric studies today grapple with this historic legacy.[12]

Apart from the two Sanitary Commission studies, the army surgeon general ordered the creation of an encyclopedia of everything that doctors learned during the war, published in multiple volumes over several years as *The Medical and Surgical History of the War of the Rebellion* (MSH). Its publication constituted a milestone in the history of American printing. The volumes included chromolithographs, graphic displays of data in multiple colors, hundreds of illustrations drawn from medical photographs (published in a separate portfolio), tabular data, and case studies. Including extant records from the former Confederacy, the MSH was at once "a chronicle of medical procedures throughout the Western world of the nineteenth century, a record of thousands of unique individual experiences in battle and living with consequent disability, and a reflection of the postwar perception of the permanently impaired Civil War veteran." Data gleaned from the bodies of our veterans inform many of the larger statistical summaries in the MSH. Kircher, because of the rarity of his double amputation, appears in two lists with a capsule description of the operation. Dunphy, perhaps because his case was documented differently due to his naval service, does not appear in these lists.[13]

Some veterans whose experiences were recorded as case studies offered them to pension authorities as documentation of their wounds or injuries. These authorities found much scientific data in the case studies about the practices that healed wounds and injuries and gained some insight into why veterans later experienced debilities resulting from wartime injuries. Following the Sanitary Commission studies, the MSH constituted the second body of government statistics regarding the health of African American men. For all veterans, the MSH could be both

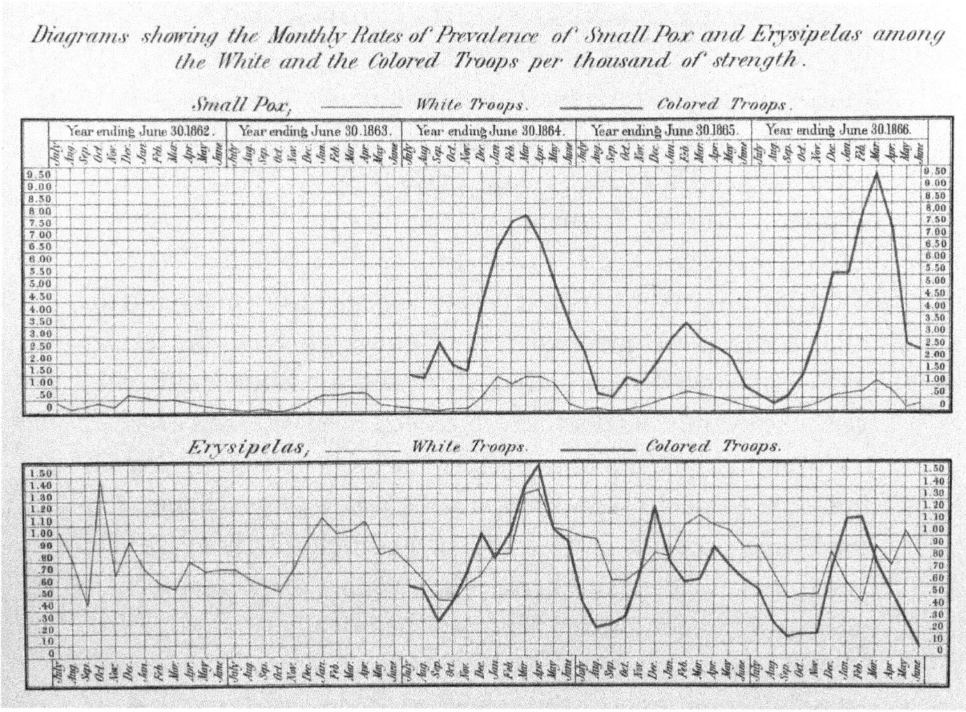

Example of tabular data about soldiers' bodies from *The Medical and Surgical History of the War of the Rebellion*. The graphs show the prevalence (by monthly cases) of smallpox and erysipelas (bacterial skin disease) among white (thin line) and black (thick line) Union troops during the war. The two diseases were combined for the graph because both were classified as "eruptive skin diseases." The data curves are printed in red. *Credit: George A. Otis, ed.,* The Medical and Surgical History of the War of the Rebellion. *Part 3, Vol. 1. (Medical History). US Government Printing Office, Washington, DC, 1876–1888. Plate is opposite p. 624.*

friend and foe. As friend, the MSH vindicated veterans' experiences and suffering. As foe, the case studies in MSH reduced their suffering to graphs and tables, thus minimizing individual experiences. Considered in the broader physical contexts of veteranhood, dialogue with pension authorities, professional and familial lives, and individual experiences suggest pathways of investigation and analysis beyond the scope of the MSH.

CONCLUSION: SEARCHING FOR MEMORY

Studies of Union veterans cite pensions in their narratives of negotiation with government agents. Frequently overlooked or underanalyzed, however, are the periodic medical examinations required by the government for veterans to receive pensions or pension increases. Each examination represents a dual vision of health, one from the perspective of the pension claimant and the other from a government-contracted physician. First, the veteran set down his wartime bodily history and subsequent suffering. Next, the examining doctor responded to the veteran's account. The examinations did not consider the body holistically but addressed the veteran's specific issues within a ratings scheme. Pension examination forms cited the current applicable law passed by Congress so that later authorities had a benchmark for interpreting an award decision according to the law at a given time. The printed forms included a diagram of the body that constituted the only extant image of the veteran's body with its afflictions. Doctors rarely tried to depict the actual wound; they used diagrams to locate and denote the size of the wound or resulting scar. Occasionally, affidavits from witnesses or other medical authorities supplemented these forms. Multiple examinations over time provide the possibility of longitudinal study and comparative analyses.

Veterans' claims as written on examination forms constitute a counternarrative to those of physicians and pension authorities. Interrogating pension records and medical examination forms allows a "language of selfhood" to emerge among the veterans examined in this book. Understanding this language—the language of another's wound—requires us to detach from the images of the era and commonly cited generalizations about disability. Mitchell's questionnaires and his correspondence with veterans provide additional counternarratives. Not bound by congressional acts or pension bureau protocols, Mitchell could and did listen to others' wounds. He listened to the body's language of nerves, making sense of its sentence fragments and applying electricity to elicit full paragraphs from veterans' bodily telegraphs. Left to pension doctors, examinations often reduced veterans' narratives of their bodies to simple equations of manual labor capacity.[14]

During the war, the army established a reserve force of wounded veterans, initially the Invalid Corps and later the Veterans Reserve Corps, to serve light-duty assignments to spare the full-bodied soldiers for active combat duty. Despite the best intentions to give disabled soldiers a way to continue their military service, their new uniforms were light blue, as if the deep blue of their previous coats had dimmed or faded, thus communicating that the inhabitant of the new uniform was reduced in manhood. Following the war, veterans wore no uniforms until the GAR permitted a shadow version of a military uniform to be worn for public events, a kepi and coat with large brass buttons emblazoned "G.A.R." Outside of these contexts, the Union veteran was visible when he achieved financial success and the resulting accolades qualified the success in relation to wartime service. Yet when historians probe these apparent Gilded Age victors to understand their thoughts, motivations, and identities, doing so "often deliver[s] a sharp warning about making inferences." The fraternal body (e.g., GAR member) coexisted with the civic body, the one active with families and businesses while enduring debility and suffering as the pensioned body. This veteran, the one in conversation with doctors and other veterans, was indeterminate, self-aware, and resisted predictions and forecasts: "Far fewer studies of the wounded and permanently disabled soldier and representations of this figure exist."[15]

During his visits to hospitals, Walt Whitman beheld the man through his suffering. Whitman saw the relationships develop between soldiers and with nurses, doctors, and orderlies. He perceived a common feature in those patients who exhibited reserves of patriotic vision, camaraderie, and self-awareness. By far, he wrote, most "of the patients are American young men, intelligent, of independent spirit, tender feelings . . . used to a hardy and healthy life." Had he encountered Huidekoper, Kircher, Dorsey/Dawson, Shields, Dunphy, or Hawkins, he would have found these qualities. He ruminated on his wartime memories with his physician, S. Weir Mitchell, late in life, both of whose writings were tinctured with the blood of the war.[16]

> The question, O me! so sad, recurring—What good amid these,
> O me,
> O life?
> Answer.
>
> That you are here—that life exists and identity,
> That the powerful play goes on, and you may contribute a verse.
>
> Walt Whitman[17]

APPENDIX A

ABSTRACT OF KEY PENSION LAWS[1]

- "[A] pension was still seen as a reward for the worthy, rather than a general entitlement . . . federal pensions provided a belated gratuity for the risks and sacrifices of soldiers and sailors during the war."[2]
- The heyday of pension awards for Civil War service occurred between 1870 and 1910 when the proportion of veterans receiving pensions leaped from 5 percent to 93 percent.[3]
- By 1893, about 42 percent of federal tax income went to veterans' pensions. As the number and dollar amount of pension claims increased, the press and legislative representatives began to criticize pensioners over fraud and corruption, questioning the distribution of government funds to the "undeserving."[4]

GENERAL LAW OF 1862

- Passed on July 22, 1861.
- Disabled, wounded volunteer soldiers to receive same disability benefits as regular army soldiers.
- 1862 expansion of law: all disabled veterans who enlisted after March 4, 1861, to receive pensions "who suffered permanent

injury or disabilities as a *direct* consequence of military service."[5]

- Disability defined as ability to perform manual labor (later more broadly interpreted to include any labor requiring "education or skill"). Statute identified "inferior" and "total" as two types of disability, left undefined.
- Mothers, widows, orphan sisters included.
- Medical examination required: The prospective pensioner required a "surgeon's certificate" as basis for initial pension award, and local physicians examined veterans for subsequent requests for increases.
- Ratings system applied to determine amount of compensation (e.g., the loss of a finger constituted a 2/8 disability, or two dollars per month for a private).
- Standard rate for a disabled private was eight dollars per month (if not totally disabled).
- Maximum allowable disability pension was twenty-five dollars per month.
- General Law amended in 1864 and 1866 to include rates for malaria, measles, and sunstroke according to equivalence to disability for wounds.
  - In 1864, Congress listed "statutory pensions" of fixed amounts for specific bodily losses, eventually expanding to fifteen.
  - In 1866, a new pensionable category of veterans needing "constant personal aid and attention" in the form of "regular aid and attendance of another person."

1870s

- Pensioners required to undergo periodic medical examinations to affirm, increase, decrease, or terminate pensions once veterans were deemed physically self-sufficient.
- Medical examiners now required to address lifestyles of veterans to identify what became labeled in 1890 "vicious

habits." Some examining doctors included race and ethnicity in assessing lifestyles and habits.

- Consolidation Act of 1873
  - Uniform scale of impairments or debilities created with accompanying ratings.
  - For the first time, pension law addressed illnesses and diseases as generally eligible.
  - Claimants who were widows and minors required to submit legal justification of pension-eligible status.
- Arrears Act of 1879
  - Lump-sum back pay available to veterans making new pension applications regarding Civil War service, resulting in large number of first-time claimants.

1880s

- Pension authorities no longer relied on physicians from the veterans' localities to conduct examinations to sustain pensions or obtain increases. Henceforth, veterans were referred to a standing three-doctor panel to conduct a "thorough and searching" examination.
- Pension panels required to discover evidence of excessive drinking, venereal diseases, or other moral lapses.
- By the late 1880s, the number of disability pensions for illness and diseases stemming from war-related maladies now superseded combat wounds and injuries.
- By 1890, the preeminent diseases for which pensions were claimed included rheumatism and cardiovascular disease.

ACT OF 1890

- Most significant change of policy since the 1862 law: origin of veteran's disability immaterial; pension awarded based on degree of inability to support self.

- To be eligible for a pension, the veteran had to have served a minimum of ninety days, be honorably discharged, and have some physical or mental ailment developing during or after military service that precluded the performance of manual labor.
- Authorized payments of six dollars or twelve dollars per month for any disability and abandoned scheme of ratings for specific debilities.
- Pensions for disabilities extended not only to disabled veterans and their familial survivors but to veterans of all wars regardless of the cause of the disability and their survivors.
- Widows no longer had to demonstrate financial need but must remain unmarried to receive a pension.

1900s

- 1904: Executive Order No. 78 under President Theodore Roosevelt eliminated the showing of medical debilities and required only an honorable discharge by service of at least ninety days.
- 1907: General Law and subsequent amendments superseded by creation of the Service and Age Pension System under which veterans no longer had to submit to medical examination; the two determining criteria were the veteran's age and service record.
- Law required veteran to be over sixty-two with graduated increases as he aged.

APPENDIX B

S. WEIR MITCHELL QUESTIONNAIRE OF VETERANS

[Page 1]

Questions should be answered as fully as possible: The circular when filled out should be mailed in the enclosed addressed envelope.

1. Name and address:
2. Age:
3. Date of amputation of limb:
4. Character of wound:
5. Interval between wound and amputation:
6. Symptoms during this period:
7. Operation:
   a. Nature of flaps, if known:
8. Symptoms following operation—shock?
   a. Duration of, if known?
   b. Hemorrhage?
   c. Pain—character?
   d. Extent?
   e. Seat?
   f. Severity? (This answer as fully as possible.)
   g. Suppuration—extent?

h. Duration?
i. Recurrence?
j. Healing, when complete?
k. When was artificial limb first worn?

9. Has the loss of your member altered the general health?
a. Have there been any alterations of pulse?
b. Body temperature?
c. Digestion?
d. Intellectual powers?
e. Disposition?
f. Or habits?

[Page 2]

g. Has there been any change in the acuteness of the special senses, i.e., hearing, sight, sense of taste?
h. What reasons have you for ascribing such alterations, if any are noted, to the injury or operation?
i. Is there any alteration in the amount of sleep or of solid or liquid nourishment required?
j. Was the amputation followed by any marked change in your ability for mental or bodily exertion?

10. Record any increase in strength and size of remaining limbs if such has been noticed.
a. Has the ability to use the remaining part been increased?

11. Does the skin of the stump differ from the rest of the body?
a. As to texture?
b. Color?
c. Temperature?
d. Growth of hair?
e. Does it sweat more or less than other surfaces of the body?

f. Is it more sensitive than other surfaces of the body as to pain; for instance, the prick of a pin?
g. How extensive is the area of the altered sensation?
h. Is it more sensitive than other surfaces of the body to touch?
i. How far does the altered sensation extend?
j. Does a touch give a sensation of pain?
k. Is there excessive sensibility to extremes of heat and cold?
  i. When applied to the part, as hot or cold water?
  ii. When dependent upon general changes in the temperature of the atmosphere, as in summer and winter?
  iii. Is there excessive sensibility to changes in the weather, as at the approach of a storm

[Page 3]

or during the prevalence of certain winds?
12. What power of movement remains in the stump?
13. What artificial appliances have been tried?
14. Which has been most satisfactory?
15. What inconveniences have attended the wearing of artificial appliances?
  a. Can they be worn continuously (excepting at night)?
16. Give length and shape of stump.
17. What alterations have taken place in its appearance since operation?
18. Are there any involuntary twitchings or spasmodic movements of the stump?
  a. What is the character of such movements?
19. When were they first noted?
  a. How often do they recur?
  b. What causes them?
  c. Are they accompanied by pain?

20. Do you still feel the lost part?
    a. If you do not feel it now, how long did you feel it after the amputation?
21. How much of the limb do you feel now, and how does the feeling differ from what it would be if the member were present?
22. Does the limb feel as if shortened?
    a. Does it feel as if in one fixed position?
    b. If not, does the apparent posture change from time to time?
    c. Has this apparent position any relation to the position of the stump?

Source: S. Weir Mitchell Papers, MSS 0241–03, box 11, Series 4.5, folder 2, Historical Medical Library, College of Physicians of Philadelphia

NOTES

1. LISTENING TO ANOTHER'S WOUND

1. "Anesthesia," *West Philadelphia Hospital Register* (Philadelphia, PA), July 25, 1863, 135.

2. E. S., "My Ether Dream," *West Philadelphia Hospital Register*, April 11, 1863, 35.

3. Ibid.

4. Cathy Caruth, *Unclaimed Experience: Trauma, Narrative, and History* (Baltimore: Johns Hopkins University Press, 1996), 8.

5. Today, these veterans might be labeled disabled or partially disabled, and the process of care and assistance available now would have been unrecognizable in the nineteenth century.

6. For instance, posttraumatic stress disorder, commonly recognized today outside of clinical practice, did not exist as a diagnosis during the Civil War or for years after, yet symptoms of the disorder are found in clinical examinations and pension documentation. Shauna Devine, *Learning from the Wounded: The Civil War and the Rise of American Medical Science* (Chapel Hill: University of North Carolina Press, 2014), 150; Hilary Daniel, Sue. S. Bornstein, and Gregory C. Kane, "Addressing Social Determinants to Improve Patient Care and Promote Health Equity: An American College of Physicians Position Paper," *Annals of Internal Medicine* 168, no. 8 (April 17, 2018): 577.

7. Brian Matthew Jordan, *Marching Home: Union Veterans and Their Unending Civil War* (New York: Liveright, 2014).

8. Lindsay Tuggle, *The Afterlives of Specimens: Science, Mourning, and Whitman's Civil War* (Iowa City: University of Iowa, 2017), 9, 64–65, 104–105.

9. Sarah Handley-Cousins, *Bodies in Blue: Disability in the Civil War North* (Athens: University of Georgia Press, 2019), 3.

10. Eric T. Dean Jr., *Shook over Hell: Post-Traumatic Stress, Vietnam, and the Civil War* (Cambridge, MA: Harvard University Press, 1997), 8, 45; American Psychiatric Association, *Diagnostic and Statistical Manual of Mental Disorders*, 5th ed. (Washington, DC: Author, 2013), PTSD criteria quoted at, accessed June 27, 2023, https://www.ncbi.nlm.nih.gov/books/NBK207191/box/part1_ch3.box16/; quotation at Caruth, *Unclaimed Experience*, 58.

11. Jess Bonnan-White, Jewelry Yep, and Melanie D. Hetzel-Riggin, "Voices from the Past: Mental and Physical Outcomes Described by American Civil War Amputees," *Journal of Trauma & Dissociation* 17, no. 1 (2016): 21, 15, respectively.

12. The federal pension authority is listed in documents as Pension Office, Bureau of Pensions, or Pension Agency. The convention throughout this study is "pension office."

13. Joanna Bourke, *Dismembering the Male: Men's Bodies, Britain and the Great War* (Chicago: University of Chicago Press, 1996), 11; italics in the original. On the "coming of age experience" for Northern soldiers, see Reid Mitchell, *The Vacant Chair: The Northern Soldier Leaves Home* (New York: Oxford University Press, 1993).

14. "True Manhood," *West Philadelphia Hospital Register*, August 29, 1863, 3.

15. Lorien Foote, *The Gentlemen and the Roughs: Manhood, Honor, and Violence in the Union Army* (New York: New York University Press, 2010), 3, 19; Elizabeth R. Varon, *Armies of Deliverance: A New History of the Civil War* (New York: Oxford University Press, 2019); Brian Craig Miller, "Manhood," in *A Companion to the Civil War*, ed. Aaron Sheehan-Dean, vol. 2 (Hoboken, NJ: Wiley Blackwell, 2014), 796; E. Anthony Rotundo, *American Manhood: Transformations in Masculinity from the Revolution to the Modern Era* (New York: Basic Books, 1993), 23; Mitchell, *Vacant Chair*, 83.

16. Allen C. Guelzo, *Gettysburg: The Last Invasion* (New York: Alfred A. Knopf, 2013), 173; Mitchell, *Vacant Chair*, 82.

17. Peter S. Carmichael, *The War for the Common Soldier* (Chapel Hill: University of North Carolina Press, 2018), chap. 1.

18. Ibid., 21; Rotundo, *American Manhood*, 10–12. Social expectations placed a premium on discipline and self-government in "that the same discipline that underlay self-government also supported manhood, and that these traits were unevenly distributed among the population." Larry M. Logue and Peter Blanck, *Race, Ethnicity, and Disability: Veterans and Benefits in Post-Civil War America* (New York: Cambridge University Press, 2010), 16. By the onset of war, young men meshed a "restrained manhood" that embodied Protestant Christianity and the identity of family and livelihood with "martial manhood," with its uncivil attributes of violence and physical endurance. See Miller, "Manhood," 802, and Amy Greenberg, *Manifest Manhood and the Antebellum American Empire* (New York: Cambridge University Press, 2005).

19. Keith M. Harris, *Across the Bloody Chasm: The Culture of Commemoration among Civil War Veterans* (Baton Rouge: Louisiana University Press, 2014), 2.

20. Ibid., 3; Union Major General Abner Doubleday, quoted in Guelzo, *Gettysburg*, 276.

21. Rotundo, *American Manhood*, 224; Fay Bound Alberti, "Bodies, Hearts, and Minds, Why Emotions Matter to Historians of Science and Medicine," *Isis* 100 (2009): 801.

22. Letter to niece Sarah from Brandy Station, March 16, 1864, in Henrietta Stratton Jaquette, ed., *Letters of a Civil War Nurse: Cornelia Hancock, 1863–1865* (Lincoln: University of Nebraska Press, 1998), 63. See also Drew Gilpin Faust, *This Republic of Suffering: Death and the Civil War* (New York: Vintage Books, 2008), chap. 5.

23. Anecdote about the Union soldiers sitting within "six paces of a rebel" from Varon, *Armies of Deliverance*, 63.

24. Devine, *Learning from the Wounded*, 29.

25. Simon Harrison, *Dark Trophies: Hunting and the Enemy Body in Modern War* (New York: Berghahn Books, 2012), 95; Leora Auslander, "Beyond Words," *American Historical Review* 110, no. 4 (October 2005): 1017; Sarah Jones Weicksel, "'Peeled' Bodies, Pillaged Homes: Looting and Material Culture in the American Civil War Era," in *Objects of War: The Material Culture of Conflict and Displacement*, ed. Leora Auslander and Tara Zahra (Ithaca, NY: Cornell University Press, 2018), 119.

26. Bourke, *Dismembering the Male*, 128, 133; Roberts Bartholow, *A Manual of Instructions for Enlisting and Discharging Soldiers* (Philadelphia: J. B. Lippincott, 1863), 165–174, quotation at 170, accessed June 27, 2023, https://archive.org/details/62430200R.nlm.nih.gov/page/n3; Sarah Jones

Weicksel, "The Dress of the Enemy: Clothing and Disease in the Civil War Era," *Civil War History* 63, no. 2 (2017): 134. "Wear flannel all over in all weathers," from Louis Le Grand, *The Military Hand-Book and Soldier's Manual of Information* (New York: Beadle, 1861), 89.

27. Bartholow, *Manual of Instructions*, 171–174.

28. Sanford B. Hunt, "The Negro as Soldier," *Anthropological Review* 7, no. 24 (January 1869): 54.

29. Bartholow, *Manual of Instructions*, 94.

30. Ibid., 95–96.

31. Dillon J. Carroll, *Invisible Wounds: Mental Illness and Civil War Soldiers* (Baton Rouge: Louisiana University Press, 2021), 65.

32. Carmichael, *War for the Common Soldier*, 289; "Introduction: The Things They Carried: War, Mobility, and Material Culture," in Auslander and Zahra, *Objects of War*, 8.

33. Kathryn Shively Meier, *Nature's Civil War: Common Soldiers and the Environment in 1862 Virginia* (Chapel Hill: University of North Carolina Press, 2013), 2.

34. Miller, "Manhood," 800; Deborah Willis, *The Black Civil War Soldier: A Visual History of Conflict and Citizenship* (New York: New York University Press, 2021), 174–178. The album resides at the Yale Collection of America Literature, Beinecke Rare Book and Manuscript Library, Randolph Linsly Simpson African-American collection, box 35, folder 1092–83.

35. Alan Trachtenberg, *Reading American Photographs: Images as History Mathew Brady to Walker Evans* (New York: Hill and Wang, 1989), 59. First Lieutenant Charles Minor Blackford, 30th Virginia Volunteers, quoted in Varon, *Armies of Deliverance*, 27; Weicksel, "'Peeled' Bodies," 119; Harrison, *Dark Trophies*, 5.

36. Jim Downs, *Sick from Freedom: African-American Illness and Suffering during the Civil War and Reconstruction* (New York: Oxford University Press, 2012), 4.

37. Bourke, *Dismembering the Male*, 31 (italics in the original); Alberti, "Bodies, Hearts, and Minds," 808; S. Weir Mitchell, George R. Morehouse, and W. W. Keen Jr., *Gunshot Wounds and Other Injuries of Nerves* (Philadelphia: J. B. Lippincott, 1864), 20; Devine, *Learning from the Wounded*, 153.

38. Private Marion C. Frost, Co. G, 89th New York Volunteers, and Corporal Chas. Chadbourne, Co. A, Eleventh US Infantry; "Deaths," *West Philadelphia Hospital Register*, February 14, 1863, 3.

39. Ibid.

40. In the flap method, the surgeon retained flaps of skin, which were secured above the amputation site. Following the removal of the limb,

the flaps were folded together below the stump so that when the wound healed, a cushion of flesh was created. This cushion in a leg wound enabled the wearing of a prosthesis that bore the weight of the upper body.

41. "Died of His Wounds," *West Philadelphia Hospital Register*, August 22, 1863, 165–166.

42. Ibid.

43. Ibid.

44. Ibid.

45. Ibid.; Michelle M. Sauer, "Touching Jesus: Christ's Side Wound & Medieval Manuscript Tradition," *Women's Literary Culture and the Medieval Canon* (University of Surrey) blog, posted January 5, 2016, accessed June 27, 2023, https://blogs.surrey.ac.uk/medievalwomen/2016/01/05/touching-jesus-christs-side-wound-medieval-manuscript-tradition; Erin Corrales Diaz, "Remembering the Veteran: Disability, Trauma, and the American Civil War, 1861–1915" (PhD diss., University of North Carolina, 2016), 158.

46. "Our Duty as Individuals in the *Present* Crisis," *West Philadelphia Hospital Register*, March 7, 1863, 15.

47. Lisa Marie Herschbach, quoted in Megan Kate Nelson, *Ruin Nation: Destruction and the American Civil War* (Athens: University of Georgia Press, 2012), 161; Suzannah Biernoff, *Portraits of Violence: War and the Aesthetics of Disfigurement* (Ann Arbor: University of Michigan Press, 2017), 4, 6; Faust, *This Republic of Suffering.*

48. Biernoff, *Portraits of Violence*, 56, 65; Bourke, *Dismembering the Male*, 44; William W. Etter, *The Good Body: Normalizing Visions in Nineteenth-Century American Literature and Culture, 1836–1867* (Newcastle upon Tyne: Cambridge Scholars, 2010), 5–11.

49. Faust, *This Republic of Suffering*, 9–10; Whitman quotation from his letter to Ralph Waldo Emerson dated January 17, 1863, quoted at Tuggle, *Afterlives of Specimens*, 8.

50. Francis Clarke, "'Honorable Scars': Northern Amputees and the Meaning of Civil War Injuries," in *Union Soldiers and the Northern Home Front: Wartime Experiences, Postwar Adjustments*, ed. Paul A. Cimbala and Randall M. Miller (New York: Fordham University Press, 2002), 366; Erin O'Connor, "'Fractions of Men': Engendering Amputation in Victorian Culture," *Comparative Studies in Society and History* 39 (1997): 744; O'Connor, *Raw Material: Producing Pathology in Victorian Culture* (Durham, NC: Duke University Press, 2000), 104; Corrales Diaz, "Remembering the Veteran," 157.

51. ADA National Network website, accessed June 27, 2023, https://adata.org/learn-about-ada; Etter, *Good Body*, 11.
52. Corrales Diaz, "Remembering the Veteran," 4.
53. Ibid., 54, 5, respectively.
54. Quoted at Corrales Diaz, "Remembering the Veteran," 20.
55. Dance theater director Alain Platel concluded that "normal" bodies do not exist and that "people with a disability have some kind of advantage over the so-called normal people, as if the disability has made them aware that there is no time to waste to make something special out of life." Platel, "Everyone Has Something to Tell," in *The Sentient Archive: Bodies, Performance, and Memory*, ed. Bill Bissell and Linda Caruso Haviland (Middletown, CT: Wesleyan University Press, 2018), 23. Quotation from Erving Goffman's *Stigma: Notes on the Management of Spoiled Identity* (London: Penguin, 1968), cited in Biernoff, *Portraits of Violence*, 3, 22–23, 65, 166; Bourke, *Dismembering the Male*, 44.
56. Trachtenberg, *Reading American Photographs*, 118.
57. Emily Dickinson, *Poems* (New York: Alfred A. Knopf, 1993), 61.
58. Martin S. Pernick, *A Calculus of Suffering: Pain, Professionalism, and Anesthesia in Nineteenth-Century America* (New York: Columbia University Press, 1985), 42, 162, respectively.
59. Frances M. Clarke, *War Stories: Suffering and Sacrifice in the Civil War North* (Chicago: University of Chicago Press, 2011), 10–11.
60. Ibid.
61. Even today, anesthesia during surgery is dangerous. In 1970, about one out of every two thousand anesthetized patients died of it. Pernick, *Calculus of Suffering*, 38–41; Susan Sontag, *Regarding the Pain of Others* (New York: Farrar, Strauss and Giroux, 2003), 42.
62. Robert I. Goler, "Loss and the Persistence of Memory: 'The Case of George Dedlow' and Disabled Civil War Veterans," *Literature and Medicine* 23, no. 1 (Spring 2004): 171; Devine, *Learning from the Wounded*, 157.
63. Sontag, *Regarding the Pain of Others*, 126.
64. "An Elementary Treatise on Human Anatomy" in Lindsay Tuggle, *Calenture* (Victoria: Cordite, 2018), 53.

2. SILAS WEIR MITCHELL (1829–1914)

1. Part of the scapula next to the head of the humerus.
2. Today, denoted thoracic vertebra T8.
3. S. Weir Mitchell, "On the Diseases of Nerves, Resulting from Injuries," in *Contributions Relating to the Causation and Prevention of Diseases,*

ed. Austin Flint (New York: US Sanitary Commission, 1867), 448–451 (Case 31). Also described under Case 31 in Mitchell et al., *Gunshot Wounds*, 148–152.

4. Per Dunglison, "difficulty of deglutition," or the act of swallowing.

5. Per Dunglison, "acute lancinating pain in one side of the chest increased by inspiration."

6. John H. Packard, *A Manual of Minor Surgery* (Philadelphia: J. B. Lippincott, 1863), 15; S. D. Gross, *A Manual of Military Surgery* (Philadelphia: J. B. Lippincott, 1862), 63. Although I quote from Robley Dunglison's *Medical Lexicon* to explicate nineteenth-century medical terms, to translate them into twenty-first-century equivalents, I relied on Alice Roberts, ed., *The Complete Human Body: The Definitive Visual Guide*, 2nd ed. (New York: Dorling Kindersley, 2016).

7. Mitchell notes from July 5, 1863, "On the Diseases of Nerves," 448.

8. The muscle over the shoulder joint.

9. Per Dunglison, a blister is "any substance which, when applied to the skin, irritates it, and occasions a serous [bloody] secretion, raising the epidermis, and inducing a vesicle [the blister]."

10. At war's end, Mitchell concluded, "Conia, atropia, and daturia [now called datura, otherwise known as jimson weed or thorn apple, known to have analgesic value] have no power to lessen pain when used subdermally. . . . Morphia thus used is of the utmost value to relieve pain, and is most potent, in certain forms of neuralgia, the nearer it is applied to the seat of the suffering." S. Weir Mitchell, George R. Morehouse, and W. W. Keen Jr., "On the Antagonism of Atropia and Morphia, Founded upon Observations and Experiments Made at the U.S.A. Hospital for Injuries and Diseases of the Nervous System," *American Journal of the Medical Sciences* 50, no. 99, New Series (July 1865): 67–76.

11. Quotations at Mitchell notes from July 5, 1863, "On the Diseases of Nerves," 450, 449, respectively.

12. Sometimes called Spanish Fly, a vesicant derived from flies of the order Coleoptera.

13. Muscles governing forearm, hand.

14. Ibid., 450.

15. To distinguish between the two Mitchells, "Mitchell" denotes Silas Weir Mitchell. His son is referred to by his full name.

16. John K. Mitchell, *Remote Consequences of Injuries of Nerves, and Their Treatment* (Philadelphia: Lea Brothers, 1895), 73–78.

17. Mitchell et al., *Gunshot Wounds*, 3.

18. Now viewed as a form of shock, reflex paralysis referred to the "collapse [of the nerves] from being in proximity of an explosion without any sign of external injury." James L. Stone, "W. W. Keen: America's Pioneer Neurological Surgeon," *Neurosurgery* 17, no. 6 (1985): 1000.

19. William S. Middleton, "Turner's Lane Hospital" (the Fielding H. Garrison Lecture delivered at the thirty-eighth annual meeting of the American Association for the History of Medicine, Philadelphia, April 30, 1965), *Bulletin of the History of Medicine* 40 (1966): 41.

20. Bonnie Ellen Blustein, *Preserve Your Love for Science: Life of William A. Hammond, American Neurologist* (Cambridge: Cambridge University Press, 1991), 49; also 47–72 regarding the Philadelphia work on wounded nerves; S. Weir Mitchell, *Injuries of Nerves and Their Consequences* (Philadelphia: J. B. Lippincott, 1872), 10; Frank R. Freemon, "The First Neurological Research Center: Turner's Lane Hospital during the American Civil War," *Journal of the History of the Neurosciences* 2 (1993): 137; Mitchell et al., *Gunshot Wounds*, 9–10; Nancy Cervetti, *S. Weir Mitchell, 1829–1914: Philadelphia's Literary Physician* (University Park: Pennsylvania State University Press, 2012), 68.

21. Freemon, "First Neurological Research Center," 139; Stone, "W. W. Keen," 999.

22. Mitchell, *Injuries of Nerves*, 13.

23. Mitchell et al., *Gunshot Wounds*, 143; Middleton, "Turner's Lane Hospital," 35; Mitchell, *Injuries of Nerves*, 10–11.

24. Caruth, *Unclaimed Experience*, 4, 7, 11; Daniel Goldberg, "'What They Think of the Causes of So Much Suffering': S. Weir Mitchell, John Kearsley Mitchell, and Ideas about Phantom Limb Pain in Late 19th c. America," *Spontaneous Generations: A Journal for the History and Philosophy of Science*, 8, no. 1 (2016): 28.

25. Mitchell, *Injuries of Nerves*, 139, 136, respectively.

26. Cervetti, *S. Weir Mitchell*, 71; Mitchell, *Injuries of Nerves*, 39; Elaine Scarry, *The Body in Pain: The Making and Unmaking of the World* (New York: Oxford University Press, 1985), 4–5.

27. Caruth, *Unclaimed Experience*, 61; Christina Cavedon, *Cultural Melancholia: US Trauma Discourses Before and After 9/11* (Boston: Brill, 2015), 40; S. Weir Mitchell, *Clinical Lessons on Nervous Diseases* (Philadelphia: Lea Brothers, 1897), 26.

28. Ibid., 26–27, 59.

29. Mitchell, *Injuries of Nerves*, 65.

30. The muscles extending from forearm to thumb.

31. Ibid., 292, 295; Cervetti, *S. Weir Mitchell*, 76; Mitchell et al., *Gunshot Wounds*, 112.

32. The term *causalgia* was suggested by Mitchell's colleague, Robley Dunglison. Mitchell, *Injuries of Nerves*, 13, 39, 41, respectively; Mitchell et al., *Gunshot Wounds*, 101; D. J. Canale, "Civil War Medicine from the Perspective of S. Weir Mitchell's 'The Case of George Dedlow,'" *Journal of the History of the Neurosciences* 11, no. 1 (2002): 14.

33. Mitchell et al., *Gunshot Wounds*, 86, 103, 105.

34. S. Weir Mitchell, "Clinical Lecture on Nervousness in the Male," *Medical News and Library* 35 (December 1877): 178; Mitchell, *Injuries to Nerves*, 201.

35. Mitchell et al., *Gunshot Wounds*, 106; quotation from W. W. Keen, S. Weir Mitchell, and George R. Morehouse, "On malingering, Especially in Regard to Simulation of Diseases of the Nervous System," *American Journal of Medical Science* 48 (October 1864): 377 (italics in the original).

36. Mitchell et al., "Antagonism of Atropia and Morphia," 68–69; Case 31, in Mitchell et al., *Gunshot Wounds*, 151.

37. Mitchell et al., *Gunshot Wounds*, 134; Professor B. Howard Rand of Central High School in Philadelphia, a school boasting perhaps the best physical sciences laboratory in the city, loaned Mitchell the galvanometer and other apparatuses.

38. Cervetti, *S. Weir Mitchell*, 111; Mitchell et al., *Gunshot Wounds*, 144–145, 71, respectively; Mitchell, *Injuries of Nerves*, 10–11.

39. Stone, "W. W. Keen," 474; Paul Gillmore, "Romantic Electricity, or the Materiality of Aesthetics," *American Literature* 76, no. 3 (September 2004): 483.

40. Keen, in *S. Weir Mitchell . . . Memorial Addresses and Resolutions* (Philadelphia: privately printed, 1914), 14; Owen Wister, "Owen Wister Views Life of Dr. S.W. Mitchell," *Philadelphia Press*, April 15, 1914.

41. Anna Robeson Burr, *Weir Mitchell: His Life and Letters* (New York: Duffield, 1929), 105; S. Weir Mitchell letters to Elizabeth K. Mitchell, MSS 2/0241-03, Series 3.4, Historical Medical Library, College of Physicians of Philadelphia.

42. Cervetti, *S. Weir Mitchell*, 74; S. Weir Mitchell, "EDM," in *The Collected Poems of S. Weir Mitchell* (New York: Century, 1896), 270.

43. Devine, *Learning from the Wounded*, 137–138.

44. Rotundo, *American Manhood*, 208; Bobby A. Wintermute, *Public Health and the U.S. Military: A History of the Army Medical Department 1818–1917* (New York: Routledge, 2011), 45, 47.

45. Wintermute, *Public Health*, 21, 23; Stuart McConnell, *Glorious Contentment: The Grand Army of the Republic, 1865–1900* (Chapel Hill: University of North Carolina Press, 1992), 222.

46. Lindsey Grubbs, "'Her Sex Points to Hysteria': Diagnostic Narratives in a Student Notebook," *Fugitive Leaves* blog, accessed December 5, 2023, http://histmed.collegeofphysicians.org/her-sex-points-to-hysteria; Lisa Herschbach, "'True Clinical Fictions': Medical and Literary Narratives from the Civil War Hospital," *Culture, Medicine and Psychiatry* 19 (1995): 192.

47. Quoted at Cervetti, *S. Weir Mitchell*, 68.

48. Charles W. Burr, *S Weir Mitchell: Physician, Man of Science, Man of Letters, Man of Affairs* (Philadelphia: College of Physicians of Philadelphia, 1920), 112; Cervetti, *S. Weir Mitchell*, 88ff.

49. Tuggle, *Afterlives of Specimens*, 64–65; Walt Whitman, *The Wound Dresser*, ed. Richard Maurice Buck (Boston: Small, Maynard, 1898), 64, quoted from a letter to his mother, April 15, 1863.

50. Mitchell et al., *Gunshot Wounds*, 20; McConnell, *Glorious Contentment*, 222.

51. Mitchell et al., *Gunshot Wounds*, 115; see Case #28, 128ff.; Mitchell, *Injuries of Nerves*, 10–11. The Invalid Corps consisted of soldiers not fit for field service. They wore a distinctive uniform and responded to the army chain of command. See S. Weir Mitchell, "Some Personal Recollections of the Civil War," *Transactions of the College of Physicians of Philadelphia* 27 (Third Series, 1905): 93.

52. Mitchell et al., *Gunshot Wounds*, 63.

53. S. Weir Mitchell Papers, Turner's Lane Hospital, case and follow-up studies of peripheral nerve disorders, MSS 2/241-03, Series 1, folder 5, Historical Medical Library, College of Physicians of Philadelphia.

54. Mitchell, *Injuries of Nerves*, 66.

55. Ibid., 145, 364.

56. Clarke, *War Stories*, 22, 146; Mitchell et al., *Gunshot Wounds*, 157.

57. S. Weir Mitchell, "The Medical Department in the Civil War," *Journal of the American Medical Association* 62, no. 19 (May 9, 1914): 1448; letter to mother, September 15, 1863, in Whitman, *Wound Dresser*, 116; letter to Mrs. Abby Price, October 11, 1863, in same volume, 127.

58. Cervetti, *S. Weir Mitchell*, 55; Anne M. Stiles, "'The Intimate Language of Friendship with Men': Same-Sex Attraction in the Civil War Fiction of S. Weir Mitchell," *Literature and Medicine* 32, no. 1 (Spring 2014): 195.

59. Ibid., 195, 208.

60. Bourke, *Dismembering the Male*, 133; Stiles, "Intimate Language," 202.

61. Eric T. Dean Jr., *Shook over Hell: Post-Traumatic Stress, Vietnam, and the Civil War* (Cambridge, MA: Harvard University Press, 1997), 117.

62. Per Dunglison: "A condition in which the system of nutrition is evidently depraved. A bad habit of body, chiefly the result of scorbutic, cancerous, tuberculous or venereal diseases when in their advanced stage."

63. Bartholow, *Manual of Instructions*, 23, 21, 17, respectively; Dean, *Shook over Hell*, 117–119; Carroll, *Invisible Wounds*, 93ff.

64. Mitchell, "Clinical Lecture," 179, 183, 180, respectively.

65. Bourke, *Dismembering the Male*, 78, 91; Carmichael, *War for the Common Soldier*, 135.

66. "Malingering" and "Abraham man" appear in Dunglison's *Medical Lexicon*. See also Keen et al., "On Malingering," 368.

67. Ibid., 373, 371, respectively.

68. Mark S. Micale, *Hysterical Men: The Hidden History of Male Nervous Illness* (Cambridge, MA: Harvard University Press, 2008), 102.

69. Ibid., 193; Dean, *Shook over Hell*, 27. Mitchell's most recent biographer takes a contrary view, stating that Mitchell's appropriation of hysteria to men's pain responses effectively desexed the term, whereupon "hysteria [became] a disease of the nervous system, impartial to sex and requiring neither emasculation nor a faulty uterus to thrive." Cervetti, *S. Weir Mitchell*, 84.

70. Micale, *Hysterical Men*, 60; Mitchell, *Clinical Lessons*, 21; Mitchell, *Injuries of Nerves*, 62.

71. Mitchell, *Clinical Lessons*, 104–106, 242.

72. Ibid., 183; Devine, *Learning from the Wounded*, 154.

73. Mitchell Papers, MSS2/241-03 box 11, Series 4.5, folder 1–6.

74. Mitchell Papers, MSS2/241-03 box 11, Series 4.5, folder 2–19.

75. John K. Mitchell, *Remote Consequences*, 14; Devine, *Learning from the Wounded*, 156.

76. Per Dunglison, "Debility or impaired activity of the nerves."

77. Mitchell, *Remote Consequences*, 223–228.

78. Ken Kryvoruka, "A Neurologist's Wartime Medical Breakthroughs," *Washington Times*, November 25, 2000, B3; Keen, in *S. Weir Mitchell . . . Memorial Addresses*, 16.

79. Devine, *Learning from the Wounded*, 140–142; Keen, in *S. Weir Mitchell . . . Memorial Addresses*, 16.

80. Quoted in Burr, *Weir Mitchell*, 105.

81. Cervetti, *S. Weir Mitchell*, 76.

82. Eric J. Pappert, "Philadelphia Infirmary for Nervous Diseases: America's Original Model of Institutional Neurology," *Neurology* 50, no. 6 (1998): 1847–1853; Mitchell, "Medical Department," 1445. This essay appeared in print four months after Mitchell died.

83. "On Slain Collegians," Herman Melville, *The Battle-Pieces of Herman Melville*, ed. Hennig Cohen (New York: Thomas Yoseloff, 1964), 144.

3. ELECTRIC AGONY

1. Joseph S. Davis case notes, Silas Weir Mitchell Papers, Z10 40 Series 1, folder 4, Item 1.

2. Gillmore, "Romantic Electricity," 474.

3. Devine, *Learning from the Wounded*, 137.

4. Gillmore, "Romantic Electricity," 476.

5. Ibid., 483.

6. Ronald Melzack, "Phantom Limbs," *Scientific American* 266 (April 1992): 120–126; *Whitmanweb*, accessed June 28, 2023, https://iwp.uiowa.edu/whitmanweb/en/writings/song-of-myself/section-27; Gillmore, "Romantic Electricity," 479.

7. Chauncy Hare Townshend, *The Three Gates* (London: Chapman and Hall, 1861), xxvii; quotations from "The Clock," 292, and "Parting," 188.

8. "Influence of the Telegraph upon Literature," *United States Democratic Review* (May 1848): 410.

9. "Influence of Telegraph," 411, 413; William F. Channing, "On the Municipal Electric Telegraph; Especially in Its Application to Fire Alarms," *American Journal of Science and Arts* 13, 2nd ser. (January 1852): 58–59.

10. Stella Pratt-Smith, *Transformations of Electricity in Nineteenth-Century Literature and Science* (Farnham: Ashgate, 2016), 38, 69; Gillmore, "Romantic Electricity," 472.

11. Goler, "Loss and the Persistence of Memory," 175. See also Iwan Rhys Morus, "Galvanic Cultures: Electricity and Life in the Early Nineteenth Century," *Endeavour* 22, no. 1 (1998): 7–11.

12. Faraday quoted in William F. Channing, *The Medical Application of Electricity*, 5th ed. (Boston: Thomas Hall, 1859), 4–5.

13. Alfred C. Garratt, *Guide for Using Medical Batteries* (Philadelphia: Lindsay and Blakiston, 1867), 7.

14. Julius Althaus, *A Treatise on Medical Electricity, Theoretical and Practical* (Philadelphia: Lindsay and Blakiston, 1860), 1; Beard quotation at R.

Gregory Lande, *Psychological Consequences of the American Civil War* (Jefferson, NC: McFarland, 2017), 194.

15. Gillmore, "Romantic Electricity," 474; Channing, *Medical Applications*, 9; Mitchell, *Injuries of Nerves*, 43; Mitchell et al., *Gunshot Wounds*, 71.

16. Mitchell et al., *Gunshot Wounds*, 8.

17. Dean P. Currier, *A Guide to Electrotherapy Instruments and History of Their American Makers* (West Conshohocken, PA: Infinity, 2005), 30.

18. Mitchell, "On the Diseases of Nerves," 451; Channing, *Medical Applications*, quotations at 16 and 45, respectively.

19. Blustein, *Preserve Your Love for Science*, 127; Mitchell, "On the Diseases of Nerves," 454.

20. Mitchell et al., *Gunshot Wounds*, 136; Mitchell, "On the Diseases of Nerves," 454–455.

21. Per Dunglison, a large, thick muscle at the calf that "extend[s] the foot on the leg, and the leg on the foot."

22. Mitchell et al., *Gunshot Wounds*, 128–129.

23. Ibid.

24. Gerard L'E. Turner, *Nineteenth-Century Scientific Instruments* (London: Sotheby, 1983), 173; Currier, *Electrotherapy Instruments*, 2–6, 19; Margaret Rowbottom and Charles Susskind, *Electricity and Medicine: History of Their Interaction* (San Francisco: San Francisco Press, 1984), 16–17.

25. Rowbottom and Susskind, *Electricity and Medicine*.

26. Mitchell and his contemporaries used water to enhance conductivity in their therapies.

27. Channing, *Medical Applications*, 32.

28. Per Dunglison, tissue includes "the various parts, which, by their union, form the organs; and are . . . anatomical elements. Histological anatomy is the anatomy of the tissues, which are the seat of the investigations of the pathological anatomist."

29. Mitchell, "On the Diseases of Nerves," 454; Currier, *Electrotherapy Instruments*, 23–25.

30. Rowbottom and Susskind, *Electricity and Medicine*, 72; Mitchell, "On the Diseases of Nerves," 453; Mitchell et al., *Gunshot Wounds*, 14; Channing, *Medical Applications*, 34–35, 44.

31. Mitchell, "On the Diseases of Nerves," 452, 454; Mitchell et al., *Gunshot Wounds*, 141, 187.

32. Mitchell, "On the Diseases of Nerves," 453; Channing, *Medical Applications*, 15.

33. Mitchell et al., *Gunshot Wounds*, 144, 156.

34. Ibid., 115, 187–188.

35. Sometimes called "nickel silver," an alloy of zinc, nickel, and copper.

36. Franklin Spencer Edmonds, *History of Central High School of Philadelphia* (Philadelphia: J. B. Lippincott, 1902), 179–183. Rand taught chemistry at Central High School from 1859 to 1864 and thereafter taught at Jefferson Medical College, Philadelphia; Mitchell et al., *Gunshot Wounds,* 134, 185; Willem D. Hackmann, "Thermopile," in *Instruments of Science: An Historical Encyclopedia,* ed. Robert Bud and Deborah Jean Warner (New York: Garland, 1998), 618–619.

37. D. Appleton, *The American Annual Encyclopedia and Register of Important Events of the Year 1867,* vol. 7 (New York: D. Appleton, 1868), 292; Willem D. Hackmann, "Galvanometer," in *Instruments of Science,* 257–259; Turner, *Nineteenth-Century Scientific Instruments,* 200.

38. Mitchell et al., *Gunshot Wounds,* 138; Mitchell, "On the Diseases of Nerves," 453.

39. Channing, *Medical Applications,* 15; Mitchell et al., *Gunshot Wounds,* 142; Currier, *Electrotherapy Instruments,* 31. The unreliable currents obtained with magneto-electric machines were identified as a chronic drawback almost twenty years before the war. See George M. Beard and A. B. Rockwell, *The Medical Use of Electricity* (New York: William Wood, 1847), 62.

40. Mitchell, "On the Diseases of Nerves," 452–453.

41. Mitchell, "Clinical Lecture," 183; Devine, *Learning from the Wounded,* 144–188.

42. Mitchell, *Remote Consequences,* 235; Melzack, "Phantom Limbs," 125.

43. Quoted in Devine, *Learning from the Wounded,* 148.

44. S. Weir Mitchell, "Phantom Limbs," *Lippincott's Magazine of Popular Literature and Science* 7 (December 1871): 566.

45. Mitchell, *Remote Consequences,* 234.

46. Ibid., 231–232.

47. Laura McWhirter, Alan Carson, and Jon Stone, "The Body Electric: A Long View of Electrical Therapy for Functional Neurological Disorders," *Brain, a Journal of Neurology* 138 (2015): 1119. Today, electrical stimulation exists in a variety of medical contexts, from stimulating peripheral nerves to bone growth in cancer patients. The more sophisticated technology that serves a comparable purpose is transcranial magnetic stimulation, or TMS.

48. Pappert, "Philadelphia Infirmary," 1850; Rowbottom and Susskind, *Electricity and Medicine,* 113.

49. Mitchell, *Remote Consequences,* 228; also known as Kelvin's galvanometer, distinguished by using a light beam that is deflected by the

electric current and thus places a spot of light onto a scale. See S. Weir Mitchell, "On the Transmission of Electric Influence across the Middle Line of the Body," pamphlet (New York: Putnam's Sons, 1877), reprint from *Transactions of the American Neurological Association* (1877).

50. Mitchell, *Injuries of Nerves*, 10–11, 250.

51. Mitchell et al., *Gunshot Wounds*, 85–86.

52. Channing, *Medical Application of Electricity*, 6.

53. Lisa A. Long, *Rehabilitating Bodies: Health, History, and the American Civil War* (Philadelphia: University of Pennsylvania Press, 2004), 31, 33.

54. McWhirter et al., "Body Electric," 1119.

55. Devine, *Learning from the Wounded*, 144; Elan D. Louis, Stacy Horn, and Lisa Anne Roth, "The Neurologic Content of S. Weir Mitchell's Fiction," *Neurology* 66, no. 3 (February 14, 2006): 406; Mitchell et al., *Gunshot Wounds*, 137.

4. HENRY ADOLPH KIRCHER (1841–1908)

1. Henry A. Kircher, letter to mother, January 3, 1863, in Earl J. Hess, ed., *A German in the Yankee Fatherland: The Civil War Letters of Henry Kircher* (Kent, OH: Kent State University Press, 1983), 47.

2. Ibid., 145; Mary Bobbitt Townsend, *Yankee Warhorse; A Biography of Major General Peter Osterhaus* (Columbia: University of Missouri Press, 2010), 136–144.

3. Guelzo, *Gettysburg*, 279; Consolidated Service Record (CSR) for Henry Adolph Kircher, National Archives and Records Administration (NARA). The quoted discussion between Kircher and Spiegelhalter that follows comes from the Casualty Report, CSR; Mitchell questionnaire for Kircher, MSS2-0241-03, Series 4.5, box 11, folder 2–6, Historical Medical Library, College of Physicians of Philadelphia.

4. Gross, *Manual of Military Surgery*, 75.

5. United States Pension Office, *Roster of All Regimental Surgeons and Assistant Surgeons* (Washington, DC, 1882), 127–129. Kohly and Bruckner duly appear in the *Roster of All Regimental Surgeons*, but the Casualty Report lists one other doctor, apparently "D. Newell" of the 31st Missouri. No such name appears in any official listing, but a Horace Newell is listed as assistant surgeon in the 32nd Missouri, which combined with the 31st in November 1864. The 32nd was present at Ringgold Gap; Gross, *Manual of Military Surgery*, 81.

6. Proximity of the medial epicondyle of the humerus.

7. Proximity of the medial condyle of the tibia.

8. Packard, *Manual of Minor Surgery*, 87–89. This manual was endorsed by the army surgeon general for army use.

9. Ibid., 280.

10. Ibid., 30–35.

11. Per Dunglison, "Formation or secretion of pus. . . . It is a frequent termination of inflammation, and may occur in almost any of the tissues."

12. Ibid., 32–34, 110–111, 280–283.

13. Laurann Figg and Jane Farrell-Beck, "Amputation in the Civil War: Physical and Social Dimensions," *Journal of the History of Medicine and Allied Sciences* 48, no. 4 (October 1993): 457; figures derived from *The Medical and Surgical History of the War of the Rebellion*, Surgical History, part 3, vol. 2, Joseph K. Barnes, ed. (Washington, DC: US Government Printing Office, 1883), 877. Note that the precise number of amputations will never be known; records are uneven and inconsistently created.

14. Kircher's surgeries are listed in *Medical and Surgical History*, Surgical History, part 2, vol. 2 (1876), 727, 883; part 3, vol. 2 (1883), 250; Hess, *German in the Yankee Fatherland*, 149.

15. Letter from father to Kircher, December 14, 1863, Hess, *German in the Yankee Fatherland*, 150.

16. Whitman, *Wound Dresser*, 38.

17. Carmichael, *War for the Common Soldier*, 80.

18. Regulations from Julian J. Chisholm, *A Manual of Military Surgery* (Richmond, VA: West & Johnston, 1861), 416–419; Brian Craig Miller, *Empty Sleeves: Amputation in the Civil War South* (Athens: University of Georgia Press, 2015), 18, 33, 124.

19. Pernick, *Calculus of Suffering*, 143, 232ff.

20. Carmichael's study notes that the psychological consequences of warfare generally were suffered privately: "There was no conversation, no confiding, and no attempt to understand. It appears that the soldier was left in isolation to brood in his thoughts." Carmichael, *War for the Common Soldier*, 144.

21. William L. Burton, *Melting Pot Soldiers: The Union's Ethnic Regiments* (Ames: Iowa State University Press, 1988), 107–108; Logue and Blanck, *Race, Ethnicity, and Disability*, 89–92.

22. Quoted in Hess, *German in the Yankee Fatherland*, 5.

23. Pernick, *Calculus of Suffering*, 4–7.

24. Hess, *German in the Yankee Fatherland*, 26; letter to mother (March 2, 1863), 74; letter to father (April 19, 1863), 92.

25. Nelson, *Ruin Nation*, 4, 196.

26. John Ordronaux, *Manual of Instruction for Military Surgeons, on the Examination of Recruits and Discharge of Soldiers* (New York: Van Nostrand, 1863), 21–22; Kim E. Nielsen, *A Disability History of the United States* (Boston: Beacon, 2012), 89.

27. *Medical and Surgical History*, part 3, vol. 2, 883.

28. Miller, *Empty Sleeves*, 4, 124; Foote, *Gentlemen and the Roughs*, 55–58.

29. Descriptive Roll, 12th Missouri Infantry, Adjutant General's Office, Jefferson City, MO, quoted in Hess, *German in the Yankee Fatherland*, 7. Unless otherwise noted, all discussion of Kircher's pension correspondence comes from his official pension record, hereafter cited as Pension File (PF), NARA.

30. *Belleville Weekly Advocate*, April 22, 1864, quoted in Hess, *German in the Yankee Fatherland*, 154.

31. Figg and Farrell-Beck, "Amputation in the Civil War," 465, 468.

32. From 1863 until subsequent revisions after the war, the government authorized fifty dollars to recompense a lost hand, foot, or a leg. Ibid., 460, 463.

33. Ibid., 462; Nelson, *Ruin Nation*, 217–218.

34. Nelson, *Ruin Nation*, 212, 220.

35. Handwritten affidavit, St. Clair County, September 24, 1864, PF.

36. Twenty dollars in 1864 equates to $377 today, which buys 5.3 percent of what it could buy in 1864. Twenty-four dollars in 1872 equates to $583 today, which buys 4 percent of what it could buy then. Monetary equivalents are contingent on many variables and are therefore approximate. Throughout this book, equivalency computations come from the Consumer Price Indicator Inflation Computer accessed June 28, 2023, https://www.in2013dollars.com/.

37. *Belleville Weekly Advocate*, November 18, 1864; "Claim for an Invalid Pension" application, December 29, 1864.

38. "Dr. Bly's Artificial Leg," *The Shelf* blog, Harvard Library Collections, accessed November 8, 2021, https://blogs.harvard.edu/preserving/2014/01/13/dr-blys-artificial-leg/.

39. Douglas Bly, "A Remarkable Invention in Artificial Legs," pamphlet (Rochester, NY: Curtis, Butts, 1862).

40. Guy R. Hasegawa, *Mending Broken Soldiers: The Union and Confederate Programs to Supply Artificial Limbs* (Carbondale: Southern Illinois University Press, 2012), 21–23, 32, 42, 76.

41. Ibid., 13.

42. Hess, *German in the Yankee Fatherland*, 159; *Belleville Weekly Advocate*, March 17, 1865, March 20, 1865, and September 28, 1865.

43. Hess, *German in the Yankee Fatherland*, 159.

44. US passport issued February 27, 1869, Henry A. Kircher, roll *158, December 1, 1863, to March 3, 1869*, NARA; United States Census 1870, roll M593_280, 354A, Belleville, St. Clair, IL.

45. Application for an artificial limb, August 9, 1870, to be forwarded to the Surgeon General, Washington, DC, PF.

46. Staatsarchiv Hamburg, Hamburg, Deutschland; *Hamburger Passagierlisten*; microfilm no.: *K_1717; Kircher traveled Erste Kajüte or First Cabin*; sworn statement before Charles Becker, Clerk, Circuit Court, Rec'd Pension Office August 4, 1874; Increase of Invalid Pension application, August 26, 1874, PF.

47. *Belleville Weekly Advocate*, July 10, 1874; December 25, 1874; January 22, 1875.

48. Ibid., January 20, 1877, July 13, 1877; Hess, *German in the Yankee Fatherland*, 160.

49. Hess, *German in the Yankee Fatherland*; *Belleville Weekly Advocate*, July 27, 1877.

50. Equivalent to $1,015 today, which buys only 3.5 percent of what it could buy in 1877.

51. Statement before Louis C. Starkel, Clerk of County Court, October 1, 1877; Examining Surgeon's Certificate in the Case of an Applicant for Increase of Pension, November 8, 1877, PF.

52. *Belleville Weekly Advocate*, January 25, 1878; December 13, 1878.

53. Sworn statement before Charles Becker, Clerk, Circuit Court, St. Clair County, July 28, 1879, PF.

54. *Belleville Weekly Advocate*, April 9, 1880.

55. Ibid., May 7, 1880; Hess, *German in the Yankee Fatherland*, letter to Bertha dated April 18, 1880, 160–161; 1880 Census, Belleville, St. Clair, IL, roll 247, 335D.

56. Figg and Farrell-Beck, "Amputation in the Civil War," 468.

57. Equates to $1,045 today, which buys 3.4 percent of what it bought in 1881.

58. Declaration for an Increase of an Invalid Pension, April 14, 1881; Examining Surgeon's Certificate in the Case of an Applicant for Increase of Pension, May 17, 1881; Increase Invalid Pension, June 20, 1881, PF.

59. *Belleville Weekly Advocate*, August 13, 1880; January 8, 1886; March 14, 1884.

60. Ibid., November 2, 1883.

61. Surgeon's Certificate, November 10, 1886, PF.

62. Sworn statement before Phillip Rhein, Clerk, County Court, June 29, 1887, attached to Amended Petition, stamped as received by Pension Office July 5, 1887, PF.

63. Figg and Farrell-Beck, "Amputation in the Civil War," 464.

64. *Belleville Weekly Advocate*, April 6, 1888; letter to John G. Black, Commissioner of Pensions re: Pension Certificate 36243, August 8, 1888, PF.

65. Increase form, August 16, 1888, PF.

66. Reissue to Correct Rate Invalid Pension, July 25, 1889, PF; *Belleville Weekly Advocate*, November 8, 1889.

67. Ibid., February 15, 1889; November 28, 1890; November 20, 1891.

68. Goldberg, "'What They Think of the Causes of So Much Suffering,'" 32.

69. Bonnan-White et al., "Voices from the Past," 26; *Belleville Weekly Advocate*, November 2, 1883.

70. Ibid., April 20, 1894; March 13, 1896.

71. Ibid., obituary, January 10, 1896.

72. United States Census 1900, Belleville Ward 1, St. Clair, IL, 17.

73. Letter from Pennebaker & Jones, Attorneys and Counselors, Washington, DC, December 2, 1902, PF.

74. *Belleville Weekly Advocate*, June 21, 1904.

75. *Belleville Illinois Illustrated* (St. Louis: Reid-Fitch, 1905), 49, 62.

76. "H.A. Kircher Dead"; "Widely Known Business Man and Banker Succumbed to Pneumonia at His Home This Afternoon," *Belleville Weekly Advocate*, May 1, 1908.

77. Obituary, *Belleville News Democrat*, May 2, 1908.

78. Pensioner Dropped form, United States Pension Agency, Chicago, September 4, 1908, PF.

79. Cassandra S. Crawford, *Phantom Limb: Amputation, Embodiment, and Prosthetic Technology* (New York: New York University Press, 2014), 4.

80. *A Treatise on Marks' Patent Artificial Limbs with Rubber Hands and Feet* (New York: A. A. Marks, 1888), 100.

81. Moyra Williams Schauffler, "Nature for Its Guide: An Object-Centered Analysis of Nineteenth-Century Mechanized and Anatomically Analogous Artificial Limbs," *Surgeon's Call/Journal of the National Museum of Civil War Medicine* 25, no. 2 (2020): 10–11.

82. Ibid., 5–6; Hasegawa, *Mending Broken Soldiers*, 12–13.

83. Nancy Cervetti, "S. Weir Mitchell Representing 'a Hell of Pain': From Civil War to Rest Cure," *Arizona Quarterly* 59, no. 3 (Autumn 2003): 81.

84. Mitchell, "Phantom Limbs," 567.

85. The vestibular system consists of sensory apparatuses in the inner ear that control balance, motion, and bodily orientation and movement.

86. Hasegawa, *Mending Broken Soldiers*, 78; Catherine J. Stevens, "We Dance What We Remember," in Bissell and Haviland, *Sentient Archive*, 91.

87. Hasegawa, *Mending Broken Soldiers*, 77; Lisa Herschbach, "Prosthetic Reconstructions: Making the Industry, Re-Making the Body, Modelling the Nation," *History Workshop Journal* 44 (Autumn 1997): 24, 36; O'Connor, *Raw Material*, 130. O'Connor also argues that prostheses are "a functional model of selfhood in place of a shattered ideal of wholeness," (105).

88. "Three Generation Store," *Hardware Dealer's Magazine*, New York, July 1914 issue, 136; *Belleville Weekly Advocate*, March 1, 1916.

89. "Lee in the Capitol," in Melville, *Battle-Pieces*, 193.

5. RICHARD DOWNEY DUNPHY (1841?–1904)

1. Coal Heaver was Dunphy's rank and rating.

2. The circumstances of the amputation and Dunphy's recovery come from the medical questionnaire he completed for S. Weir Mitchell, Mitchell Papers, MSS 2-0241-03, Series 4.5, box 11, folder 2, item 49.

3. This narrative of the Battle of Mobile Bay derives from the navy's history, including the after-action reports of August 5 and 12, 1864, by Rear Admiral Farragut, found at the Naval History and Heritage Command website, accessed June 30, 2023, https://www.history.navy.mil/content/history/nhhc/research/library/online-reading-room/title-list-alphabetically/b/battle-of-mobile-bay-selected-documents.html; on the coal heaver's duties, see Coal Heaver, accessed June 30, 2023, https://news.usni.org/2014/12/03/brief-list-old-obscure-obsolete-u-s-navy-jobs; Michael C. Adams, *Living Hell: The Dark Side of the Civil War* (Baltimore: Johns Hopkins University Press, 2014), 81.

4. US Naval Enlistment Rendezvous, 1855–1891, list D, *U.S. Navy Pensions Index, 1861–1910* (database online). Provo, UT, USA: Ancestry.com Operations Inc., 2008. Although the navy may have recorded Dunphy's age as twenty in 1863, he was certainly older. His tombstone in Vallejo, California, gives his birth year as 1842; military records are mostly consistent in recognizing his birth year as 1841; his Medal of Honor citation states the year as 1840.

5. Richard D. Dunphy PF. Dunphy's pension file runs almost 160 pages and includes the detailed history of his pension reviews and upgrades and, after his death, his widow's pension claims.

6. *Civil War Medal of Honor Recipients*. Medal of Honor Citations, United States Army Center of Military History, accessed June 30, 2023, https://www.army.mil/medalofhonor/citations1.html.

7. *Passenger Lists of Vessels Arriving at New York, New York, 1820–1897*. Microfilm Publication M237, roll 160, line: 29, NAI: 6256867. Records of the US Customs Service, Record Group 36, NARA.

8. Handley-Cousins, *Bodies in Blue*, 2; Etter, *Good Body*, 164.

9. Micale, *Hysterical Men*, 281; Nelson, *Ruin Nation*, 197, 202.

10. Equivalent to $466 today, which buys 5.4 percent of what it could buy in 1866.

11. War of 1861 claim for an invalid pension, January 20, 1866, PF.

12. James Marten, *Sing Not War: The Lives of Union & Confederate Veterans in Gilded Age America* (Chapel Hill: University of North Carolina Press, 2011), 20.

13. Nelson, *Ruin Nation*, 238.

14. Richard D. Dunphy letter to Gideon Welles, Gilder Lehrman Collection # GLC08655, New York Historical Society. Dunphy may not have been the victim of an administrative oversight in not having received his medal. The Mare Island Historic Park Foundation has a letter from Admiral Farragut to the secretary of the navy stating that the medal would not be awarded because Dunphy was expected to die from wounds. See letter from Farragut to Gideon Welles, February 15, 1866, Mare Island Historic Foundation, quoted in Kevin Lavery, "Richard D. Dunphy: The Measure of Honor," *Gettysburg Compiler*, November 8, 2013, accessed June 30, 2023, https://gettysburgcompiler.org/2013/11/08/richard-d-dunphy-the-measure-of-honor/.

15. Enumeration of the Inhabitants of the Town of Menomonee, Waukesha, Wisconsin, June 1, 1855; Dunphy repeatedly asserted during his postwar life that he was the only surviving double amputee of the war. This is untrue. *The Medical and Surgical History of the War of the Rebellion*, part 3, vol. 2, 882–884, lists Union and Confederate double amputees, many of whom survived the war; Memorial No. 3, *Wisconsin Session Laws* (Madison, WI: Atwood & Rublee, 1868), 225; *U.S. City Directories, 1822–1995* (database online; Provo, UT, USA: Ancestry.com Operations, Inc., 2011). Information on Dunphy's marriage comes from a notarized statement re: pension claim of Catherine Dunphy, from H. T. Dunphy and Mary J. Henry, PF.

16. O'Connor, "'Fractions of Men,'" 742–777; Goler, "Loss and the Persistence of Memory," 167, 169; Etter, *Good Body*, 163–167.

17. "Form of application for an Artificial Limb, or for Commutation for the same; to be forwarded to the Surgeon General, Washington, D.C.," June 7, 1870; "Certification from the Bureau of Medicine + Surgery" that Dunphy had received prosthetic limbs, October 12, 1870, PF. On not wearing prosthetic limbs, see Figg and Farrell-Beck, "Amputation in the Civil War," 454–475.

18. Dunphy's employment at the navy yard was noted in the *Indianapolis Journal*, February 13, 1887, and the *Indiana Herald* (Huntington, IN), February 16, 1887. The 1870 census found Dunphy living in a boarding house, owning no real estate and personal property valued at $800, his occupation given as "discharged soldier." From United States Census 1870, *San Francisco Ward 1, California*, roll M593_79, 136A. *On the Soldiers' Messenger Corps*, see Larry M. Logue and Peter Blanck, *Heavy Laden: Union Veterans, Psychological Illness, and Suicide* (New York: Cambridge University Press, 2018), 73.

19. Etter, *Good Body*, 170. For an analysis of poses and settings of disabled veterans in cartes de visite, see 163–167.

20. Handley-Cousins, *Bodies in Blue*, 5, 7.

21. Logue and Blanck, *Race, Ethnicity, and Disability*, 2.

22. Leonard Kriegel, "Uncle Tom as Tiny Tim: Reflections on the Cripple as Negro," *American Scholar* 38, no. 3 (Summer 1969): 413–416.

23. Ibid.; Logue and Blanck, *Race, Ethnicity, and Disability*, 11.

24. In 1872, $31.25 equated to $759 today, which buys 4.1 percent of what it bought in 1872. Fifty dollars in 1874 equates to $1,299 today, which buys 3.8 percent of what it bought in 1874.

25. Sworn, notarized statement of George W. McGill dated July 27, 1874, PF.

26. *Sacramento Bee* (CA, July 18, 1874); "(Navy) War of 1861. Act of July 14, 1862" form dated August 5, 1874, PF. We do not know if Dunphy's brief sojourn in an asylum was at a state hospital. The leading cause of admittance to state hospitals for veterans at this time was alcoholism or, rather, "mental illness supposedly caused by intemperance." See Carroll, *Invisible Wounds*, 207.

27. Equates to $2,132 today, which buys 3.4 percent of what it bought in 1878.

28. Logue and Blanck, *Race, Ethnicity, and Disability*, 18.

29. United States Census *1880, Vallejo Ward 1, Enumeration District 151, Solano County, California*, roll 83, 317A; Genealogy Trails History Group, Solano, California Genealogy Trails, accessed June 30, 2023, https://genealogytrails.com/cal/solano/1883pensioners.html.

30. Marten, *Sing Not War*, 57; *Indianapolis Journal*, February 13, 1887. *Indiana Herald*, same date, also carried the story and criticism of the Democratic administration; *Santa Cruz Surf*, Santa Cruz, CA, February 17, 1887.
31. Ibid.
32. Equates to $3,219 today, which buys 3.1 percent of what it bought in 1889.
33. Invalid Pension form dated February 14, 1889, PF.
34. Many histories of science demarcate the "second scientific revolution" to include a spectrum of disciplines shaped by scientific thinking between about 1800 and 1950. See Stephen G. Brush, *The History of Modern Science: A Guide to the Second Scientific Revolution, 1800–1950* (Ames: Iowa State University Press, 1988); Micale, *Hysterical Men*, 5–6, 37.
35. Mitchell, "Phantom Limbs," 564–565.
36. Mitchell, *Injuries of Nerves*, 342; medical terms defined in Dunglison, *Medical Lexicon*.
37. Dunphy's questionnaire, Mitchell Papers.
38. Mitchell, *Injuries of Nerves*, 342–343.
39. Ibid., 348, 350.
40. Ibid., 349, 361.
41. This proviso first showed up in 1866 pension legislation. Logue and Blanck, *Race, Ethnicity, and Disability*, 19; Jordan, *Marching Home*, 154–156.
42. J. H. Shepard letter to Pension Agent Jesse B. Fuller, September 25, 1899, PF.
43. Bureau of Pensions, Law Division letter to Chief, Special Examinations Division, October 5, 1899, PF.
44. Bureau of Pensions letter to E. G. Hursh, Special Examiner, San Francisco, October 5, 1899, PF.
45. Logue and Blanck, *Race, Ethnicity, and Disability*, 18, 32; Donald R. Shaffer, *After the Glory: The Struggles of Black Civil War Veterans* (Lawrence: University Press of Kansas, 2004), 46.
46. Notarized affidavit of Catherine M. Dunphy, October 7, 1899, PF.
47. "Business men of the town of Vallejo" letter to Commissioner of Pensions, October 7, 1899, PF.
48. J. H. Shepard letter to Pensions Agent Office, San Francisco, October 11, 1899; Pensions Agent Office, San Francisco, letter to Commissioner of Pensions, October 11, 1899; Deposition F of James Topley, October 13, 1899; Deposition C by Julia Borland, October 12, 1899, PF.
49. Deposition A by Catherine M. Dunphy, October 12, 1899, PF.
50. Deposition B by Mary E. Dunphy, October 12, 1899, PF.
51. Deposition E by Platon M. G. Vallejo, MD, October 13, 1899, PF.

52. Sworn statement of Richard D. Dunphy, October 20, 1899, PF.

53. E. G. Hursh report to Commissioner H. Clay Evans, October 30, 1899, PF.

54. United States Census 1900, Vallejo Ward 1, enumeration district 151, Solano County, California, 3; "Victim's Body—Brutal Murder of Edward D. Stanton by James W. Dunphy," *San Francisco Call*, September 28, 1901.

55. "James Dunphy Set at Liberty," *San Francisco Call*, December 19, 1901.

56. "Armless Veteran," *San Francisco Call*, August 20, 1903.

57. Quotations from "Veteran Badly Wounds Two of His Old Comrades," *San Francisco Call*, October 17, 1903, and "Two Army Veterans at Vallejo Have Close Call in a Melee Brought About by Drink," *San Francisco Chronicle*, October 17, 1903, respectively. Other coverage of the incident and aftermath: "Stabbed Veterans Many Times," *Oakland Tribune* (CA), October 17, 1903; *San Francisco Call*, November 7, 1903; and "Judge Says Accused Is Sane," *San Francisco Examiner*, November 10, 1903.

58. Published notices gave Dunphy's age as sixty-two or sixty-five.

59. Dunglison uses the Latin term for senility, *senectus*, to mean "The last period of life, commencing according to some, at 60 years of age. . . . It is characterized by progressive diminution of the physical and moral faculties."

60. Dunphy Certificate of Death, Department of Health, City and County of San Francisco, November 24, 1904. The document gives Dunphy's birth date as December 12, 1841. Obituaries and death notices appeared in the *San Francisco Call*, November 24, 1904, 14, and the *San Francisco Chronicle*, November 25, 1904, 13. Quotation from the *Chronicle*. Information regarding Dunphy's burial apparel from the invoice of the California Undertaking Company, November 24, 1904, PF.

61. Pensioner Dropped, U.S. Pension Agency, November 28, 1904; "Record of Proof of Marriage of Widow to Soldier," December 5, 1904; affidavit of Elizabeth Hall and Michael Hall in support of Catherine Dunphy, January 16, 1905; notarized statement of Catherine Dunphy, January 25, 1905; Bureau of Pensions document titled, "The principal point at issue: dependence," February 11, 1905, PF.

62. Deposition A, Case of Catherine Dunphy, April 20, 1905; Deposition B, Case of Catherine Dunphy, statement of Henry Dunphy, April 20, 1905; Deposition C, C. H. Hyde, Case of Catherine Dunphy, April 20, 1905, PF.

63. Credibility report from US Navy pension examiner to Commissioner of Pensions, April 21, 1905, PF.

64. Equates to $269 today, which buys 3 percent of what it bought in 1905.

65. Widow's Pension Form, Catherine Dunphy, claimant, May 9, 1905, PF; "Government Drops Unpopular Employee—Dismisses Mare Island Workman Who Informed on Foreman," *San Francisco Call*, August 24, 1905.

66. Equates to $391 today, which buys 3.1 percent of what it bought in 1909.

67. Pension Dropped form for Catherine Dunphy, December 12, 1909, PF.

68. Michael W. Shaefer, "'Really, Though, I'm Fine,' Civil War Veterans and the Psychological Aftereffects of Killing," in *The Civil War in Popular Culture: Memory and Meaning*, ed. Lawrence A. Kreiser Jr. and Randal Allred (Lexington: University of Kentucky Press, 2013), 11–23.

69. Logue and Blanck, *Race, Ethnicity, and Disability*, 37.

70. Handley-Cousins, *Bodies in Blue*, 5.

71. Brendan Riley, "Tough Times for Armless Civil War Vet in Vallejo," *Times-Herald* (Vallejo, CA), November 10, 2019.

6. PRESTLEY DORSEY/DAWSON (1842?–1907)

1. United States Colored Troops, within the army's administrative parlance during the war, encompassed infantry, cavalry, and artillery units. This work follows the convention of the wartime carded records in designating regiments.

2. Letter to Miss Margaret Weld, near Petersburg, July 1, 1864, in Sarah Swan Weld Blake, *Diaries and Letters of Francis Minot Weld, M.D. with a Sketch of His Life* (Boston: privately published, 1925), 158.

3. Eric Ledell Smith, letter of May 26, 1864, "The Civil War Letters of Quartermaster Sergeant John C. Brock, 43rd Regiment, United States Colored Troops," in *Pennsylvania's Civil War*, ed. William Blair and William Pencak (University Park: Pennsylvania State University Press, 2001), 151; letter of June 5, 1864, in Smith, "Civil War Letters," 152.

4. Letter to Miss Margaret Weld, near Petersburg, July 1, 1864; Blake, *Diaries and Letters*, 163.

5. Ibid., 160; letter of July 16, 1864, in Smith, "Civil War Letters," 155; Kelly D. Mezurek, *For Their Own Cause: The 27th United States Colored Troops* (Kent, OH: Kent State University Press, 2016), 113–117.

6. Packard, *Manual of Minor Surgery*, 195, 215.

7. The result of the medical examination and the accompanying "Volunteer Enlistment" form are found in Dawson's CSR; Muster Roll, Company H, 43rd USCT, April 22, 1864, CSR.

8. *P. falciparum* and *P. vivax* were the prevalent strains of malaria during the war. A feature of the latter is the recurrence of relapses weeks or

months following the original infection. Dawson's hospital stays for malaria argue for the latter variant, but it is impossible to be certain. Dawson was possibly reinfected by another Anopheles bite months following the original one.

9. Susan Sontag, *Illness as Metaphor* (New York: Vintage Books, 1979), 3.

10. The Centers for Disease Control and Prevention maintains an extensive website on all facets of malaria and its complex coevolution in the bodies of mosquitoes and people: accessed January 27, 1922, https://www.cdc.gov/malaria/about/biology/index.html; Meier, *Nature's Civil War*, 14–15.

11. Todd L. Savitt, "Black Health on the Plantation: Masters, Slaves, and Physicians," in *Science and Medicine in the Old South*, ed. Ronald L. Numbers and Todd L. Savitt (Baton Rouge: Louisiana State University Press, 1989), 337.

12. Joseph Janvier Woodward, *Outlines of the Chief Camp Diseases of the United States Armies as Observed during the Present War: A Practical Contribution to Military Medicine* (Philadelphia: J. B. Lippincott, 1863), 28.

13. Ibid., 30 (italics in the original), 34, 39–40.

14. Andrew McIlwaine Bell, *Mosquito Soldiers: Malaria, Yellow Fever, and the Course of the American Civil War* (Baton Rouge: Louisiana State University Press, 2010), 12, 13, 83; Savitt, "Black Health," 329, 339. Defining disease has never been simple. Even in the twenty-first century, we construct, deconstruct, and reconstruct what disease is. "It is not simply a less than optimum physiological state. The reality is obviously a good deal more complex; disease is at once a biological event, a generation-specific repertoire of verbal constructs reflecting medicine's intellectual and institutional history, an occasion of and potential legitimation for public policy, an aspect of social role and individual—intrapsychic—identity, a sanction for cultural values, and a structuring element in doctor and patient interactions," from Charles E. Rosenberg, "Framing Disease: Illness, Society, and History," in *Framing Disease: Studies in Cultural History*, ed. Charles E. Rosenberg and Janet Golden (New Brunswick, NJ: Rutgers University Press, 1992), xiv; Etter, *Good Body*, 90–93.

15. Woodward, *Outlines of the Chief Camp Disease*, 37.

16. Report of Surgeon Edward Barry Dalton, US Volunteers, and Chief Medical Officer, Depot Field Hospital, Army of the Potomac, City Point, VA, December [31], 1864. Online at *The Petersburg Project*, accessed January 28, 2022, http://www.petersburgproject.org/depot-hospital-at-city-point.html. The Hospital Muster Roll of USA Hospital for Colored Troops, Army of the Potomac, City Point, VA, gives Dawson's admission

date of September 10, whereas a letter from the Surgeon General's Office to the Adjutant General, US Army dated February 19, 1886, gives an admission date of September 27. The latter document gives Dawson's name as Prestley Dorsey, PF; Varon, *Armies of Deliverance*, 387.

17. Jane Stuart Woolsey, *Hospital Days: Reminiscence of a Civil War Nurse*, intro. Daniel John Hoisington (Roseville, MN: Edinborough, 2007), 95; Mezurek, *For Their Own Cause*, 181–183.

18. Quoted in Joseph T. Glatthaar, *Forged in Battle: The Civil War Alliance of Black Soldiers and White Officers* (New York: Free Press, 1990), 218.

19. *Medical and Surgical History*, Medical History, Part III, Volume I, 701: Case 52, Private Noah Davis, Co. C, 8th USCI; Margaret Humphreys, *Intensely Human: The Health of the Black Soldier in the American Civil War* (Baltimore: Johns Hopkins University Press, 2008), 120.

20. Ibid., 126; Christopher Waldrep, *Vicksburg's Long Shadow: The Civil War Legacy of Race and Remembrance* (New York: Rowman & Littlefield, 2005), 11.

21. Humphreys, *Intensely Human*, 130.

22. Ibid., 120, 130; quotation at 139.

23. "Report of the Provost-Marshal-General's Office," March 17, 1866, in United States War Department, *A Compilation of the Official Records of the Union and Confederate Armies* (Washington, DC: US Government Printing Office, 1889–1901), vol. 5, Series 3:669.

24. Glatthaar, *Forged in Battle*, 233.

25. What can we surmise about this surname, on the assumption that Dawson had been reared in enslavement, probably in Maryland? One document in Dawson's pension file, Deposition E by John H. Dawson, Presley's son, dated May 12, 1909, states that the elder Dawson recalled his father reminiscing about two places in Maryland that he had enjoyed before the war, one of which may have been Taneytown, Carroll County, although the identification seems improbable. If true, and Dawson lived near there before joining the army, he could have traversed the distance to his enlistment location of about seventy-five miles without encountering large cities.

26. Author's recorded interview with Thomas Dawson, March 18, 2017, Philadelphia, PA.

27. C. M. Hopkins, *Atlas of Fifteen Miles around Baltimore Including Howard Co, Maryland* (Philadelphia: F. Bourguin's, 1878), accessed June 21, 2023, http://www.historicmapworks.com/Map/US/18356/Title+Page/Baltimore+and+Howard+County+1878/Maryland/.

28. Robert A. Hagaman, "Personal Battles: The Lives of Maryland's Black Civil War Veterans, 1840–1920" (PhD diss., Northern Illinois University, 2004), 11, 22–23.

29. Herbert G. Gutman, *The Black Family in Slavery and Freedom 1750–1925* (New York: Pantheon Books, 1976), 236; Shaffer, *After the Glory*, 100.

30. I am indebted to genealogical researcher Patricia Guida, who strenuously, but fruitlessly, tried to find Prestley Dorsey in early slave schedules.

31. A then-popular medicine for pain and a diaphoretic made from ipecac and opium.

32. Reid Mitchell, *The Vacant Chair: The Northern Soldier Leaves Home* (New York: Oxford University Press, 1993), 68; letter to Miss Margaret Weld, Camp near Manassas Junction, May 3, 1864, in Blake, *Diaries and Letters*, 152.

33. Humphreys, *Intensely Human*, 68; Sharla M. Fett, *Working Cures: Healing, Health, and Power on Southern Slave Plantations* (Chapel Hill: University of North Carolina Press, 2002), 49.

34. Typho-malaria, according to assistant surgeon Joseph Janvier Woodward, is not easy to distinguish from malarial fevers but generally included a range of symptoms for which "the malarial element" predominated, or where "the typhoid element" predominated in concert with malarial fever, or where "the scorbutic element" occasionally predominated. See Woodward, *Outlines of the Chief Camp Diseases*, 77ff.

35. Humphreys, *Intensely Human*, 46; Downs, *Sick from Freedom*, 34; Margaret Humphreys, *Marrow of Tragedy: The Health Crisis of the American Civil War* (Baltimore: Johns Hopkins University Press, 2013), 93; Meier, *Nature's Civil War*, 19.

36. Humphreys, *Intensely Human*, 37; Mitchell, *Vacant Chair*, 68.

37. Rosenberg, "Framing Disease," xxii; Etter, *Good Body*, 90–97.

38. Woodward, *Outline of the Chief Camp Diseases*, 11–20; Devine, *Learning from the Wounded*, 99–100.

39. Savitt, "Black Health," in Numbers and Savitt, *Science and Medicine in the Old South*, 329; Downs, *Sick from Freedom*, 11. On the South's "epidemiological distinctiveness," see K. David Patterson, "Disease Environments of the Antebellum South," in Numbers and Savitt, *Science and Medicine in the Old South*, 152; Bourke, *Dismembering the Male*, 60.

40. Elizabeth Barnaby Keeney, "Unless Powerful Sick: Domestic Medicine in the Old South," in Numbers and Savitt, *Science and Medicine in the Old South*, 276; Fett, *Working Cures*, 39; Elliott J. Gorn, "Black Magic: Folk Beliefs of the Slave Community," in Numbers and Savitt, *Science and Medicine in the Old South*, 298, 300.

41. Fett, *Working Cures*, 199; Gretchen Long, *Doctoring Freedom: The Politics of African American Medical Care in Slavery and Emancipation* (Chapel Hill: University of North Carolina Press, 2012), 15, 118; Gorn, "Black Magic," 304; Humphreys, *Intensely Human*, 69.

42. David I. Harrower and Thomas J. Wieckowski, eds., *A Spectacle for Men and Angels: A Documentary Narrative of Camp William Penn and the Raising of Colored Regiments in Pennsylvania* (Conshohocken, PA: Infinity, 2013).

43. Glatthaar, *Forged in Battle*, 227.

44. Ibid., 237.

45. I will maintain the use of Dawson to refer to Prestley Dorsey/Dawson, his army name. "Blowing the Smoke Outen' His Eyes," *Denton Journal*, June 28, 1924.

46. Hagaman, *Personal Battles*, 102, 111.

47. Telephone interview with Jack Walsh, president, Caroline County Historical Society, May 13, 2020.

48. Sworn statement of the clerk for the Circuit Court, Caroline County, May 15, 1909, PF; Hagaman, *Personal Battles*, 163.

49. Certified copy of the marriage record from the clerk, Circuit Court, Queen Anne County, August 11, 1908, PF; United States Census 1870, District 2, Caroline, Maryland, roll M593_581, 153B.

50. United States Census 1880, Henderson, Caroline, MD, roll 506, 129D, enumeration district, 001; Caroline County Land Deeds LH 6, Liber 44 of 364, 365.

51. Shaffer, *After the Glory*, 123–124; Corrales Diaz, "Remembering the Veteran," 117; Logue and Blanck, *Race, Ethnicity, and Disability*, 37; Carroll, *Invisible Wounds*, 159; Varon, *Armies of Deliverance*, 280; Jean Franzino, "'Harmonies of Form and Color': Race and the Prosthetic Body in Civil War America," *Literature and Medicine* 38, no. 1 (Spring 2020): 57.

52. Marten, *Sing Not War*, 23; Holly A. Pinheiro Jr. *The Families' Civil War: Black Soldiers and the Fight for Racial Justice* (Athens: University of Georgia Press, 2022), 11; Logue and Blanck, *Heavy Laden*, 154.

53. Declaration for Original Pension, August 29, 1885, PF.

54. Card "Ex'r. Invalid. No. '548786' Acts of July 14, 1862, and March 3, 1873," PF.

55. "Appendix A: Union Army Pensions and Civil War Records," in Dora L. Costa, *The Evolution of Retirement: An American Economic History, 1880–1990* (Chicago: University of Chicago Press 1998), 198.

56. Ibid., 203; Logue and Blanck, *Heavy Laden*, 118.

57. Logue and Blanck, *Race, Ethnicity, and Disability*, 37, 49, 61, 63.

58. Ibid., 80; Gutman, *Black Family in Slavery and Freedom*, 14.

59. Jordan, *Marching Home*, 156.

60. Letter, Surgeon General's Office to Adjutant General, US Army, February 19, 1886; letter, War Department to Pension Office re: Prestley Dawson, February 24, 1886, PF.

61. Equates to $192.96 today, which buys 3.1 percent of what it bought in 1890.

62. Invalid Card for Presley Dawson, October 12, 1891; application dated July 8, 1890, PF.

63. Letter, Board of Pensions, Finance Division, to Presley Dawson, September 5, 1894, PF.

64. Bureau of Pensions form re: case 668017, Presley Dawson, September 21, 1896, PF.

65. Bureau of Pensions questionnaire to Presley Dawson, November 20, 1897, PF; United States Census 1900, Church Hill, Queen Anne, Maryland, 6, Enumeration District 0058, FHL microfilm 1240626.

66. Equates to $266.05 today, which buys 3.0 percent of what it bought in 1903.

67. "Pension Certificates Issued," *Times* (Philadelphia, PA), March 25, 1902; "Pensions Issued," *Baltimore Sun* (MD), March 6, 1903.

68. Deed of sale by Eli Kenton and wife to "P. Dorsey and wife," the land described in Liber C.W.H. No. 65 folio 414, the deed found at 68 f. 597, the mortgage record at 7 f. 274–275. Dawson evidently paid $300 down and carried a $700 mortgage. Dawson never lived on the property, as the deed shows that the mortgage transferred to three nonrelated persons in succession, beginning in 1904. These assignees paid the remaining balance on the mortgage as rent. The sale was fully satisfied in 1909, whereupon Dawson's wife would have enjoyed a clear title.

69. Surgeon's Certificate for "Presley Dawson," Pension Claim 668017, February 24, 1904, PF.

70. Per Dunglison, rheumatism was "a kind of shifting phlegmasia [inflammation] or neuralgia [a generic name for a cluster of diseases, each characterized by extreme pain], sometimes seated in the muscles, sometimes in the parts surrounding the joints; and at others, within them." Rheumatism is subdivided into acute and chronic varieties.

71. Probably the medial condyle of the tibia, part of the thickened upper end of the tibia just below the patella.

72. Dunglison defines periosteum as "a fibrous, white, resisting medium, which surrounds the bones every where [*sic*], except the teeth . . . and the

parts of the bone covered with cartilage. . . . The periosteum unites the bones to the neighboring parts."

73. Per Dunglison, "An osseous tumour which forms at the surface of bones."

74. Nielsen, *Disability History*, 83–86.

75. Ibid., 42, 64; Handley-Cousins, *Bodies in Blue*, 29; "Black Americans were also deemed biologically incapable of true independence, and even free blacks were often considered dependent members of white households," from Handley-Cousins, 13.

76. Ibid., 66, 74; Logue and Blanck, *Race, Ethnicity, and Disability*, 109.

77. W. Fitzhugh Brundage, "Race, Memory, and Masculinity: Black Veterans Recall the Civil War," in *The War Was You and Me: Civilians in the American Civil War*, ed. Joan E. Cashin (Princeton: Princeton University Press, 2002), 141; Shaffer, *After the Glory*, 2–4, quotation at 5.

78. In comparison with Maryland, Pennsylvania had six black posts and thirty-six integrated ones. Barbara A. Gannon, *The Won Cause: Black and White Comradeship in the Grand Army of the Republic* (Chapel Hill: University of North Carolina Press, 2011), 204–206, 219–220.

79. Ibid., 4; Donald R. Shaffer, "'I Would Rather Shake Hands with the Blackest Nigger in the Land': Northern Black Civil War Veterans and the Grand Army of the Republic," in Cimbala and Miller, *Union Soldiers and the Home Front*, 444.

80. Today, physicians award lower disability ratings to black people with consequent smaller disability compensation. Gannon, *Won Cause*, 6; Logue and Blanck, *Race, Ethnicity, and Disability*, 148, 151.

81. Gannon, *Won Cause*, 48; Long, *Doctoring Freedom*, 90; Hagaman, *Personal Battles*, 39.

82. Letter of Sgt. John C. Brock, March 9, 1865, quoted in Smith, "Civil War Letters," 162.

83. Carmichael, *War for the Common Soldier*, 67.

84. Pinheiro, *Families' Civil War*, 112.

85. Mezurek, *For Their Own Cause*, 234.

86. David Silkenat, *Moments of Despair: Suicide, Divorce, & Debt in Civil War Era North Carolina* (Chapel Hill: University of North Carolina Press, 2011), 87.

87. "Under Act of June 27, 1890. Increase" pension application of Mary J. Dawson, #548086, April 6, 1907; "Declaration for Widow's Pension Acts of June 27, 1890, and May 9, 1900," application of Mary J. Dawson, April 10, 1907, PF. At this time, the five children living with Janey, all over age

twenty-one, included William H., Mary E., Samuel P., John H., and Arline B.

88. Letter of Commissioner, Southern Division, Bureau of Pensions re: Wid. Orig. 867,651, October 24, 1908, PF.

89. Department of the Interior/Bureau of Pensions form for completion by widow; a questionnaire to Mrs. Mary J Dawson, Ingleside, MD, October 28, 1908, PF; Pinheiro, *Families' Civil War*, 141.

90. Although pension officials identified still-living veterans of Dawson's company, none were contacted.

91. Affidavit of Charles Lewis before the justice of the peace, Queen Anne County, February 4, 1909; General Affidavit by Peter Groose, Goldsboro, Caroline County, MD, March 2, 1909; letter of Dr. James E. Graham, March 12, 1909; Widow's Pension Application, Mary J. Dawson, April 23, 1909, PF.

92. Bureau of Pensions card re: claim 867651, pension certificate 668017, April 27, 1909, PF. The same document notes that hospital records bear the veteran's name as Presley Dorsey and Prestley Dorsley.

93. Notice of Special Examination, May 12, 1909. Depositions in the pension file include Deposition B, Mary J. Dawson, May 12, 1909; Deposition E, John H. Dawson, May 12, 1909; Deposition F, Charles H. Reese, May 12, 1909; Deposition G, William Brown, May 11, 1909; Deposition H, Hannah Brown, May 11, 1909; Deposition I, James A. Brown, May 11, 1909; Deposition J, Annie M. Hutchins, May 13, 1909; Deposition K, William J. Hutchings [*sic*], May 13, 1909; Deposition L, Peter Goose [*sic*], May 13, 1909; Deposition M, Tennessee Dawson, May 13, 1909, PF.

94. Deposition B, Mary J. Dawson, May 12, 1909; Claimant's Final Statement, Mary J. Dawson pension claim, May 12, 1909, PF.

95. Deposition L, Peter Goose, May 13, 1909; Deposition M, Tennessee Dawson, May 13, 1909, PF.

96. Letter of R. P. Fletcher, Special Examiner, to Commissioner of Pensions, May 18, 1909, PF.

97. Widow's Pension form per Act of June 27, 1890, re: claim of Mary J. Dawson (filed by attorney Garrett), May 21, 1909. Dawson's pension file "Index Sheet, claim #867,651" lists affidavits filed in 1907 and 1908, which are included in the file. Affidavits were sworn by William J Colman, Charles H. Reses or Reese, Francis D. Thomas, James Brown, William Rochester, William Hutchens, Anna Hutchens, and Dr. James Graham, who attended Dawson's death. Except for the physician, all signed with an X; PF.

98. Letter from Commissioner of Pensions to Auditor, War Department, October 17, 1910, PF.

99. Letter from Bureau of Pensions Commissioner re Civil War Division Widow's Original #867,651 claim of Mary J. Dawson, June 30, 1911; letter from Civil War Division, Bureau of Pensions, to John Wainwright & Co., Wilmington, DE, May 17, 1912, PF.

100. According to Dunglison, apoplexy was a term generally "employed to signify interstitial hemorrhage, or every effusion of blood, which occurs suddenly into the substance of an organ or tissue." Most commonly, cerebral hemorrhage was indicated.

101. Logue and Blanck, *Race, Ethnicity, and Disability*, 11.

102. Meier, *Nature's Civil War*, 2.

103. Waldrep, *Vicksburg's Long Shadow*, 91; Daryl Black, "Relics of Reunion: Souvenirs and Memory at Chickamauga and Chattanooga National Military Park, 1889–1895," in Kreiser and Allred, *Civil War in Popular Culture*, 56.

104. Gannon, *Won Cause*, 22; Carmichael, *War for the Common Soldier*, 73.

105. Shaffer, *After the Glory*, 52–54.

106. Mezurek, *For Their Own Cause*, 233; Waldrep, *Vicksburg's Long Shadow*, 86.

107. Benjamin Apthorp Gould, *Investigations in the Military and Anthropological Statistics of American Soldiers* (New York: US Sanitary Commission, 1869); J. H. Baxter, comp., *Statistics, Medical and Anthropological, of the Provost-Marshal's Bureau* (Washington, DC: US Government Printing Office, 1875); Lundy Braun, "Spirometry, Measurement, and Race in the Nineteenth Century," *Journal of the History of Medicine and Allied Sciences* 60, no. 2 (2005): 135–169. On the definition of black bodies as inherently diseased, see the discussion of *Cachexia Africana* in Rana A. Hogarth, *Medicalizing Blackness: Making Racial Difference in the Atlantic World, 1780–1840* (Chapel Hill: University of North Carolina Press, 2017); Leslie A. Schwalm, *Medicine, Science & Making Race in Civil War America* (Chapel Hill: University of North Carolina Press, 2023), 8, 55, 66.

7. JOHN SHIELDS (1839–1923)

1. Letter by Shields to the *Maunch Chunk Gazette*, July 15, 1862, repr. in Irvin C. Myers, *We Might as Well Die Here: The 53rd Pennsylvania Veteran Infantry* (Shippensburg, PA: White Mane, 2004), 25–27; Samuel P. Bates, *History of Pennsylvania Volunteers, 1861*, vol. 2 (Harrisburg, PA: B. Singerly, State Printer, 1869), 92–94.

2. Description by a witness, quoted in Guelzo, *Gettysburg*, 300.
3. Ibid., 295, 299; Bates, *History of Pennsylvania Volunteers*, 95–96.
4. Guelzo, *Gettysburg*, 277–278, 293.
5. "Thyroid" comes from the Greek word *thyreos*, meaning "shield-shaped." Vocal cords attach to the upper part of this cartilage, the thyroid prominence or Adam's apple.
6. Unless otherwise noted, medical data derive from Shields's CSR and PF. I also quote from John K. Mitchell's examination of Shields in the 1890s, which includes details of his wounding gleaned from army medical records. See Case XLVI, Mitchell, *Remote Consequences of Injuries of Nerves*, 182–184.
7. Per Dunglison, emphysema referred to crackling or bubbling noises accompanying the escape of air into adjacent tissues. "Injuries of the larynx, trachea, or lungs; fractures of ribs, or wounds penetrating into the chest, are the most frequent causes . . . owing to the air escaping from the air passages."
8. Among the large Irish immigrant community, a branch of the secret society of coal miners, the Molly Maguires, became active. A society with obscure origins in Ireland, the Maguires had established themselves in several Irish communities in the eastern United States where they committed violent acts. Several convicted members were hanged in Mauch Chunk in the 1870s. Perhaps Shields's move to New Jersey during that decade was influenced by a desire to distance himself from these events.
9. 7th Census of the United States 1850, roll M432_762, 343B; 8th Census of the United States 1860, roll M653_1092, 671.
10. A South American tree that produces a resin used as an anti-inflammatory agent that aids healing.
11. Gross, *Manual of Military Surgery*, 131. Documentation of Shields's two hospitalizations for gonorrhea appear in only one record, Bureau of Pensions request to the War Department for "full military and medical history of [Captain John Shields]," July 11, 1899, PF.
12. Surgeons Certificate for sick leave, August 3, 1863, PF.
13. Equates to $373 today, which buys about 18 percent of what it bought in 1864. This year experienced an atypically high inflation rate of 24.6 percent.
14. Goldberg, "'What They Think of the Causes of So Much Suffering,'" 36.
15. Mitchell, *Injuries of Nerves*, 65.
16. Mitchell et al., *Gunshot Wounds*, 49.
17. Mitchell, *Injuries of Nerves*, 65–66.

18. Marten, *Sing Not War*, 25–26; Rotundo, *American Manhood*, 20.

19. Examining Surgeon's Certificate, April 7, 1864; affidavit given May 21, 1864, PF.

20. Marten, *Sing Not War*, 82; Logue and Blanck, *Race, Ethnicity, and Disability*, 90.

21. 9th Census of the United States 1870, roll M593_1320, 322B.

22. Surgeon's Certificate, November 10, 1873, PF.

23. Surgeon's Certificates, February 22, 1876, and September 19, 1877, PF.

24. 10th Census of the United States 1880, roll 787, 144B, enumeration district 073; Raritan, Hunterdon Co, NJ; State Census, NJ, New Jersey State Archive, State Census of New Jersey, 1885, Film No. 26.

25. Both photographs appear in Myers, *We Might As Well Die Here*.

26. McConnell, *Glorious Contentment*, 192, 209–210.

27. Rotundo, *American Manhood*, 233, 246.

28. Theda Skocpol, *Protecting Soldiers and Mothers: The Political Origins of Social Policy in the United States* (Cambridge, MA: Harvard University Press, 1992), 3.

29. Declaration for the Increase of an Invalid Pension, December 18, 1889, PF.

30. Per Dunglison, "varicose distillation of the veins of the scrotum and spermatic cord.... It appears under the form of a soft, doughy, unequal, knotty, compressible and indolent tumour."

31. Shields letter to S. Weir Mitchell, February 3, 1890; A. Parish, MD, letter to S. Weir Mitchell, November 5, 1890. S. Weir Mitchell Papers, College of Physicians of Philadelphia, MSS 2/241-03, Series 4, box 11, folder 1, Items 6 and 9.

32. Undated handwritten notes about John Shields, S. Weir Mitchell Papers Z10 40, Series 2, folder 1, Item 2; letter of G. E. de Schweinitz to S. Weir Mitchell, February 10, 1890, S. Weir Mitchell Papers MSS 2/241-03 Series 2, folder 41, Item 1.

33. Surgeon's Certificate, June 18, 1890, PF.

34. John K. Mitchell, with notes by Dr. Parish; Case # XLVI, "Buckshot through left side of larynx and neck; tracheotomy; late weakness of right arm; absence of sweat on right face, neck, and arm; sensitiveness to heat," in Mitchell, *Remote Consequences*, 185–186.

35. Ibid.

36. Equates to $758 today, which buys 3 percent of what it could buy in 1891.

37. Dated March 17, 1891, PF.

38. Photograph PX337, "Erection of Soldiers Monument on Main St., Flemington," Hunterdon County Historical Society, Flemington, NJ.

39. Records spell the name as both Connett and Connet.

40. James P. Snell, comp., *History of Hunterdon and Somerset Counties, New Jersey* (Philadelphia: Everts & Peck, 1881), 335–337.

41. "The G.A.R. Adjourns," *Courier-Post* (Camden, NJ), February 10, 1894; "Politics in the State," *Camden Daily Telegram*, October 17, 1894.

42. E. E. Bice and John L. Connet, *Flemington, New Jersey, Illustrated* (privately printed, 1898), no pagination, accessed July 3, 2023, https://babel.hathitrust.org/cgi/pt?id=loc.ark:/13960/t9h41zh5d&view=1up&seq=36.

43. Physician's Affidavit of E. D. Leidy, MD, December 20, 1898, PF.

44. "History of the New Jersey Memorial Home for Disabled Soldiers, Sailors, Marines and Their Wives," undated typescript (no author), Vineland Historical & Antiquarian Society, Vineland, NJ.

45. Surgeon's Certificate, March 11, 1899. Handwritten note states that X-ray was filed on April 4, 1899. The quotation from Shields asserting that the X-ray has been mailed appears on a cover note by Shields to the commissioner of pensions. The X-ray apparently no longer survives.

46. Bureau of Pensions questionnaire to John Shields, July 8, 1899; Bureau of Pensions request to the War Department, July 11, 1899 (reply August 5, 1899); Bureau of Pensions internal order for a medical examination, August 15, 1899, PF.

47. Surgeon's Certificate, November 8, 1899, PF.

48. Increase Invalid Pension form, August 8, 1899, rejected November 24, 1899, PF.

49. 12th Census of the United States 1900, 15, enumeration district 0020, microfilm 1240981.

50. "Legislature's Work," *Morning Post* (Camden, NJ), January 30, 1900.

51. McConnell, *Glorious Contentment*, 25; Mark A. Tabbert and William D. Moore, eds., *Secret Societies in America: Foundational Studies in Fraternalism* (New Orleans: Cornerstone Books, 2011), vii, accessed July 3, 2023, https://www.academia.edu/3479334/Secret_Societies_in_America_Foundational_Studies_of_Fraternalism.

52. McConnell, *Glorious Contentment*, 21; Harris, *Across the Bloody Chasm*, 44.

53. McConnell, *Glorious Contentment*, 102, 192, 222, 237; Jordan, *Marching Home*, 60, 95, 111; Jordan quotes "deadly addiction" from Jonathan Shay, *Odysseus in America: Combat Trauma and the Trials of Homecoming* (New York: Simon & Schuster, 2003), 87.

54. Jordan, *Marching Home*, 73; McConnell, *Glorious Contentment*, 89–93, 104. Quotations at 92–93.

55. Sarah F. Rose, *No Right to Be Idle: The Invention of Disability, 1840s–1930s* (Chapel Hill: University of North Carolina Press, 2017), 2; Marten, *Sing Not War*, 21, 27–30; quotation at 27.

56. "Work on the Tunnel," *New York Tribune*, July 8, 1900; "Report of the Managers of the Home, etc, for the Year Ending October 31st, 1905" (Trenton, NJ: MacCrellish & Quigley, State Printers, 1906), not paginated.

57. "G.A.R. National Encampment," *Morning Post*, August 22, 1901.

58. Death certificate for Anna M. Curran, September 5, 1904, PF.

59. "General Law Declaration for the Increase of an Invalid Pension," Shields application of September 17, 1904; sworn statement, "Additional Evidence: Claim of John Shields," November 8, 1904, PF.

60. Marten, *Sing Not War*, 17; Peter Blanck, "Civil War Pensions and Disability," *Ohio State Law Journal* 62, no. 1 (2001): 202; Dora L. Costa, *The Evolution of Retirement: An American Economic History, 1880–1900* (Chicago: University of Chicago Press, 1998), 197.

61. Peter Blanck, Claudia Linares, and Chen Song, "Evolution of Disability in Late 19th Century America: Civil War Pensions for Union Army Veterans with Musculoskeletal Conditions," *Behavioral Sciences and the Law* 20 (2002): 683; Figg and Farrell-Beck, "Amputation in the Civil War," 473.

62. Logue and Blanck, *Race, Ethnicity, and Disability*, 7; Blanck et al., "Evolution of Disability," 684; Jordan, *Marching Home*, 149.

63. Logue and Blanck, *Race, Ethnicity, and Disability*, 18, 20; Blanck et al., "Evolution of Disability," 685.

64. Handley-Cousins, *Bodies in Blue*, 49.

65. Blanck, "Civil War Pensions and Disability," 200–204; Handley-Cousins, *Bodies in Blue*, 3.

66. Christopher T. Baer, "A General Chronology of the Pennsylvania Railroad Company Its Predecessors and Successors and Its Historical Context" (April 2015 edition), accessed December 12, 2023, https://docplayer.net/101870294-A-general-chronology-of-the-pennsylvania-railroad-company-its-predecessors-and-successors-and-its-historical-context-by-christopher-t.html; "Bergen Hill Tunnels," *Evening Record and Bergen County Herald* (Hackensack, NJ) March 14, 1905.

67. "Asks Bankruptcy for Railroad Contractors," *Patterson Morning Call* (NJ), January 19, 1906; Baer, "General Chronology of the Pennsylvania Railroad Company"; "New Construction Company," *Passaic Daily News*,

December 28, 1906 (includes the quotation); "Flemington," *Trenton Evening Times*, January 12, 1907.

68. Letter from commissioner of pensions to the Hon. Ira W. Wood, House of Representatives, January 31, 1907; John Shields application for a new certificate, April 8, 1907, PF.

69. "Captain Shields Chooses," *Evening Journal* (Vineland), January 30, 1908; "Delegation Received a Sudden, Startling Jolt," *Morning Call* (Paterson, NJ), February 8, 1908; W. Rex McCrosson, "The Story of Fifty Odd Years of the New Jersey Memorial Home for Soldiers, Sailors, Marines Their Wives & Widows" mimeographed typescript, 1952 with a 1957 supplement, unpaginated. McCrosson, a former superintendent of the home, combed thousands of primary documents to abstract them into a chronological history of the institution. In addition to providing a timeline of milestones from the home's founding until the 1950s, he summarized and abstracted various discussions about the home's finances, management and administration, and personnel. After compiling this document, he or someone else evidently destroyed the primary sources. The document exists at the Vineland Historical & Antiquarian Society.

70. By the time Shields became commandant, about 5 percent of living veterans resided in government-sponsored homes. Marten, *Sing Not War*, 13, 15, 159; Jeffrey W. McClurken, *Take Care of the Living: Reconstructing Confederate Veteran Families in Virginia* (Charlottesville: University of Virginia Press, 2009), 119; quotation at Marten, 13; Skocpol, *Protecting Soldiers and Mothers*, 65, 102.

71. "Old Soldiers Make a Kick," *Camden Post-Telegram* (*Morning Post*), April 17, 1907.

72. McCrosson, "Story of Fifty Odd Years."

73. Ibid.

74. Ibid; 13th Census of the United States 1910, roll T624_875l, 22A, enumeration district 0114.

75. McCrosson, "Story of Fifty Odd Years."

76. Letter, John Shields to the commissioner of pensions, November 29, 1910, PF.

77. Letter, Civil War Division, Bureau of Pensions, to John Shields, December 3, 1910, PF.

78. Letter, John Shields to Thomas B. Holmes, Commissioner of Public Reports, January 5, 1911; quoted in McCrosson, "Story of Fifty Odd Years."

79. Physician's affidavit by John D. Halsey, MD, on behalf of John Shields, June 14, 1911; Invalid Pension Reissue, May 16, 1911; Pension Increase Form, May 16, 1911, PF.

80. Surgeon's Certificate, August 2, 1911, PF.

81. Letter, John Shields to commissioner of pensions, August 4, 1911; letter, Civil War Division, Bureau of Pensions, to Examining Secretary, Millville, NJ, August 7, 1911, PF.

82. Letter, Civil War Division, Bureau of Pensions, to John Shields, September 9, 1911, PF.

83. McCrosson, "Story of Fifty Odd Years."

84. Declaration for Pension, May 16, 1912; General affidavit of John D. Halsey, MD, June 22, 1912; letter, Civil War Division to John Shields, June 17, 1912, PF.

85. Equates to $889 today, which buys almost 4 percent of what it bought in 1912.

86. General affidavit, Edward P. Southwick and Samuel S. Weaver, June 22, 1912, PF.

87. Memoranda, Board of Review, Bureau of Pensions, certificate 29, 121, July 8 and July 9, 1912; Memorandum re John Shields by the Chief Dalton, Board of Review, July 17, 1912, PF.

88. McCrosson, "Story of Fifty Odd Years."

89. Equates to $786 today, which buys 5.1 percent of what it bought in 1918.

90. The pension file form for the 1912 increase to thirty dollars monthly carries an endorsement to increase it to forty dollars, effective June 10, 1918; general affidavit, Edward P. Southwick and Samuel S. Weaver, June 22, 1912, PF.

91. Marriage license, John Shields and Lydia Bontecou, Cecil County, Maryland, November 13, 1918, PF.

92. Letter, John Shields to commissioner of pensions, January 2, 1919; letter, John Shields to commissioner of pensions, January 23, 1919, PF.

93. Letter, Civil War Division, Bureau of Pensions, to John Shields, January 29, 1919; Declaration for the Increase of an Invalid Pension, February 17, 1919, which recognized Shields's expressed need for "the constant care of an attendant"; letter, John Shields to commissioner of pensions, March 3, 1919, PF.

94. Sworn statement of John S. Halsey, MD, March 12, 1919; letter, Civil War Division, Bureau of Pensions, to John Shields, March 26, 1919, PF.

95. Letter, E. C. Hutchinson to commissioner of pensions, May 1, 1919; letter, deputy commissioner of pensions to E. C. Hutchinson, May 2, 1919, PF.

96. 14th Census of the United States 1920, roll T625_1027, 17B, enumeration district 133; Clayton, Gloucester Co, NJ; Declaration for Pension, May 11, 1920; sworn statements of John Shields, Lydia Shields, May 24, 1920, PF.

97. Letter, Charles Franklin Fisler to commissioner of pensions, June 9, 1920, PF.

98. Equates to $1,035 today, which buys 7 percent of what it purchased in 1920; letter, Walter E. Edge, United States Senate, to commissioner of pensions, June 21, 1920; letter, J. Ellis Paulin to Bureau of Pensions, Washington, DC, July 10, 1920. The pension office responded to Edge that Shields was receiving forty-two dollars a month and awaited further medical evidence of the need for a personal assistant; letter, Civil War Division, Bureau of Pensions, to Walter E. Edge, July 7, 1920, PF.

99. Certificate of Medical Examination, August 16, 1920; letter, J. Ellis Paulin to Bureau of Pensions, Washington, DC, September 9, 1920, PF.

100. Certificate and Record of Death, John Shields, August 27, 1923, Department of Health of the State of New Jersey, PF.

101. "Captain John Shields Dead," *Camden Post-Telegram,* August 29, 1923; *Hunterdon Republican,* September 5, 1923 (under "Obituary").

102. Letter, Lydia Bontecou Shields to commissioner of pensions, September 1, 1923; Declaration of a Widow for Accrue Pension, September 12, 1923; Accrued Pension Increase, September 14, 1923; sworn statements of Josephine A. Hurd, Elizabeth Kemmerer, October 17, 1923; sworn statements of James Dugan, Mary Dugan, October 25, 1923; letter, Lydia Bontecou Shields to Bureau of Pensions, November 7, 1923; letter, commissioner, Widow Division, Bureau of Pensions, November 16, 1923; sworn statements of Edward P. and Emma J. Southwick, November 26, 1923; sworn statements of Thomas K. and Nettie Eastburn, December 7, 1923; PF.

103. Blanck, "Civil War Pensions and Disability," 12.

104. Etter, *Good Body,* 154, 164; quotation from Leonard Kriegel, "Uncle Tom as Tiny Tim: Reflections on the Cripple as Negro," *American Scholar* 38, no. 3 (Summer 1969): 41; Blanck, "Civil War Pensions and Disability," 3; Bourke, *Dismembering the Male,* 251; Dean, *Shook over Hell,* 145.

105. Ibid.; Rose, *No Right to Be Idle,* 3.

106. Ibid., 111; Etter, *Good Body,* 198.

107. Shaffer, *After the Glory,* 137; Logue and Blanck, *Race, Ethnicity, and Disability,* 130–132; Etter, *Good Body,* 218.

108. Quoted in Myers, *We Might As Well Die Here,* 24–25.

8. THOMAS R. HAWKINS (1840–1870)

1. Hawkins's middle name, if he had one, was not recorded.

2. Frequently caricatured in the press because of his heavy-lidded cross-eyed appearance, Butler had conceived of the "contraband of war" policy for rejecting pleas from Confederate opponents to return escaped enslaved people.

3. James M. Paradis, *Strike the Blow for Freedom: The 6th United States Colored Infantry in the Civil War* (Shippensburg, PA: White Mane, 1998), 53–55; Memorandum, War Department/Adjutant General's Office to Commissioner of Pensions re Thomas R. Hawkins, May 20, 1865, PF.

4. My account derives primarily from three sources: George W. Williams, *A History of the Negro Troops in the War of the Rebellion 1861–1865* (New York: Harper & Brothers, 1888), 250–255; Paradis, *Strike the Blow for Freedom*, 69–79; James S. Price, *The Battle of New Market Heights* (Charleston, SC: History Press, 2011), 41–66. Fleetwood's recollection appeared in his obituary for Hawkins, "Thomas R. Hawkins, Late Sergeant Major, 6th U.S.C. Infantry," *New Era* (Washington, DC), March 10, 1870.

5. The battle is recounted in Donald Scott Sr., *Camp William Penn 1863–1865* (Atglen, PA: Schiffer Military History, 2012), 144–146, 148–150; Williams, *History of the Negro Troops*, 252–254; Price, *Battle of New Market Heights*, 56–59.

6. Edgerton quotation at Price, *Battle of New Market Heights*, 56; Duncan quotation at Price, 60.

7. Fleetwood quotation at Price, *Battle of New Market Heights*, 63.

8. Dean, *Shook over Hell*, 55–56.

9. "Flag Presentation at Camp William Penn," *Christian Recorder*, September 5, 1863. Quotation at Scott, *Camp William Penn*, 121.

10. McMurray, Wilkes quotations at Paradis, *Strike the Blow for Freedom*, 71.

11. Certificate of Discharge for Thomas R. Hawkins, May 20, 1865; letter, Christian A. Fleetwood to Rev. Dr. Septimus Justin, March 2, 1870, PF. Most histories of the New Market Heights battle have Hawkins and Kelly retiring from the field with the colors. Hawkins's wounds, however, were temporarily disabling, and Fleetwood's assertion that he remained on the battlefield for hours until rescued has the authority of an eyewitness account.

12. Butler quotation at Williams, *History of the Negro Troops*, 255.

13. Paradis, *Strike the Blow for Freedom*, 76; Butler quotation at Paradis, 79.

14. Letter, J. H. Franz, Asst Surgeon, to Brig. Gen. Shepley, Commanding District of Eastern Virginia, October 4, 1864, MMN #76607, Maine Historical Society, Maine Memory Network, accessed June 27, 2023, https://www.mainememory.net/media/pdf/76607.pdf.

15. Thomas Longmore, *A Treatise on Gunshot Wounds* (Philadelphia: J. B. Lippincott, 1862), quotations at 53, 16, respectively.

16. Ibid., 54.

17. Ibid., 105.

18. Varon, *Armies of Deliverance*, 145; Carmichael, *War for the Common Soldier*, 85, 134.

19. Bartholow, *Manual of Instructions for Enlisting and Discharging Soldiers*, 163–164; Substitute Volunteer Enlistment Form [signed by the provost marshal and commissioner of the board (same person) and board surgeon], August 4, 1863, PF. Further details about Passmore Henry are found in census and draft records: United States Census 1870, Philadelphia Ward 4 District 12, 2nd enumeration district, Philadelphia, PA, roll M593_1418, 394A; Philadelphia City Directory, 1867, Ancestry.com. US, City Directories, 1822–1995 [database online] (Lehi, UT, USA: Ancestry.com Operations, Inc., 2011); US Civil War Draft Registration Records, 1863–1865, NARA Collection Consolidated Enrollment Lists, 1863–1865, NAI 4213514, archive vol. no. 3 of 6. Christian Fleetwood recalled Hawkins's entrance into the Union Army without mention of his serving as a substitute for another. Fleetwood wrote, "Making his escape through the Southern lines in 1863, [Hawkins] knelt down and kissed the first Union soil his foot pressed, and vowed his young life to the cause of liberty." "Thomas R. Hawkins," *New Era* (see n. 3).

20. Walt Whitman, *Memoranda during the War*, ed. Peter Coviello (New York: Oxford University Press, 2004), 44.

21. Dorothy Roberts, *Killing the Black Body: Race, Reproduction, and the Meaning of Liberty* (New York: Pantheon Books, 1997), 9, 23.

22. The exception was photographs of maimed but recovering soldiers taken for the army surgeon general's office.

23. Corrales Diaz, "Remembering the Veteran," 5; Bourke, *Dismembering the Male*, 210.

24. Harrison, *Dark Trophies*, 10, 95.

25. Ibid., 20, 43.

26. Richard M. Reid, ed., *Medicine in a Black Regiment: The Civil War Diary of Burt G. Wilder, 55th Massachusetts* (Boston: University of Massachusetts Press, 2010), 25; Shaffer, *After the Glory*, 26–27; letter, Tillman

Valentine to Annie Valentine, December 26, 1863, quoted in Jonathan W. White, Katie Fisher, and Elizabeth Wall, eds., "The Civil War Letters of Tillman Valentine, Third U.S. Colored Troops," *Pennsylvania Magazine of History and Biography* 139 (April 2015): 181.

27. Mezurek, *For Their Own Cause*, 81. The description of Hawkins as mulatto appeared in Schedule 2, a list of persons who died in the Second Ward, Washington, DC, in the year ending June 1, 1870, from *Federal Mortality Census Schedules, 1850–1880, and Related Indexes, 1850–1880*, collection T655, roll number 5; United States Census 1870, Washington Ward 2, Washington, DC, 19, NARA.

28. Letter, Fleetwood to Septimus Justin. Kelly and Fleetwood were awarded their medals on April 6, 1865. Edgerton received the Medal of Honor for the same action on March 30, 1898. From the US Army Medal of Honor website, accessed June 27, 2023, https://www.army.mil/medalofhonor/index.html.

29. Certificate of Discharge, May 20, 1865, PF.

30. Invalid Pension No. 13464, dated June 13, 1865, PF.

31. Equates to approximately ninety-five dollars today, which buys about 6 percent of what it bought in 1865.

32. Pension certificate, July 5, 1865, PF; Hawkins's job as a messenger appears alongside his name in *Federal Mortality Census Schedules*, collection T655, roll number 5; United States Census 1870, Washington Ward 2, DC, 19; "Thomas R. Hawkins," *New Era* (see n. 3).

33. Marriage certificate for Thomas R. Hawkins and Julia B. Landre, PF. Augusta eventually reached the rank of lieutenant colonel, the highest rank held by an African American during the war, and later became the first black professor of medicine in the United States, the first black head of a hospital and, eventually, the first black officer to be buried at Arlington National Cemetery. Abbott was the first black physician to be granted a license to practice in Canada.

34. Moorland-Spingarn Research Center, Howard University, "Fifteenth Street Presbyterian Church, Washington, DC" (2015) Manuscript Division Finding Aids, 74, accessed June 27, 2023, https://dh.howard.edu/finaid_manu/74; Joseph Thomas Kelly, "Rev. John C. Smith, D.D., and Other Pioneer Presbyterian Ministers of Washington," *Records of the Columbia Historical Society, Washington, DC* 24 (1922): 118–135, accessed June 27, 2023, https://www.jstor.org/stable/40067162?seq=1; Jonathan W. White, *A House Built by Slaves: African American Visitors to the Lincoln White House* (New York: Rowman & Littlefield, 2022), 39, 59.

35. Hunt, "Negro as Soldier," 40–41, 45; Downs, *Sick from Freedom*, 6, 166–168.

36. Surgeon's Examination for an Increase of Pension; November 10, 1868; Application for Increase of Invalid Pension, November 11, 1868, PF.

37. Equates to approximately $371 today, which buys about 5 percent of what it bought in 1868.

38. Surgeon's Examination for an Increase of Pension, January 26, 1869; Claim for an Invalid Pension, July 6, 1869; PF.

39. Corrales Diaz, "Remembering the Veteran," 115, 173–174.

40. W. Fitzhugh Brundage, "Race, Memory, and Masculinity: Black Veterans Recall the Civil War," in *The War Was You and Me: Civilians in the American Civil War*, ed. Joan E. Cashin (Princeton, NJ: Princeton University Press, 2002), 137; Shaffer, *After the Glory*, 38, 41.

41. Dunglison's definition: Phthisis pulmonalis is "a . . . progressive emaciation of every part of his body. . . . It consists in the formation of tubercules in the lungs, which sooner or later soften and break down." Symptoms include a "sense of uneasiness in the chest, with severe fits of coughing, or a short and dry cough with dyspnoea." These symptoms intensify and become more frequent. "The expectoration is evidently purulent, with fever in the evening, and circumscribed redness of the cheeks; wasting . . . sweats early in the morning." In the final stages, the sufferer exhibits "small pulse, pungent heat . . . diarrhea. The weakness becomes extreme, and the patient exhausted." Most secondary works on Hawkins mistakenly list his cause of death as cancer.

42. Scott, *Camp William Penn*, 152; Claim for Widow's Pension, No. 143,042, in case of Julia B. Hawkins, May 25, 1870, PF.

43. Sworn statement of Edwin H. Grant, MD, May 20, 1870, PF.

44. Julia's ten-dollar pension equates to about $223 today, which buys about 5 percent of what it bought in 1870.

45. Pension certificate for Julia B. Hawkins, June 18, 1870; PF; United States Census 1870, Washington Ward 2, District of Columbia, roll M593_123, 386B; sworn statement by Alexander T. Augusta before the Justice of the Peace, DC, November 19, 1870, PF.

46. Guardianship document for Julia B. Grant, Supreme Court for the District of Columbia, May 26, 1874; marriage license for Henry Lee Grant and Julia B. Hawkins, April 2, 1874; Declaration for Pension of Children under Sixteen years of age, June 4, 1874; Pension Certificate for Thomas V. Hawkins, September 7, 1874, granting him eight dollars monthly through October 23, 1883; sworn statements by Christian A. Fleetwood and George D. Johnson, August 29, 1874, PF.

47. Death certificate for Henry Fleetwood Grant, December 8, 1904; Declaration for Remarried Widow's Pension, November 8, 1916; sworn statement of Julia B. Grant to the Bureau of Pensions, June 8, 1917; sworn statements of Francis J. Grimké and E. D. Wilson, MD, June 8, 1917; Pension Certificate for Julia B. Grant, August 2, 1917 (effective November 10, 1916); handwritten note, Disbursing Office, Bureau of Pensions, July 11, 1919; PF. Again, the pension documents reveal the continuing intersection of the Hawkins-Grant families with the larger intellectual milieu of black Washington. Grimké, a founder of the National Association for the Advancement of Colored People, began his ministry at the Fifteenth Street Presbyterian Church. His aunts, Sara Grimké and her sister, Angelina Grim, were famous abolitionists of the Civil War era. Francis Grimké was married to diarist, educator, and abolitionist Charlotte Forten of Philadelphia.

48. Equivalent to approximately $322 today, which buys about 4 percent of what it bought in 1916.

49. Bureau of Pensions request to the Finance Division re: audit, July 2, 1917; PF.

50. Dean, *Shook over Hell*, 27; Judith Pizarro, Roxanne Cohen Silver, and JoAnn Prause, "Physical and Mental Health Costs of Traumatic War Experiences Among Civil War Veterans," *Archives of General Psychiatry* 63 (February 2006): 194–198; Carroll, *Invisible Wounds*, 67.

51. Paradis, *Strike the Blow for Freedom*, 94.

52. Letter, Fleetwood to Septimus Justin.

9. HENRY SHIPPEN HUIDEKOPER (1839–1918)

1. Henry M. Rogers, "Henry Shippen Huidekoper," *Harvard Graduates Magazine* 27 (March 1919): 325; Thomas Chamberlin, *History of the One Hundred and Fiftieth Regiment Pennsylvania Volunteers* (Philadelphia: J. B. Lippincott, 1895), 107–109.

2. Chamberlin, *History of the One Hundred and Fiftieth Regiment*, 110–111.

3. Ibid., 110; Henry S. Huidekoper, "A Short Story of the First Day's Fight at Gettysburg," pamphlet (Philadelphia: Bicking Print, 1906), 4–5.

4. Chamberlin, *History of the One Hundred and Fiftieth Regiment*, 111–112.

5. Ibid., 113; St. Clair Augustin Mulholland, *The Story of the 116th Regiment Pennsylvania Volunteers in the War of the Rebellion* (Philadelphia: F. McManus Jr., 1903), 128.

6. Chamberlin, *History of the One Hundred and Fiftieth Regiment*, 112–113, 15–18; *The War of the Rebellion: Official Records of the Civil War* [OR] Serial 043, chap. 39, 347, "The Gettysburg Campaign," "Report of Lieutenant Colonel Henry S. Huidekoper," no. 67, accessed July 3, 2023, https://ehistory.osu.edu/books/official-records.

7. The record does not specify which leg was hit.

8. Chamberlin, *History of the One Hundred and Fiftieth Regiment*, 118–119, 122; Huidekoper, "Short Story of the First Day's Fight"; Mulholland, *Story of the 116th Regiment*, 128; "If the 1st Corps and 11th Corps together could hug that long ridgeline, with the McPherson farm at its center, then Meade and the others would have time to collect the rest of the Army of the Potomac and stride to their rescue; if not, there was always Cemetery Hill (and Steinwehr's division) as the fallback." From Guelzo, *Gettysburg*, 165.

9. Chamberlin, *History of the One Hundred and Fiftieth Regiment*, 121–122; letter of Roy Stone, Commanding Second Brigade, Third Division, First Army Corps at Gettysburg, supporting the Huidekoper Medal of Honor nomination, May 1, 1902, Huidekoper scrapbook, Union League Legacy Foundation, Philadelphia.

10. Chamberlin, *History of the One Hundred and Fiftieth Regiment*, 123; Huidekoper letter to S. Weir Mitchell, "In matter of loss of limb," February 10, 1906, Mitchell Papers, MSS 2/241-3/Series 4.5, box 11.

11. Chamberlin, *History of the One Hundred and Fiftieth Regiment*, 124; Henry S. Huidekoper, "Historic Church and Hospital on the Battlefield of Gettysburg," undated pamphlet (publisher unknown, 1916), Gettysburg National Military Park Collections. The unnamed editor of the pamphlet notes that it was published posthumously and reprints a letter from Huidekoper, dated November 23, 1916, to Chas. F. McKenna, member of the Gettysburg Battlefield Memorial Commission.

12. Huidekoper, "Historic Church."

13. Ibid.

14. Ibid.; Huidekoper's last published reminiscence about Gettysburg contains no conversation between Ewell and himself. By the time Huidekoper died, however, a story circulated (possibly encouraged by Huidekoper) that when a staff officer called down that the Union forces were on the verge of defeat, Ewell said, "We've licked the Yankees," and Huidekoper "spoke up angrily in denial." See Rogers, "Henry Shippen Huidekoper."

15. Huidekoper, "Historic Church."

16. Ibid.

17. Henry S. Huidekoper, "Personal Notes and Reminiscences of Lincoln," pamphlet (Philadelphia: Bicking Print, 1896), 5.

18. Ibid.

19. Ibid., 9.

20. Welsh-born Owens had a controversial military career. Just before the Gettysburg battle began, Owens was relieved of command of the Philadelphia Brigade because of disciplinary problems in the regiment. In 1864, he was discharged from the army possibly due to nonfeasance of duty or cowardice; Huidekoper letter to Mitchell, "In matter of loss of limb"; Huidekoper, "Historic Church."

21. Medical Certificate, July 29, 1863; letter, Huidekoper to Brigadier-General G. Thomas, Adjutant General United States Army, July 29, 1863; Medical Certificate prepared by John T. Ray, MD, Meadville, Pennsylvania; CSR.

22. Special Order No. 475, Adjutant General, War Department, Washington, DC, to Huidekoper, October 23, 1863. CSR; Huidekoper, "Personal Notes," 12.

23. Chamberlin, *History of the One Hundred and Fiftieth Regiment*, 166.

24. Ibid., 165, 180; Special Order No. 13, Headquarters First Army Corps, Army of the Potomac, CSR.

25. Marten, *Sing Not War*, 27–30; Francis Clarke, "Honorable Scars," in Cimbala and Miller, *Union Soldiers and the Home Front*, 379.

26. Clarke, "'Honorable Scars.'"

27. S. Weir Mitchell, "Phantom Limbs," *Lippincott's Magazine of Popular Literature and Science* 7 (December 1871): 565; Clarke, "'Honorable Scars,'" 390.

28. Figg and Farrell-Beck, "Amputation in the Civil War," 473.

29. Mitchell, "Phantom Limbs," 566–567.

30. S. Weir Mitchell, "The Case of George Dedlow," *Atlantic Monthly* 18, no. 105 (July 1866): 2–4.

31. Ibid., 4–5.

32. Ibid., 6.

33. Ibid., 6–8.

34. Herschbach, "'True Clinical Fictions,'" 199; Mitchell, "Case of George Dedlow," 1–11. Mitchell describes the story as having no "scientific value whatsoever" but value "as a psychological statement," 1; Cervetti, "S. Weir Mitchell," 80.

35. Cervetti, "S. Weir Mitchell," 86; Corrales Diaz, "Remembering the Veteran," 10; Mitchell, "Case of George Dedlow," 11; Goler, "Loss and the Persistence of Memory," 162, 171.

36. Mitchell, "Case of George Dedlow," 11.

37. Herschbach, "True Clinical Fictions," 185, 192; on animal magnetism, see Doris V. Falk, "Poe and the Power of Animal Magnetism," *Publications of the Modern Language Association* 84, no. 3 (May 1969): 536.

38. O'Connor, *Raw Material*, 104, 114, 125; Clarke, "'Honorable Scars,'" 363; Louis et al., "Neurologic Content of S. Weir Mitchell's Fiction," 403.

39. Equates to $566 today, which buys about 5.3 percent of what it could buy in 1864.

40. Adjutant General's Office, receipt of pension application form, May 20, 1864; Claim for an Invalid Pension, May 27, 1864, PF.

41. Royden Keith Yerkes, *The History of Saint Luke's Church, Germantown, Philadelphia* (Philadelphia: privately published, 1912), 34, accessed July 3, 2023, https://archive.org/details/historyofsaintluooyerk/mode/2up; John Thomas Scharf and Thompson Westcott, *History of Philadelphia, 1609–1884*, vol. 2 (Philadelphia: L. H. Everts, 1884), 1350–1351; *History of Northampton County, Pennsylvania*, part 5, chap. 43 (Pennsylvania: Peter Fritts, 1877), 185–186, accessed July 3, 2023, http://files.usgwarchives.net/pa/northampton/history/local/davis/davis20.txt.

42. United States Census 1850, Meadville, Crawford County, PA, roll M432_770, 169A; United States Census 1860, Meadville, roll M653_1099, 529; "Great Fire at Meadville: Destruction of Huidekoper's Woolen Mills—Loss About $100,000," *Cleveland Daily Leader*, November 6, 1865.

43. Brian Matthew Jordan, "Living Monuments: Union Veteran Amputees and Embodied Memory of the Civil War," *Civil War History* 57, no. 2 (June 2011): 139.

44. United States Census 1870, Meadville Ward 2, Crawford, PA, roll M593_1330, 285A; Rogers, "Henry Shippen Huidekoper," 326; Headquarters, National Guard of Pennsylvania, Adjutant General's Office, General Order No. 35, November 6, 1895, Union League Legacy Foundation.

45. Rogers, "Henry Shippen Huidekoper," 326; "Peace Prevailing," *Pittsburgh Post-Gazette*, July 30, 1877; *Biographies of Notable Americans, 1904* (database online) (Provo, UT, USA: Ancestry.com Operations Inc., 1997), accessed July 3, 2023, https://www.ancestry.com/search/collections/2022/.

46. Henry S. Huidekoper, "'Gettysburg': A Lecture Delivered by Gen. H. S. Huidekoper, before the Society of Inquiry of Meadville Theological School, Monday Evening, January 13, 1873," *Daily Republican* (Meadville, PA), January 18, 1873; United States Census 1880, Philadelphia, PA; Record of Appointment of Postmasters, 1832-September 30, 1971, Records of the

Post Office Department, Record Group 28, series M841, roll number 112, NARA.

47. "More Monuments: The Unveiling of the Soldier's Statue at Germantown PA: The Parade," *National Tribune* (Washington, DC), July 12, 1883.

48. The archive of the Union League Legacy Foundation maintains a file and scrapbook on member Huidekoper, including newspaper clippings and other ephemera relating to his activities. The file also includes MOLLUS membership paperwork.

49. "Hard Nuts to Crack," *Chicago Tribune,* November 26, 1885.

50. A bony projection of the scapula over the head of the humerus and nestled against the clavicle. Per Dunglison, "The process which terminates the spine of the scapula, and is articulated with the clavicle."

51. Per Dunglison: "A morbid enlargement of a nerve. Applied to subcutaneous, circumscribed, and highly painful tumours formed on the tissue of the nerves."

52. Equates to $1,403 today, which buys about 3.2 percent of what it bought in 1887.

53. Form 3–217 re: pension increase claim of Huidekoper, June 23, 1887; medical examination for increase of pension #29, 153, May 25, 1887, PF.

54. "He's got the glove," *Peninsula Enterprise* (Accomac, VA), quoted from *Philadelphia Record,* February 20, 1897.

55. "Never Heard Complaints: A Telephone Man with a Conveniently Deaf Ear," *New York Times,* December 11, 1887; Rogers, "Henry Shippen Huidekoper," 326; Huidekoper obituary in an undated, unnamed Meadville newspaper in the Huidekoper scrapbook, Union League.

56. "Maimed Soldiers' League," *National Soldier's Tribune* (Washington, DC), March 6, 1890.

57. Henry S. Huidekoper, "Oration by . . . at the Reunion of the Survivors of the 150th Regiment, Pennsylvania Volunteers at Gettysburg, Penna., August 13th, 1894"; "Statue of General Reynolds: The Oration at Unveiling Ceremonies at Gettysburg Delivered by Gen. Huidekoper," *New York Times,* July 2, 1899; Headquarters, National Guard of Pennsylvania, Adjutant General's Office, General Order No. 35, November 6, 1895, Huidekoper scrapbook, Union League.

58. Whitman, *Wound Dresser,* letter to mother, April 26, 1864, 168.

59. United States Census 1900, Philadelphia Ward 22, roll 1464, 7A, enumeration district 0509; The Huidekoper scrapbook at the Union League contains the advertisement for the relief map (dated 1901) and an advertising brochure.

60. "Gen. Huidekoper's Opinion of Those Who Kiss King's Hand," undated, unsourced newspaper article, Huidekoper scrapbook, Union League.

61. Copy of letter from Roy Stone, Commanding Second Brigade, Third Division, First Army Corps at Gettysburg, July 1, 1863, to the Secretary of War, Huidekoper scrapbook, Union League.

62. Copy of letter of Major General Oliver Howard, Commanding 1st, 3rd, & 11th Corps at Gettysburg, July 1, 1863, to the Secretary of War, December 24, 1902, Huidekoper scrapbook, Union League.

63. Equates to about $1,895 today, which buys 2.9 percent of what it bought in 1902.

64. Letter, Huidekoper to Commissioner of Pensions, March 7, 1903; Increase Invalid Pension form, April 29, 1903; Invalid Card, May 5, 1903, PF.

65. Copy of letter from Chief, Record and Pension Office, War Department, to Major General O. O. Howard, October 13, 1903; copy of letter from Assistant Secretary of War Robert Shaw Oliver to Col. Henry S. Huidekoper, cc to Col John P. Nicholson; Huidekoper scrapbook, Union League.

66. Letter, Huidekoper to Col. John P. Nicholson, Huidekoper scrapbook, Union League.

67. Huidekoper letter to Mitchell, "In matter of loss of limb."

68. Ibid.

69. Ibid.

70. Ibid., Dean, *Shook over Hell*, 106; Caruth, *Unclaimed Experience*, 100; Jonathan W. White, *Midnight in America: Darkness, Sleep, and Dreams during the Civil War* (Chapel Hill: University of North Carolina Press, 2017), 183; Goldberg, "'What They Think of the Causes of So Much Suffering,'" 28; Tuggle, *Afterlives of Specimens*, 124.

71. Mitchell, "Phantom Limbs," 564; Corrales Diaz, "Remembering the Veteran," 107; William James, "Consciousness of Lost Limbs," *Proceedings of the American Society for Psychical Research* 1 (1888): 249–258, accessed July 3, 2023, https://psychclassics.yorku.ca/James/lostlimbs.htm; Goler, "Loss and the Persistence of Memory," 174.

72. For Mitchell's discussion of phantoms as tricksters, see Mitchell, "Phantom Limbs," 365–366; James, "Consciousness of Lost Limbs"; Melzack, "Phantom Limbs," 121. Note that phantom sensations do not exclusively occur with amputations; laceration or destruction of nerves can evoke the same phenomena.

73. Crawford, *Phantom Limb*, 9, 12.

74. Tuggle, *Afterlives of Specimens*, 76; Melzack, "Phantom Limbs," 120; Clarke, "'Honorable Scars.'"

75. Crawford, *Phantom Limb*, 33; Robert S. Feldman, "Current Theories and Treatments Related to Phantom Limb Pain," *Orthotics and Prosthetics* 35, no. 3 (1981): 26–30; V. S. Ramachandran and Sandra Blakeslee, *Phantoms of the Brain: Probing the Mysteries of the Human Mind* (New York: William Morrow, 1999); Tuggle, *Afterlives of Specimens*, 103–104; Melzack, "Phantom Limbs," 120–121.

76. Frederic Huidekoper enjoyed a career as influential and prestigious as Henry's, "leaving an honorable record as a soldier, as a business man of high repute . . . and as a leader and adviser of men in great enterprises." Frederic and Herman were the only other brothers to serve in the army, however brief, as enlistees in the 58th Pennsylvania Militia, Company F, which mustered for one month only to defend the state in case of invasion, Frederic as company captain, Herman as a private. Rogers, "Henry Shippen Huidekoper," 325; *Pennsylvania, U.S., Civil War Muster Rolls, 1860–1869* (database online). Provo, UT (Ancestry.com Operations, Inc., 2015); United States Census 1910, Philadelphia Ward 7, roll T624_1389, 5B, enumeration district 0102, FHL microfilm 1375402.

77. "Pennsylvania at Gettysburg: A State Memorial to the Soldiers Who Fought There," *National Tribune*, April 29, 1909; letter from Huidekoper as president, Gettysburg Battlefield Memorial Commission, July 11, 1910, re: date of the memorial dedication, Huidekoper scrapbook, Union League.

78. "The Field at Gettysburg," *Star* (Reynoldsville, PA), October 13, 1910.

79. "Address of General H. S. Huidekoper, president of the Gettysburg Battlefield Memorial Commission, on September 27th, 1910, tendering to Governor Edwin S. Stuart the monument erected at Gettysburg to the Pennsylvania soldiers who fought there in 1863," Huidekoper scrapbook, Union League. "Of all the battlefields, Gettysburg is among the most important. . . . With over nine hundred individual monuments dedicated by the first decades of the twentieth century, the battlefield clearly stood apart from others in importance. Many Union veterans retrospectively recognized Gettysburg as the war's turning point." Quoted from Harris, *Across the Bloody Chasm*, 98.

80. "Address of General H. S. Huidekoper."

81. An obituary noted that Emma Huidekoper had been "widely known socially, and in her younger days was one of the belles of the city." From "Mrs. Henry S. Huidekoper," *Public Ledger* (Philadelphia), December 30, 1912; notice in *Tribune-Republican*, no date or place of publication, re: the memorial tablet; "Industrial School News," source and date not given, re: reunion dinner; Huidekoper scrapbook, Union League.

82. "Unveiling on Appomattox Day," *Star-Independent* (Harrisburg, PA), November 19, 1914; "Repairing State Monument." *Harrisburg Telegraph*

(Harrisburg, PA), August 4, 1915; Rogers, "Henry Shippen Huidekoper," 327.

83. Equates to $1,907 today, which buys 3.4 percent of what it bought in 1915.

84. Anti-German sentiment was common as the United States prepared to enter World War I. This reference alludes to the worthlessness of German ultimatums.

85. Form 3–1638 Pension Increase dated June 6, 1916; certificate 29, 153, stamped at top, "Medal of Honor Roll Act Apr 27, 1916"; Invalid Pension form, stamped "Medal of Honor Roll," October 12, 1916; letter, Huidekoper to Disbursing Officer, Pension Office, Washington, DC, June 19, 1918; letter, Commissioner, Pension office, to Huidekoper, August 6, 1918. All documents from PF.

86. Undated, unsourced newspaper obituary; "Funeral of General H. S. Huidekoper," newspaper clipping, source and date not noted; both in Huidekoper scrapbook, Union League; Huidekoper burial record of Kirk & Ice, Undertakers of Germantown, Philadelphia, Historic Pennsylvania Church and Town Records, Historical Society of Pennsylvania, Philadelphia, PA.

87. Jordan, "Living Monuments," 104, 136, 151–152.

88. Herschbach, "True Clinical Fictions," 196.

89. Huidekoper, "Historic Church" (italics in the original).

90. Richard L. Ashhurst, "Address to the Survivors' Association of the 150th Regiment, Pennsylvania Volunteers. Read at Gettysburg, Sept. 25, 1896," pamphlet (Philadelphia: Allen, Lane & Scott, 1896), 6, 12–13, accessed July 3, 2023, https://archive.org/details/addresstosurvivoooashh/mode/2up; Tuggle quotation from her poem "The Northern Road," *Calenture*, 37.

91. Typed form, Commissioner G. M. Saltzgaber, Finance Division, Dept. of Interior, Office of Pensions to J. H. Devine, Philadelphia, January 11, 1919; Office of Pensions form, Pensioner Dropped, certificate 29153, January 16, 1919. Both documents in PF.

10. THE WIND OF THEIR PLACE AND TIME

1. "On the Slain Collegians," in Melville, *Battle-Pieces of Herman Melville*, 143.

2. Not all respondents to the Mitchells' survey bore Civil War injuries or wounds; three experienced amputation following various accidents in nonmilitary contexts. For information about the study of the questionnaires, see Bonnan-White et al., "Voices from the Past," 17. In the 1890s, the

federal government tried to elicit data from veterans in need of health services. By then, the government had either rejected or could not adjudicate more than 250,000 claims for assistance because living witnesses could not be found to testify to applicants' needs and verify wartime disability. The government therefore conducted its own survey to identify living veterans and establish their whereabouts. No evidence shows that government agencies serving veterans knew about the Mitchells' study or incorporated clinical questions in any special census of veterans. Logue and Blanck, *Heavy Laden*, 205.

3. Foote, *Gentlemen and the Roughs*, 119.

4. Whitman, *Memoranda*, 37–38.

5. Letter, Walt Whitman to Ralph Waldo Emerson, January 17, 1863, *The Collected Writings of Walt Whitman; The Correspondence, Vol. 1, 1842–67*, ed. Edwin Haviland Miller (New York University Press, 1961), 69.

6. Whitman, *Memoranda*, 45.

7. Letter, Walt Whitman to Ralph Waldo Emerson, 69; Tuggle, *Afterlives of Specimens*, 8.

8. Carroll, *Invisible Wounds*, 239.

9. Etter, *Good Body*, 95, 100; On the definition of Black bodies as inherently diseased, see the discussion of *Cachexia Africana* in Hogarth, *Medicalizing Blackness*.

10. Logue and Blanck, *Heavy Laden*, 11, 104, 157, 217.

11. Whitman, *Memoranda*, 125.

12. Gould, *Investigations in the Military and Anthropological Statistics*; Baxter, *Statistics, Medical and Anthropological*; Braun, "Spirometry, Measurement, and Race."

13. Etter, *Good Body*, 198, 201; *Medical and Surgical History*; Kircher listing appears in the *Surgical History*, part 2, vol. 2, 727, and part 3, vol. 2, 883.

14. Etter, *Good Body*, 220; Handley-Cousins, *Bodies in Blue*, 135.

15. Logue and Blanck, *Heavy Laden*, 84; Etter, *Good Body*, 149.

16. Whitman, *Wound Dresser*, 2.

17. Walt Whitman, "O me! O life!" from Whitman, *Drum-Taps: The Complete 1865 Edition*, ed. Lawrence Kramer (New York: New York Review of Books, 2015), 121.

APPENDIX A

1. Peter Blanck, "Civil War Pensions and Disability," *Ohio State Law Journal* 62, no. 1 (2001): 109–238; Peter Blanck, Claudia Linares, and Chen Song, "Evolution of Disability in Late 19th Century America: Civil War Pensions for Union Army Veterans with Musculoskeletal Conditions,"

Behavioral Sciences and the Law 20 (2002): 681–697; Brian Matthew Jordan, *Marching Home: Union Veterans and Their Unending Civil War* (New York: Liveright, 2014), 149–156; Larry M. Logue and Peter Blanck, *Race, Ethnicity, and Disability: Veterans and Benefits in Post-Civil War America* (New York: Cambridge University Press, 2010), 18–32; John William Oliver, "History of Civil War Military Pensions, 1861–1885," *Bulletin of the University of Wisconsin* 844 (1917): 55–111; Holly A. Pinheiro Jr., *The Families' Civil War: Black Soldiers and the Fight for Racial Justice* (Athens: University of Georgia Press, 2022), 111–129; Theda Skocpol, "America's First Social Security System: The Expansion of Benefits for Civil War Veterans," *Political Science Quarterly* 108 (1993): 85–116.

2. Donald R. Shaffer, *After the Glory: The Struggles of Black Civil War Veterans* (Lawrence: University Press of Kansas, 2004), 123.

3. Blanck et al., "Evolution of Disability in Late 19th Century America," 685.

4. Ibid.

5. Ibid., 684.

BIBLIOGRAPHY

ARCHIVES

Belleville Public Library, Illinois
Henry A. Kircher file
Gettysburg National Military Park Library and Research Center, Pennsylvania
Henry S. Huidekoper file
Historical Medical Library, The College of Physicians of Philadelphia
S. Weir Mitchell papers, follow-up studies of patients with nerve injuries, 1863–1906, MSS 2/241-03, Series 4.5
Turner's Lane Hospital; case and follow-up studies of peripheral nerve disorders, including correspondence addressed to S. W. Mitchell: Philadelphia, 1861–1892, Z10 40
United States Army. *West Philadelphia Hospital Register.* Philadelphia: General Hospital, 1863–1865
Hunterdon County Historical Society, Flemington, New Jersey
John Shields file
National Archives and Records Administration
Civil War Consolidated Service Records
Civil War Federal Military Pension Files
United States Census, 1850–1920
The Union League Legacy Foundation, Philadelphia
Henry S. Huidekoper member scrapbook
Vineland Historical & Antiquarian Society, Vineland, New Jersey
John Shields file

NEWSPAPERS

Belleville Advocate (IL)
Belleville Illinois Illustrated
Belleville News Democrat
Camden Daily Telegram (NJ)
Camden Post-Telegram (NJ)
Chicago Tribune (IL)
Cleveland Daily Leader (OH)
Courier-Post (Camden, NJ)
The Daily Republican (Meadville, PA)
Denton Journal (MD)
Evening Journal (Vineland, NJ)
The Evening Record and Bergen County Herald (Hackensack, NJ)
Hardware Dealer's Magazine (NY)
Harrisburg Telegraph (PA)
Hunterdon Republican (NJ)
Indiana Herald (Huntington, IN)
Indianapolis Journal (IN)
The Mauch Chunk Gazette (PA)
The Morning Post (Camden, NJ)
The National Tribune (*The National Soldier's Tribune*) (Washington, DC)
New Era (Washington, DC)
The New York Times
New York Tribune
Oakland Tribune (CA)
Passaic Daily News (NJ)
The Patterson Morning Call (NJ)
Peninsula Enterprise (Accomac, VA)
Pittsburgh Post-Gazette (PA)
Public Ledger (Philadelphia, PA)
Sacramento Bee (CA)
San Francisco Call (CA)
San Francisco Chronicle (CA)
San Francisco Examiner (CA)
Santa Cruz Surf (CA)
The Star (Reynoldsville, PA)
The Star-Independent (Harrisburg, PA)
Trenton Evening Times (NJ)

PRIMARY PUBLISHED SOURCES

Althaus, Julius. *A Treatise on Medical Electricity, Theoretical and Practical.* Philadelphia: Lindsay and Blakiston, 1860.

Appleton, D. *The American Annual Encyclopedia and Register of Important Events of the Year 1867.* Vol. 7. New York: D. Appleton, 1868.

Ashhurst, Richard L. "Address to the Survivors' Association of the 150th Regiment, Pennsylvania Volunteers. Read at Gettysburg, Sept. 25, 1896." Pamphlet. Philadelphia: Allen, Lane & Scott, 1896.

Bartholow, Roberts. *A Manual of Instructions for Enlisting and Discharging Soldiers.* Philadelphia: J. B. Lippincott, 1863.

Bates, Samuel P. *History of Pennsylvania Volunteers, 1861–5.* 5 vols. Harrisburg, PA: B. Singerly, State Printer, 1869–1871.

Baxter, J. H., comp. *Statistics, Medical and Anthropological, of the Provost-Marshal's Bureau . . . etc.* Washington, DC: US Government Printing Office, 1875.

Beard, George M., and A. B. Rockwell. *The Medical Use of Electricity.* New York: William Wood, 1847.

Bice, E. E., and John L. Connet. *Flemington, New Jersey, Illustrated.* Privately printed, 1898.

Blake, Sarah Swan Weld. *Diaries and Letters of Francis Minot Weld, M.D. with a Sketch of His Life.* Boston: privately published, 1925.

Bly, Douglas. "A Remarkable Invention in Artificial Legs." Pamphlet. Rochester, NY: Curtis, Butts, 1862.

Chamberlin, Thomas. *History of the One Hundred and Fiftieth Regiment Pennsylvania Volunteers.* Philadelphia: J. B. Lippincott, 1895.

Channing, William F. *The Medical Application of Electricity.* 5th ed. Boston: Thomas Hall, 1859.

———. "On the Municipal Electric Telegraph; Especially in Its Application to Fire Alarms." *American Journal of Science and Arts* 13, 2nd ser. (January 1852): 58–83.

Chisholm, Julian J. *A Manual of Military Surgery.* Richmond, VA: West & Johnston, 1861.

Dickinson, Emily. *Poems.* New York: Alfred A. Knopf, 1993.

Dunglison, Robley. *Medical Lexicon: Dictionary of Medical Science.* Philadelphia: Henry C. Lea, 1868.

Flint, Austin, ed. *Contributions Relating to the Causation and Prevention of Diseases.* New York: US Sanitary Commission, 1867.

Garratt, Alfred C. *Guide for Using Medical Batteries.* Philadelphia: Lindsay and Blakiston, 1867.

Gould, Benjamin Apthorp. *Investigations in the Military and Anthropological Statistics of American Soldiers.* New York: US Sanitary Commission, 1869.

Gross, S. D. *A Manual of Military Surgery.* Philadelphia: J. B. Lippincott, 1862.

Harrower, David I., and Thomas J. Wieckowski, eds. *A Spectacle for Men and Angels: A Documentary Narrative of Camp William Penn and the Raising of Colored Regiments in Pennsylvania.* Conshohocken, PA: Infinity, 2013.

Hess, Earl J., ed. *A German in the Yankee Fatherland: The Civil War Letters of Henry Kircher.* Kent, OH: Kent State University Press, 1983.

History of Northampton County, Pennsylvania. Part 5. Pennsylvania: Peter Fritts, 1877.

Hopkins, C. M. *Atlas of Fifteen Miles around Baltimore Including Howard Co, Maryland.* Philadelphia: F. Bourguin's, 1878.

Huidekoper, Henry S. "Historic Church and Hospital on the Battlefield of Gettysburg." Updated Pamphlet. Publisher unknown, 1916. Gettysburg National Military Park Collections.

———. "Personal Notes and Reminiscences of Lincoln." Pamphlet. Philadelphia: Bicking Print, 1896.

———. "A Short Story of the First Day's Fight at Gettysburg." Pamphlet. Philadelphia: Bicking Print, 1906.

Hunt, Sanford B. "The Negro as Soldier." *Anthropological Review* 7, no. 24 (January 1869): 40–54.

"Influence of the Telegraph upon Literature." *United States Democratic Review* 22 (May 1848): 409–413.

James, William. "Consciousness of Lost Limbs." *Proceedings of the American Society for Psychical Research* 1 (1888): 249–258.

Jaquette, Henrietta Stratton, ed. *Letters of a Civil War Nurse: Cornelia Hancock, 1863–1865.* Lincoln: University of Nebraska Press, 1998.

Keen, W. W., S. Weir Mitchell, and George R. Morehouse. "On Malingering, Especially in Regard to Simulation of Diseases of the Nervous System." *American Journal of Medical Science* 48 (October 1864): 367–394.

Le Grand, Louis. *The Military Hand-Book and Soldier's Manual of Information.* New York: Beadle, 1861.

Longmore, Thomas. *A Treatise on Gunshot Wounds.* Philadelphia: J. B. Lippincott, 1862.

The Medical and Surgical History of the War of the Rebellion. Edited by George A. Otis. 6 vols. Washington, DC: US Government Printing Office, 1876–1888.

Melville, Herman. *The Battle-Pieces of Herman Melville*. Edited by Hennig Cohen. New York: Thomas Yoseloff, 1964.

Mitchell, John K. *Remote Consequences of Injuries of Nerves, and Their Treatment*. Philadelphia: Lea Brothers, 1895.

Mitchell, S. Weir. "The Case of George Dedlow." *Atlantic Monthly* 18, no. 105 (July 1866): 1–11.

———. "Clinical Lecture on Nervousness in the Male." *Medical News and Library* 35 (December 1877): 177–183.

———. *Clinical Lessons on Nervous Diseases*. Philadelphia: Lea Brothers, 1897.

———. *The Collected Poems of S. Weir Mitchell*. New York: Century Press, 1896.

———. "The Early History of Instrumental Precision in Medicine. An Address before the Second Congress of American Physicians and Surgeons, September 23, 1891." Pamphlet. New Haven, CT: Tuttle, Morehouse & Taylor, 1892.

———. *Injuries of Nerves and Their Consequences*. Philadelphia: J. B. Lippincott, 1872.

———. "The Medical Department in the Civil War." *Journal of the American Medical Association* 62, no. 19 (May 9, 1914): 1445–1450.

———. "On the Transmission of Electric Influence across the Middle Line of the Body." Pamphlet. New York: Putnam's Sons, 1877. Reprint from *Transactions of the American Neurological Association* (1877).

———. "Phantom Limbs." *Lippincott's Magazine of Popular Literature and Science* 7 (December 1871): 563–569.

———. "Some Personal Recollections of the Civil War." *Transactions of the College of Physicians of Philadelphia* 27, Third Series (1905): 87–94.

Mitchell, S. Weir, George R. Morehouse, and W. W. Keen Jr. *Gunshot Wounds and Other Injuries of Nerves*. Philadelphia: J. B. Lippincott, 1864.

———. "On the Antagonism of Atropia and Morphia, Founded upon Observations and Experiments Made at the U.S.A. Hospital for Injuries and Diseases of the Nervous System." *American Journal of the Medical Sciences* 50, no. 99, New Series (July 1865): 67–76.

Mulholland, St. Clair Augustin. *The Story of the 116th Regiment Pennsylvania Volunteers in the War of the Rebellion*. Philadelphia: F. McManus Jr., 1903.

Ordronaux, John. *Manual of Instruction for Military Surgeons, on the Examination of Recruits and Discharge of Soldiers*. New York: Van Nostrand, 1863.

Packard, John H. *A Manual of Minor Surgery*. Philadelphia: J. B. Lippincott, 1863.

Powell, William Henry, ed. *Officers of the Army and Navy Who Served in the Civil War*. Philadelphia: L. R. Hamersly, 1893.

Reid, Richard M., ed. *Medicine in a Black Regiment: The Civil War Diary of Burt G. Wilder, 55th Massachusetts*. Boston: University of Massachusetts Press, 2010.

S. Weir Mitchell . . . Memorial Addresses and Resolutions. Philadelphia: privately printed, 1914.

Townshend, Chauncy Hare. *The Three Gates*. London: Chapman and Hall, 1861.

A Treatise on Mark's Artificial Limbs with Rubber Hands and Feet. New York: A. A. Marks, 1888.

United States Pension Office. *Roster of All Regimental Surgeons and Assistant Surgeons*. Washington, DC: United States Pension Office, 1882.

United States War Department. *A Compilation of the Official Records of the Union and Confederate Armies*. Washington, DC: US Government Printing Office, 1889–1901.

Whitman, Walt. *The Collected Writings of Walt Whitman; The Correspondence, Vol. 1, 1842–67*. Edited by Edwin Haviland Miller. New York: New York University Press, 1961.

———. *Drum-Taps: The Complete 1865 Edition*. Edited by Lawrence Kramer. New York: New York Review of Books, 2015.

———. *Memoranda during the War*. Edited by Peter Coviello. New York: Oxford University Press, 2004.

———. *The Wound Dresser*. Edited by Richard Maurice Buck. Boston: Small, Maynard, 1898.

Wister, Owen. "Owen Wister Views Life of Dr. S.W. Mitchell." *Philadelphia Press*, April 15, 1914.

Woodward, Joseph Janvier. *Outlines of the Chief Camp Diseases of the United States Armies as Observed during the Present War: A Practical Contribution to Military Medicine*. Philadelphia: J. B. Lippincott, 1863.

Woolsey, Jane Stuart. *Hospital Days: Reminiscence of a Civil War Nurse*. Intro by Daniel John Hoisington. Roseville, MN: Edinborough, 2007.

SECONDARY SOURCES

Abraham, Nicolas, and Maria Torok. *The Shell and the Kernel: Renewals of Psychoanalysis*. Vol. 1. Edited and translated by Nicolas T. Rand. Chicago: University of Chicago Press, 1968.

Adams, Michael C. *Living Hell: The Dark Side of the Civil War*. Baltimore: Johns Hopkins University Press, 2014.

Alberti, Fay Bound. "Bodies, Hearts, and Minds, Why Emotions Matter to Historians of Science and Medicine." *Isis* 100 (2009): 798–810.

Auslander, Leora. "Beyond Words." *American Historical Review* 110, no. 4 (October 2005): 1015–1045.

Auslander, Leora, and Tara Zahra, eds. *Objects of War: The Material Culture of Conflict and Displacement*. Ithaca, NY: Cornell University Press, 2018.

Bell, Andrew McIlwaine. *Mosquito Soldiers: Malaria, Yellow Fever, and the Course of the American Civil War*. Baton Rouge: Louisiana State University Press, 2010.

Biernoff, Suzannah. *Portraits of Violence: War and the Aesthetics of Disfigurement*. Ann Arbor: University of Michigan Press, 2017.

Bilby, Joseph G. "Uncommon Soldiers, Vignettes from the War between the States." *Military Images* 14, no. 6 (May–June 1993): 10–11.

Bissell, Bill, and Linda Caruso Haviland, eds. *The Sentient Archive: Bodies, Performance, and Memory*. Middletown, CT: Wesleyan University Press, 2018.

Blair, William, and William Pencak, eds. *Pennsylvania's Civil War*. University Park: Pennsylvania State University Press, 2001.

Blanck, Peter. "Civil War Pensions and Disability." *Ohio State Law Journal* 62, no. 1 (2001): 109–238.

Blanck, Peter, Claudia Linares, and Chen Song. "Evolution of Disability in Late 19th Century America: Civil War Pensions for Union Army Veterans with Musculoskeletal Conditions." *Behavioral Sciences and the Law* 20 (2002): 681–697.

Blustein, Bonnie Ellen. *Preserve Your Love for Science: Life of William A. Hammond, American Neurologist*. Cambridge: Cambridge University Press, 1991.

Bonnan-White, Jess, Jewelry Yep, and Melanie D. Hetzel-Riggin. "Voices from the Past: Mental and Physical Outcomes Described by American Civil War Amputees." *Journal of Trauma & Dissociation* 17, no. 1 (2016): 13–34.

Bourke, Joanna. *Dismembering the Male: Men's Bodies, Britain and the Great War.* Chicago: University of Chicago Press, 1996.

Braun, Lundy. "Spirometry, Measurement, and Race in the Nineteenth Century." *Journal of the History of Medicine and Allied Sciences* 60, no. 2 (2005): 135–169.

Brush, Stephen G. *The History of Modern Science: A Guide to the Second Scientific Revolution, 1800–1950.* Ames: Iowa State University Press, 1988.

Bud, Robert, and Deborah Jean Warner, eds. *Instruments of Science: An Historical Encyclopedia.* New York: Garland, 1998.

Burr, Anna Robeson. *Weir Mitchell: His Life and Letters.* New York: Duffield, 1929.

Burr, Charles W. *Affairs.* Philadelphia: College of Physicians of Philadelphia, 1920.

Burton, William L. *Melting Pot Soldiers: The Union's Ethnic Regiments.* Ames: Iowa State University Press, 1988.

Canale, D. J. "Civil War Medicine from the Perspective of S. Weir Mitchell's 'The Case of George Dedlow.'" *Journal of the History of the Neurosciences* 11, no. 1 (2002): 11–18.

Carmichael, Peter S. *The War for the Common Soldier.* Chapel Hill: University of North Carolina Press, 2018.

Carroll, Dillon J. *Invisible Wounds: Mental Illness and Civil War Soldiers.* Baton Rouge: Louisiana State University Press, 2021.

Caruth, Cathy. *Unclaimed Experience: Trauma, Narrative, and History.* Baltimore: Johns Hopkins University Press, 1996.

Cashin, Joan E., ed. *War Matters: Material Culture in the Civil War Era.* Chapel Hill: University of North Carolina Press, 2018.

———, ed. *The War Was You and Me: Civilians in the American Civil War.* Princeton, NJ: Princeton University Press, 2002.

Cavedon, Christina. *Cultural Melancholia: US Trauma Discourses Before and After 9/11.* Boston: Brill, 2015.

Cervetti, Nancy. "S. Weir Mitchell Representing 'a Hell of Pain': From Civil War to Rest Cure." *Arizona Quarterly* 59, no. 3 (Autumn 2003): 69–96.

———. *S. Weir Mitchell, 1829–1914: Philadelphia's Literary Physician.* University Park: Pennsylvania State University Press, 2012.

Cetina, Judith Gladys. "A History of Veterans' Homes in the United States, 1811–1930." PhD diss., Case Western Reserve University, 1977.

Cimbala, Paul A., and Randall M. Miller, eds. *Union Soldiers and the Northern Home Front: Wartime Experiences, Postwar Adjustments.* New York: Fordham University Press, 2002.

Clarke, Frances M. *War Stories: Suffering and Sacrifice in the Civil War North*. Chicago: University of Chicago Press, 2011.

Corrales Diaz, Erin. "Remembering the Veteran: Disability, Trauma, and the American Civil War, 1861–1915." PhD diss., University of North Carolina, 2016.

Costa, Dora L. *The Evolution of Retirement: An American Economic History, 1880–1900*. Chicago: University of Chicago Press, 1998.

Crawford, Cassandra S. *Phantom Limb: Amputation, Embodiment, and Prosthetic Technology*. New York: New York University Press, 2014.

Cullen, Jim. *The Civil War in Popular Culture: A Reusable Past*. Washington, DC: Smithsonian Institution Press, 1995.

Currier, Dean P. *A Guide to Electrotherapy Instruments and History of Their American Makers*. West Conshohocken, PA: Infinity, 2005.

Daniel, Hilary, Sue. S. Bornstein, and Gregory C. Kane. "Addressing Social Determinants to Improve Patient Care and Promote Health Equity: An American College of Physicians Position Paper." *Annals of Internal Medicine* 168, no. 8 (April 17, 2018): 577–578.

Dean, Eric T., Jr. *Shook over Hell: Post-Traumatic Stress, Vietnam, and the Civil War*. Cambridge, MA: Harvard University Press, 1997.

Devine, Shauna. *Learning from the Wounded: The Civil War and the Rise of American Medical Science*. Chapel Hill: University of North Carolina Press, 2014.

Downs, Jim. *Sick from Freedom: African-American Illness and Suffering during the Civil War and Reconstruction*. New York: Oxford University Press, 2012.

Earnest, Ernest. *S. Weir Mitchell: Novelist and Physician*. Philadelphia: University of Pennsylvania Press, 1950.

Edmonds, Franklin Spencer. *History of Central High School of Philadelphia*. Philadelphia: J. B. Lippincott, 1902.

Etter, William M. *The Good Body: Normalizing Visions in Nineteenth-Century American Literature and Culture, 1836–1867*. Newcastle upon Tyne: Cambridge Scholars, 2010.

Falk, Doris V. "Poe and the Power of Animal Magnetism." *Publications of the Modern Language Association* 84, no. 3 (May 1969): 536–546.

Faust, Drew Gilpin. *This Republic of Suffering: Death and the Civil War*. New York: Vintage Books, 2008.

Feldman, Robert S. "Current Theories and Treatments Related to Phantom Limb Pain." *Orthotics and Prosthetics* 35, no. 3 (1981): 26–30.

Fett, Sharla M. *Working Cures: Healing, Health, and Power on Southern Slave Plantations*. Chapel Hill: University of North Carolina Press, 2002.

Figg, Laurann, and Jane Farrell-Beck. "Amputation in the Civil War: Physical and Social Dimensions." *Journal of the History of Medicine and Allied Sciences* 48, no. 4 (October 1993): 454–475.

Foote, Lorien. *The Gentlemen and the Roughs: Manhood, Honor, and Violence in the Union Army*. New York: New York University Press, 2010.

Foucault, Michel. *The Birth of the Clinic*. London: Routledge, 1989.

Franzino, Jean. "'Harmonies of Form and Color': Race and the Prosthetic Body in Civil War America." *Literature and Medicine* 38, no. 1 (Spring 2020): 51–87.

Freemon, Frank R. "The First Neurological Research Center: Turner's Lane Hospital during the American Civil War." *Journal of the History of the Neurosciences* 2 (1993): 135–142.

Gannon, Barbara A. *The Won Cause: Black and White Comradeship in the Grand Army of the Republic*. Chapel Hill: University of North Carolina Press, 2011.

Gillmore, Paul. "Romantic Electricity, or the Materiality of Aesthetics." *American Literature* 76, no. 3 (September 2004): 467–494.

Glatthaar, Joseph T. *Forged in Battle: The Civil War Alliance of Black Soldiers and White Officers*. New York: Free Press, 1990.

Goldberg, Daniel. "'What They Think of the Causes of So Much Suffering': S. Weir Mitchell, John Kearsley Mitchell, and Ideas about Phantom Limb Pain in Late 19th c. America." *Spontaneous Generations: A Journal for the History and Philosophy of Science* 8, no. 1 (2016): 27–54.

Goler, Robert I. "Loss and the Persistence of Memory: 'The Case of George Dedlow' and Disabled Civil War Veterans." *Literature and Medicine* 23, no. 1 (Spring 2004): 160–183.

Greenberg, Amy. *Manifest Manhood and the Antebellum American Empire*. New York: Cambridge University Press, 2005.

Guelzo, Allen C. *Gettysburg: The Last Invasion*. New York: Alfred A. Knopf, 2013.

Gutman, Herbert G. *The Black Family in Slavery and Freedom 1750–1925*. New York: Pantheon Books, 1976.

Hagaman, Robert A. "Personal Battles: The Lives of Maryland's Black Civil War Veterans, 1840–1920." PhD diss., Northern Illinois University, 2004.

Handley-Cousins, Sarah. *Bodies in Blue: Disability in the Civil War North*. Athens: University of Georgia Press, 2019.

Harris, M. Keith. *Across the Bloody Chasm: The Culture of Commemoration among Civil War Veterans*. Baton Rouge: Louisiana University Press, 2014.

Harrison, Simon. *Dark Trophies: Hunting and the Enemy Body in Modern War.* New York: Berghahn Books, 2012.

Hasegawa, Guy R. *Mending Broken Soldiers: The Union and Confederate Programs to Supply Artificial Limbs.* Carbondale: Southern Illinois University Press, 2012.

Herschbach, Lisa. "Prosthetic Reconstructions: Making the Industry, Re-Making the Body, Modelling the Nation." *History Workshop Journal* 44 (Autumn 1997): 22–57.

———. "'True Clinical Fictions': Medical and Literary Narratives from the Civil War Hospital." *Culture, Medicine and Psychiatry* 19 (1995): 183–205.

History of Northampton County, Pennsylvania. Part 5. PA: Peter Fritts, 1877.

Hogarth, Rana A. *Medicalizing Blackness: Making Racial Difference in the Atlantic World, 1780–1840.* Chapel Hill: University of North Carolina Press, 2017.

Horwitz, Tony. "Did Civil War Soldiers Have PTSD?" *Smithsonian Magazine,* January 2015. https://www.smithsonianmag.com/history/ptsd-civil-wars-hidden-legacy-180953652/.

Humphreys, Margaret. *Intensely Human: The Health of the Black Soldier in the American Civil War.* Baltimore: Johns Hopkins University Press, 2008.

———. *Marrow of Tragedy: The Health Crisis of the American Civil War.* Baltimore: Johns Hopkins University Press, 2013.

Jordan, Brian Matthew. "Living Monuments: Union Veteran Amputees and Embodied Memory of the Civil War." *Civil War History* 57, no. 2 (June 2011): 121–152.

———. *Marching Home: Union Veterans and Their Unending Civil War.* New York: Liveright, 2014.

Kelly, Joseph Thomas. "Rev. John C. Smith, D.D., and Other Pioneer Presbyterian Ministers of Washington." *Records of the Columbia Historical Society, Washington, D.C.* 24 (1922): 118–135.

Kreiser, Lawrence A., Jr., and Randal Allred, eds. *The Civil War in Popular Culture: Memory and Meaning.* Lexington: University of Kentucky Press, 2013.

Kriegel, Leonard. "Uncle Tom as Tiny Tim: Reflections on the Cripple as Negro." *American Scholar* 38, no. 3 (Summer 1969): 412–430.

Lande, R. Gregory. *Psychological Consequences of the American Civil War.* Jefferson, NC: McFarland, 2017.

Logue, Larry M., and Peter Blanck. *Heavy Laden: Union Veterans, Psychological Illness, and Suicide.* New York: Cambridge University Press, 2018.

———. *Race, Ethnicity, and Disability: Veterans and Benefits in Post-Civil War America*. New York: Cambridge University Press, 2010.

Long, Gretchen. *Doctoring Freedom: The Politics of African American Medical Care in Slavery and Emancipation*. Chapel Hill: University of North Carolina Press, 2012.

Long, Lisa A. *Rehabilitating Bodies: Health, History, and the American Civil War*. Philadelphia: University of Pennsylvania Press, 2004.

Louis, Elan D., Stacy Horn, and Lisa Anne Roth. "The Neurologic Content of S. Weir Mitchell's Fiction." *Neurology* 66, no. 3 (February 14, 2006): 403–407.

Lubar, Steven, and W. David Kingery, eds. *History from Things: Essays on Material Culture*. Washington, DC: Smithsonian Institution, 1993.

Marten, James. *Sing Not War: The Lives of Union & Confederate Veterans in Gilded Age America*. Chapel Hill: University of North Carolina Press, 2011.

Martin, David G. *Gettysburg, July 1*. Lebanon, IN: Da Capo, 1995.

McClurken, Jeffrey W. *Take Care of the Living: Reconstructing Confederate Veteran Families in Virginia*. Charlottesville: University of Virginia Press, 2009.

McConnell, Stuart. *Glorious Contentment: The Grand Army of the Republic, 1865–1900*. Chapel Hill: University of North Carolina Press, 1992.

McCrosson, W. Rex, ed. "The Story of Fifty Odd Years of the New Jersey Memorial Home for Soldiers, Sailors, Marines Their Wives & Widows." Unpublished mimeograph copy, Vineland Historical & Antiquarian Society, 1952, supplement 1957.

McWhirter, Laura, Alan Carson, and Jon Stone. "The Body Electric: A Long View of Electrical Therapy for Functional Neurological Disorders." *Brain, a Journal of Neurology* 138 (2015): 1113–1120.

Meier, Kathryn Shively. *Nature's Civil War: Common Soldiers and the Environment in 1862 Virginia*. Chapel Hill: University of North Carolina Press, 2013.

Melzack, Ronald. "Phantom Limbs." *Scientific American* 266 (April 1992): 120–126.

Mezurek, Kelly D. *For Their Own Cause: The 27th United States Colored Troops*. Kent, OH: Kent State University Press, 2016.

Micale, Mark S. *Hysterical Men: The Hidden History of Male Nervous Illness*. Cambridge, MA: Harvard University Press, 2008.

Middleton, William S. "Turner's Lane Hospital." *Bulletin of the History of Medicine* 40, no. 1 (January–February 1966): 14–42.

Miller, Brian Craig. *Empty Sleeves: Amputation in the Civil War South.* Athens: University of Georgia Press, 2015.

Mitchell, Reid. *The Vacant Chair: The Northern Soldier Leaves Home.* New York: Oxford University Press, 1993.

Morus, Iwan Rhys. "Galvanic Culture: Electricity and Life in the Early Nineteenth Century." *Endeavour* 22, no. 1 (1998): 7–11.

Myers, Irvin C. *We Might As Well Die Here: The 53rd Pennsylvania Veteran Infantry.* Shippensburg, PA: White Mane, 2004.

Nelson, Megan Kate. *Ruin Nation: Destruction and the American Civil War.* Athens: University of Georgia Press, 2012.

Nielsen, Kim E. *A Disability History of the United States.* Boston: Beacon, 2012.

Numbers, Ronald L., and Todd L. Savitt, eds. *Science and Medicine in the Old South.* Baton Rouge: Louisiana State University Press, 1989.

O'Connor, Erin. "'Fractions of Men': Engendering Amputation in Victorian Culture." *Comparative Studies in Society and History* 39 (1997): 742–777.

———. *Raw Material: Producing Pathology in Victorian Culture.* Durham, NC: Duke University Press, 2000.

Oliver, John William. "History of Civil War Military Pensions, 1861–1885." *Bulletin of the University of Wisconsin* 844 (1917): 55–111.

Page, Sebastian N. *Black Resettlement and the American Civil War.* New York: Cambridge University Press, 2021.

Pappert, Eric J. "Philadelphia Infirmary for Nervous Diseases: America's Original Model of Institutional Neurology." *Neurology* 50, no. 6 (1998): 1847–1853.

Paradis, James M. *Strike the Blow for Freedom: The 6th United States Colored Infantry in the Civil War.* Shippensburg, PA: White Mane, 1998.

Pernick, Martin S. *A Calculus of Suffering: Pain, Professionalism, and Anesthesia in Nineteenth-Century America.* New York: Columbia University Press, 1985.

Pinheiro, Holly A., Jr. *The Families' Civil War: Black Soldiers and the Fight for Racial Justice.* Athens: University of Georgia Press, 2022.

Pizarro, Judith, Roxanne Cohen Silver, and JoAnn Prause. "Physical and Mental Health Costs of Traumatic War Experiences among Civil War Veterans." *Archives of General Psychiatry* 63 (February 2006): 193–200.

Pratt-Smith, Stella. *Transformations of Electricity in Nineteenth-Century Literature and Science.* Farnham: Ashgate, 2016.

Price, James S. *The Battle of New Market Heights.* Charleston, SC: History Press, 2011.

Ramachandran, V. S., and Sandra Blakeslee. *Phantoms of the Brain: Probing the Mysteries of the Human Mind*. New York: William Morrow, 1999.

Riley, Brendan. "Tough Times for Armless Civil War Vet in Vallejo." *Times-Herald* (Vallejo, CA), November 10, 2019.

Roberts, Alice, ed. *The Complete Human Body: The Definitive Visual Guide*. 2nd ed. New York: Dorling Kindersley, 2016.

Roberts, Dorothy. *Killing the Black Body: Race, Reproduction, and the Meaning of Liberty*. New York: Pantheon Books, 1997.

Rogers, Henry M. "Henry Shippen Huidekoper." *Harvard Graduate Magazine* 27 (March 1919): 325–327.

Rose, Sarah F. *No Right to Be Idle: The Invention of Disability, 1840s–1930s*. Chapel Hill: University of North Carolina Press, 2017.

Rosenberg, Charles E., and Janet Golden, eds. *Framing Disease: Studies in Cultural History*. New Brunswick, NJ: Rutgers University Press, 1992.

Rotundo, E. Anthony. *American Manhood: Transformations in Masculinity from the Revolution to the Modern Era*. New York: Basic Books, 1993.

Rowbottom, Margaret, and Charles Susskind. *Electricity and Medicine: History of Their Interaction*. San Francisco: San Francisco Press, 1984.

Scarry, Elaine. *The Body in Pain: The Making and Unmaking of the World*. New York: Oxford University Press, 1985.

Scharf, John Thomas, and Thompson Westcott. *History of Philadelphia, 1609–1884*. Vol. 2. Philadelphia: L. H. Everts, 1884.

Schauffler, Moyra Williams. "Nature for Its Guide: An Object-Centered Analysis of Nineteenth-Century Mechanized and Anatomically Analogous Artificial Limbs." *Surgeon's Call/Journal of the National Museum of Civil War Medicine* 25, no. 2 (2020): 5–14.

Schlereth, Thomas J., ed. *Material Culture Studies in America*. Nashville, TN: American Association for State and Local History, 1982.

Schwalm, Leslie A. *Medicine, Science & Making Race in Civil War America*. Chapel Hill: University of North Carolina Press, 2023.

Scott, Donald, Sr. *Camp William Penn 1863–1865*. Atglen, PA: Schiffer Military History, 2012.

Shaffer, Donald R. *After the Glory: The Struggles of Black Civil War Veterans*. Lawrence: University Press of Kansas, 2004.

Sheehan-Dean, Aaron, ed. *A Companion to the Civil War*. 2 vols. Hoboken, NJ: Wiley Blackwell, 2014. (Essay "Manhood").

Silkenat, David. *Moments of Despair: Suicide, Divorce, & Debt in Civil War Era North Carolina*. Chapel Hill: University of North Carolina Press, 2011.

Skocpol, Theda. "America's First Social Security System: The Expansion of Benefits for Civil War Veterans." *Political Science Quarterly* 108 (1993): 85–116.

———. *Protecting Soldiers and Mothers: The Political Origins of Social Policy in the United States*. Cambridge, MA: Harvard University Press, 1992.

Smith, Pamela H., Amy R. Meyers, and Harold J. Cook, eds. *Ways of Making and Knowing: The Material Culture of Empirical Knowledge*. Ann Arbor: University of Michigan Press, 2014.

Sontag, Susan. *Illness as Metaphor*. New York: Vintage Books, 1979.

———. *Regarding the Pain of Others*. New York: Farrar, Strauss and Giroux, 2003.

Stiles, Anne M. "'The Intimate Language of Friendship with Men': Same-Sex Attraction in the Civil War Fiction of S. Weir Mitchell." *Literature and Medicine* 32, no. 1 (Spring 2014): 193–217.

Snell, James P., comp. *History of Hunterdon and Somerset Counties, New Jersey*. Philadelphia: Everts & Peck, 1881.

Stone, James L. "W. W. Keen: America's Pioneer Neurological Surgeon." *Neurosurgery* 17, no. 6 (1985): 997–1010.

Tabbert, Mark A., and William D. Moore, eds. *Secret Societies in America: Foundational Studies in Fraternalism*. New Orleans: Cornerstone Books, 2011.

Thurber, Evangeline. "The 1890 Census Records of the Veterans of the Union Army." *National Genealogical Society Quarterly* 34 (March 1946): 7–9.

Townsend, Mary Bobbitt. *Yankee Warhorse; A Biography of Major General Peter Osterhaus*. Columbia: University of Missouri Press, 2010.

Trachtnberg, Alan. *Reading American Photographs: Images as History Mathew Brady to Walker Evans*. New York: Hill and Wang, 1989.

Tuggle, Lindsay. *The Afterlives of Specimens: Science, Mourning, and Whitman's Civil War*. Iowa City: University of Iowa Press, 2017.

———. *Calenture*. Victoria, Australia: Cordite, 2018.

Turner, Gerard L'E. *Nineteenth-Century Scientific Instruments*. London: Sotheby, 1983.

Varon, Elizabeth R. *Armies of Deliverance: A New History of the Civil War*. New York: Oxford University Press, 2021.

Waldrep, Christopher. *Vicksburg's Long Shadow: The Civil War Legacy of Race and Remembrance*. New York: Rowman & Littlefield, 2005.

Weicksel, Sarah Jones. "The Dress of the Enemy: Clothing and Disease in the Civil War Era." *Civil War History* 63, no. 2 (2017): 133–150.

White, Jonathan W. *A House Built by Slaves: African American Visitors to the Lincoln White House*. New York: Rowman & Littlefield, 2022.

———. *Midnight in America: Darkness, Sleep, and Dreams during the Civil War*. Chapel Hill: University of North Carolina Press, 2017.

White, Jonathan W., Katie Fisher, and Elizabeth Wall, eds. "The Civil War Letters of Tillman Valentine, Third U.S. Colored Troops." *Pennsylvania Magazine of History and Biography* 139 (April 2015): 171–188.

Williams, George W. *A History of the Negro Troops in the War of the Rebellion 1861–1865*. New York: Harper & Brothers, 1888.

Willis, Deborah. *The Black Civil War Soldier: A Visual History of Conflict and Citizenship*. New York: New York University Press, 2021.

Wintermute, Bobby A. *Public Health and the U.S. Military: A History of the Army Medical Department 1818–1917*. New York: Routledge, 2011.

Yerkes, Royden Keith. *The History of Saint Luke's Church, Germantown, Philadelphia*. Philadelphia: privately published, 1912.

INDEX

Page numbers appearing in italics refer to illustrations.

ROBERT D. HICKS, PhD, is an independent scholar of the history of science and medicine. Formerly, he was Senior Consulting Scholar and William Maul Measey Chair for the History of Medicine at the College of Physicians of Philadelphia. For over a decade, he served as director of the Mütter Museum and Historical Medical Library at the college. He holds a doctorate in history from the University of Exeter, United Kingdom, and degrees in anthropology and archaeology from the University of Arizona. His most recent book, *Civil War Medicine: A Surgeon's Experience,* was published in 2019 by Indiana University Press.

FOR INDIANA UNIVERSITY PRESS

Lesley Bolton *Project Manager/Editor*

Tony Brewer *Artist and Book Designer*

Dan Crissman *Acquisitions Editor and Editorial Director*

Anna Francis *Assistant Acquisitions Editor*

Samantha Heffner *Marketing and Publicity Manager*

Brenna Hosman *Production Coordinator*

Katie Huggins *Production Manager*

Dan Pyle *Online Publishing Manager*

Jennifer Witzke *Senior Artist and Book Designer*